T0094411

Digitizing Diagnosis

Studies in Computing and Culture

This series publishes interdisciplinary, historically grounded works that examine our digital world in its broader sociocultural, political, economic, legal, and environmental contexts. With a global scope, it focuses on the relationships of digital technology to political economies and socioeconomic power inequalities and imbalances.

# Digitizing Diagnosis

## Medicine, Minds, and Machines in Twentieth-Century America

ANDREW S. LEA

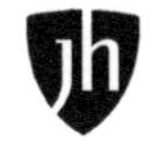

Johns Hopkins University Press
*Baltimore*

Printed in the United States of America on acid-free paper
2 4 6 8 9 7 5 3 1

Johns Hopkins University Press
2715 North Charles Street
Baltimore, Maryland 21218
www.press.jhu.edu

Library of Congress Cataloging-in-Publication Data is available.

ISBN 978-1-4214-4681-3 (hardcover)
ISBN 978-1-4214-4682-0 (ebook)

A catalog record for this book is available from the British Library.

*Special discounts are available for bulk purchases of this book. For more information, please contact Special Sales at specialsales@jh.edu.*

*For Cindy and Scott*

# CONTENTS

# ACKNOWLEDGMENTS

This book benefited from the intellectual generosity of numerous individuals spread across several institutions. I was fortunate to have the University of Oxford's Wellcome Unit for the History of Medicine as my intellectual home base as I wrote the doctoral dissertation from which this book developed. Mark Harrison shaped this book every step of the way, providing invaluable advice about my driving questions, sources, and arguments. At Oxford I also benefited from conversations with Joshua Aiken, Pietro Corsi, Kylie de Chastelain, Suzanna Fritzberg, Sam Greene, Stephen Johnston, Michael Joseph, Claas Kirchhelle, Laura Lamont, Lindsay Lee, Margaret Pelling, Steve Server, Katherine Warren, Meredith Wheeler, Courtney Wittekind, and Steve Woolgar. Particularly warm thanks must go to Erica Charters, Robert Iliffe, and Sloan Mahone, whose sharp and generous readings influenced early versions of this book. Belinda Clark's friendship and administrative support kept me both nurtured and productive.

Many others outside of Oxford contributed to this project. At the Max Planck Institute for the History of Science (MPIWG), there was a rich and vibrant institutional culture to draw from as a doctoral fellow in Department II. Robert Aronowitz, Lorraine Daston, Cathy Gere, Andrew Mendelsohn, and David Sepkoski all provided incisive feedback on this book project. Having Carsten Timmermann on my viva committee shaped this book in important ways. David Jones and Scott Podolsky read and commented on large portions of this book. Their enthusiasm for my research sustained me, and their insights improved this work immeasurably. Travis Hallett and Elizabeth Wang have been inexhaustible sources of insight, encouragement, and humor throughout this project. Emma Pierson deftly fielded some of my technical questions about mathematics and computing.

As I finished my doctorate and started medical school, I was fortunate to join a welcoming scholarly community at the Institute for the History of Medicine and the Center for the Medical Humanities and Social Medicine at Johns Hopkins. I am particularly indebted to Jeremy Greene, who read and commented on multiple versions of this work. Our conversations—about history, computing, and clinical medicine—have helped form many of the ideas presented in the book as well as my broader sense of what it means to pursue a career that bridges historical scholarship and clinical practice. This book would not be what it is were it not for his extraordinary intellectual energy and generosity. Valuable feedback on portions of this book also came from Nathaniel Comfort, Tom Özden-Schilling, Margo Peyton, and Randy Packard. Clinical leaders and mentors at Johns Hopkins, including Colleen Christmas, Graham Mooney, and Carolyn Sufrin, made the institution a supportive place to study the medical humanities in tandem with clinical medicine. Mary Chen graciously offered her design expertise and assisted in formatting the images in this book.

I cannot imagine a better place to have started my training as a physician than the internal medicine residency program at Brigham and Women's Hospital. I am grateful to Marshall Wolf, Joel Katz, and Maria Yialamas for building a residency program that doesn't just tolerate circuitous paths but celebrates them. My coresidents and patients have taught me more about medicine and the importance of history than has any course or book.

Audiences of all kinds thoughtfully engaged with this project. I am especially indebted to audiences at Oxford, MPIWG, Johns Hopkins, and Harvard, as well as those at the annual meetings of the History of Science Society, the Society for the History of Technology, and the Special Interest Group on the History of Computing, for their questions and insights.

The editors and staff at Johns Hopkins University Press have expertly shepherded this book through the publication process. I am grateful to my editor, Matt McAdam, for his enthusiasm and wise guidance. Adriahna Conway, Kait Howard, Kristina Lykke, and Juliana McCarthy also played critical roles in the making of this book. Special thanks must go to the three anonymous reviewers for the Press for their insightful comments, constructive criticism, and encouraging feedback. Joanne Haines's meticulous copyediting improved this book considerably.

Countless archivists and librarians at many institutions went above and beyond the call of duty in helping me locate critical materials for this project. This book would not have been possible without them. It also would not have been possible without generous funding from the Max Planck Society, the

Hagley Museum and Library, and the Johns Hopkins Office of Medical Student Research and Scholarship. Early portions of this project have appeared as "Computerizing Diagnosis: Keeve Brodman and the Medical Data Screen," *Isis* 110, no. 2 (2019): 228–249, and (with Jeremy A. Greene) "Digital Futures Past—The Long Arc of Big Data in Medicine," *New England Journal of Medicine* 381, no. 5 (2019): 480–485. I thank the University of Chicago Press and the Massachusetts Medical Society for permission to draw from these articles.

Above all, I am grateful to my family and friends for their love and support. My parents, Cindy Bruckner-Lea and Scott Lea, have long entertained and encouraged my peculiar academic interests. Andrew Supron came into my life as I was working on this project, and I have been nourished by his friendship and love. I couldn't have balanced the challenge of writing this book with the rigors of medical school and residency without him. Max keeps us on our toes and reminds us of what really matters.

Digitizing Diagnosis

# Introduction

Diagnosis is one of the cardinal acts of medicine. It gives name and meaning to a patient's affliction. It dictates treatment course and guides prognostication. But it does more than that; it performs social and bureaucratic work as well. It is a ritual that structures the personal relationship between physician and patient, even as it is a mechanism by which clinicians are reimbursed for their labor.[1] It is the crystallized product of the physician's artful and human skill. Indeed, for many, diagnosis is the very embodiment of "medical art." The celebrated Edinburgh physician William Cullen wrote in 1800: "Every one must acknowledge the difficulty of distinguishing diseases, but in most cases, the possibility must also be allowed; for whoever denies this, may as well deny that there is such a thing as the medical art."[2]

Beginning in the 1950s, a new actor began to participate in this once exclusively human art: the digital computer. Interdisciplinary teams of physicians, mathematicians, engineers, and philosophers began applying this new technology to the old problem of diagnosis. This book offers a history of these efforts—and of the broader questions, challenges, and transformations that arose in their wake. It explores how attempts to computerize diagnosis produced certain professional tensions, economic interests, disease constructions, cultural ideals, and material practices. Debates about how and whether to computerize diagnosis were often animated by larger debates about the nature of diagnosis and medical reasoning, the definitions of disease, and the authority as well as the identity of physicians and their patients.

In this book, I argue that the introduction of computers, and their associated material and mathematical practices, to medicine shaped the identities of patients, diseases, and physicians. As computers entered the realm of medical diagnosis for the first time, physicians began to think about their patients, diseases, and indeed themselves in new ways. These pioneers of computerized medicine distilled their patients' rich clinical presentations into standardized yes-no surveys; they translated the definitions of disease "into the standardized language of the machine"; and they carved out the areas of medicine that were suitable for human practitioners vis-à-vis those areas that they saw as better suited to the machine. In so doing, they defined anew what a disease was, and what it meant to be a patient and a clinician.

Even as I document some of the transformations wrought by the introduction of the computer into medical diagnosis, I also attend to many of the continuities that span the worlds of medicine before and after the computer. The computer was both a cause and an effect of certain ways of collecting, sorting, managing, reporting, and analyzing medical information. Through the twentieth century, physicians and medical scientists developed standardized modes of gathering and manipulating medical information as well as statistical techniques for making sense of this information. The computer's foray into medical diagnosis grew out of these earlier, paper-based tools and practices. Yet computerization also created the need for the transformation of medical information into forms that were suitable to the material conditions of the machine. The computer's emergence within medicine, moreover, created new cognitive models about what it meant for medical information to be "truly standardized."

As much as this is a story about computers, it is also fundamentally a story about the complexity of medicine. The actors in this book sought to bring medicine, in all of its unruly splendor, to heel. Their self-declared charge was to render the art of medicine a science—to circumscribe, codify, and ultimately computerize it. Where others saw artistic reasoning, they saw equations, models, and algorithms. But as I'll demonstrate, they underestimated medicine time and time again. They underestimated the complexity of medical knowledge, to be sure. But they also misjudged its social, moral, personal, cultural, and legal dimensions—and the extent to which these facets of medicine could be programmed into a computer.

Their efforts, though, were not fruitless. Even when they failed to computerize diagnosis, they succeeded remarkably in other ways. Through their engagement with medicine, some defined entire new fields within computer science. Others developed more philosophically rich understandings of medicine and medical reasoning. This book follows these stories of failure and success. It is a book about the often-peculiar people behind these efforts. It is about what happened when they thought to bring a new and curious technology into the very heart of medicine.

## Histories of Computerized Medicine

Computers have been the subjects of sustained historical inquiry for many decades.[3] More recently, historical perspectives on artificial intelligence and machine learning have also entered the scholarly literature, as have rich analyses of gender, race, and bias.[4] Despite this proliferation of scholarship on the history of computing, the introduction of computing into medicine and medical diagnosis remains an underexplored topic, eclipsed by an interest in the application of computers to other domains.[5] Just as medicine has been an underexamined topic among historians of computing, computing has been an underexamined topic among historians of medicine. Medical technology has long been a rich and productive focus within the history of medicine.[6] But until recently historians of the life sciences, medicine, and medical technology have paid insufficient attention to the emergence of digital computing in medical practice.[7]

This book bridges this divide, building upon recent histories by Joseph November, Hallam Stevens, and others.[8] It demonstrates that there is much to learn within the history of computing by refocusing on the arena of medicine. As I will show, the computer's engagements with medicine—and its intellectual, logistical, and human complexities—spawned some of the foremost technological developments and philosophical conversations within the broader field of computer science. Medicine was not just a run-of-the-mill "problem domain" for computer scientists: it was an unusually productive space, both intellectually and technologically. It was Stanford researchers' engagements with the domain of medicine, for instance, that opened up the entire computer science field of expert systems, with their creation of the MYCIN system in the 1970s.

Historians of medicine likewise have much to learn by turning to the realm of computing. Following methodological advances in the fields of software studies and critical algorithm studies, I have brought new kinds of sources to bear on topics and questions in the history of medicine: computer inputs, computer printouts, punched cards, numerical tabulations, algorithms, and code.[9] Such sources permit analysis of how, for example, the creation of computerized systems generated new definitions of disease and ways of handling medical information. By attending to unfamiliar sources, historians can better understand how computing technologies—and medicine's material grounding more broadly—have influenced the practice, experience, and work of medicine. This book thus sits in conversation with recent histories that have begun to highlight the importance of material culture to medical work and thought.[10]

## Situating Computerized Medicine in Time

The efforts outlined in this book unfolded during a period when the meaning and nature of a "computer" were in flux. From the Victorian period all the way to the 1940s, "computers" referred to humans, usually women, who performed calculations. Well before the advent of digital computers, human computers produced mathematical tables for a range of purposes, such as the improvement of navigational accuracy in eighteenth-century Britain.[11] Beginning in the late nineteenth century and continuing through the early twentieth century, a growing office-machine industry, dominated by companies like Remington Rand, Burroughs Adding Machine Company, and International Business Machines Corporation (IBM), delivered increasing numbers of mechanical aids to these human computers in the form of typewriters, adding machines, and punched-card accounting machines.[12] Hospitals and health departments were early adopters of tabulating machines, using them to track financial and medical information.[13]

Beginning in the 1940s, digital electronic computers emerged alongside their analog ancestors. These early digital computers were as much the products of collaborative teams of scientists and technicians as they were products of the broader pressures of war. Engineers, mathematicians, and cryptanalysts built one such computer, the Colossus, in 1943 to assist British intelligence officers in breaking German codes.[14] Other computing devices soon joined its ranks. Among them was the IBM Automatic Sequence Controlled Calculator, known more commonly as Harvard Mark I, which was used between 1944 and 1959 to compute tables for various branches of the American military.[15] Mark I achieved significant cultural currency owing to its status as the first fully automatic computer.[16] Once programmed by inserting "operation codes" punched onto a segment of paper tape, the machine could run computations for days on end. Such feats were enabled by an onerous paraphernalia of hardware: the machine stood fifty-one feet wide and two feet deep, weighed about five tons, relied on a five-horsepower electric motor, and was assembled from over a hundred miles of wiring and nearly a million different parts.[17]

From these earliest digital electronic systems, further improvements in computing technology did not proceed in a linear fashion—computers built just years after the Colossus and Mark I were orders of magnitude faster than their progenitors. The Electronic Numerical Integrator and Computer (ENIAC), developed in 1946 at the University of Pennsylvania, could perform five thousand operations in the time that Mark I could perform three.[18] While these capabilities gave the machine greater practical relevance, the ENIAC emerged initially as a pragmatic solution to a narrow problem: to carry out time-consuming and tedious artillery firing table calculations as a way of predicting projectile trajectories under a set of external and environmental constraints. Humans at the US Army's Ballistic Research Laboratory could only perform these laborious calculations at a certain pace, so the ENIAC's original and primary purpose was to relieve this human-resource bottleneck. Commercial mainframe computers, from Remington's UNIVAC to IBM's 700 series, followed on the heels of their military forerunners.[19] With the collective appearance of these devices through the 1940s and 1950s, machines began to supplant humans as the primary referents of the title "computer."[20]

By the 1970s, many computers only faintly resembled their precursors of two decades prior: once prohibitively expensive, computers became cheap enough (relatively speaking) to be marketed to individuals as well as institutions; once ponderous, many computers of the 1970s were no longer the size of large rooms; and once limited by the constraints of vacuum-tube switches, the computer's processing power through these decades surged with the advent of transistors. The computer, however, did not progress from the mainframe to the microcomputer in a sharp, punctuated fashion, nor did the introduction of minicomputers or microcomputers render mainframe computers immediately obsolete. Rather, this change unfolded gradually and unevenly, through the development of various intermediate technologies, stages, and sociotechnical configurations.[21] A cadre of changes across the computing landscape during the 1950s and 1960s—the development of transistors and integrated circuits, the introduction of time-sharing, the invention of the microprocessor—successively enhanced computers and computing technology along all three dimensions of cost, size, and speed. These technological innovations arrived in tandem with a changing social and intellectual environment as well as an emerging computer industry.[22] Collectively, these forces altered the computer's material form in addition to its economic, intellectual, professional, and social function. A device that had been developed in military contexts began to fan out into other domains. Medicine stood among them.

## Patient, Disease, Physician: Book Structure

This book offers a history of computerizing medical diagnosis through the prism of three case studies: the Medical Data Screen (MDS), a computer system developed to provide a snapshot of "the total patient"; HEME, a computer program designed to make diagnoses in the field of hematology; and finally, MYCIN, an early expert system that aimed to furnish advice concerning the diagnosis and treatment of bacterial infections. While far from exhaustive, these efforts were among the earliest and most widely discussed attempts to bring medical diagnosis under the remit of the digital computer. They all generated considerable discussion about whether, how, and why to apply computers to arguably the most foundational, intimate, and cerebral task of medicine—diagnosis. And yet, they all have received scant historical attention.

Each of these case studies, moreover, highlights a different facet of my argument: in the MDS, we see most clearly the computer's role in transforming the identity of the *patient*; in HEME, we see the computer reconfiguring the definition and identity of *disease*; and in MYCIN, we see debates about, and reformulations of, the identity of the *physician* in medical practice. To be sure, each of these cases demonstrates some element of all these transformations—of patient, disease, and physician identity. But each case illuminates each of these reconfigurations to different degrees.

The book proceeds both chronologically and thematically. Each section is organized around one of these case studies in the history of computerizing diagnosis and takes on one of these themes. Part I, "Patient," explores how the use of computers, and the paper-based media from which they emerged, gave rise to new conceptions of the patient. In 1947, Cornell psychiatrist Keeve Brodman and a handful of colleagues began developing what would become one of the most widely used health questionnaires of its time—the Cornell Medical Index (CMI). A rigidly standardized form, the CMI presented 195 yes-no questions designed to capture the health status of "the total patient." Over the following decades, Brodman's project of standardizing medical history-taking gradually evolved into a project of mathematizing and computerizing diagnosis: out of the CMI grew the MDS, an early computerized method of deriving diagnoses from patient data. Chapter 1 considers the creation and dissemination of the CMI: its motivating aims, surprising uses, and material grounding. It shows how the CMI mapped the patient's rich presentation onto a four-page form of binary, yes-no responses.

Chapter 2 charts the evolution of the paper-based CMI into the computer-based MDS. The chapter reconstructs the computer program's creation as well as the hopes and fears that were grafted upon it. In an era of overstretched and underresourced physicians, Brodman and his colleagues believed that these technologies would not only extend the reach of medical personnel to rural and underserved areas but also relinquish physicians from the monotonous aspects of medical practice, giving them more time to focus on the "human" aspects of care. The introduction of decision support technologies like the CMI and MDS into medical history-taking and diagnosis fueled concerns around professional deskilling, interpersonal dehumanization, and substandard care. The chapter concludes with consideration of the patient's identity as constructed by the MDS—an identity that I call "the statistical patient."

Part II, "Disease," examines how the use of computers, and material culture more generally, shapes the definitions of disease. The section explores this theme through the lens of a thirty-five-year effort to computerize the diagnosis of hematologic diseases. In 1957, a group of researchers based at the Rockefeller Institute gathered at the Radio Corporation of America (RCA) facility in Camden, New Jersey, to witness RCA's Bizmac computer render, from inputs of patient data, diagnoses of hematologic diseases. Chapter 3 follows the development and evolution of this hematology program. It shows how physicians and engineers, as they encountered novel digital media, began to represent medical information and define diseases in new ways. The chapter suggests that the process of disease definition is not just a social or intellectual process, as many historians have noted. It is a material process as well, shaped profoundly by the material media with which physicians work. Disease concepts are *corporeal*: they cohere, come apart, and reconfigure in material bodies, whether paper notebooks or magnetic tape.

As interdisciplinary teams worked to automate medical diagnosis, they repeatedly bumped up against fundamental epistemological questions. How do doctors think? What is the nature of human reasoning? Are human modes of reasoning amenable to computerization? If they are, should computers aim to mimic them? In what ways do physicians come to define and classify disease categories? Are these categories even necessary? While following the hematology program into its final decades, chapter 4 explores how computers both generated and incorporated ideas about the medical mind and its inner workings.

Part III, "Physician," uses the case of MYCIN to examine key moral and professional tensions attendant to the computer's introduction into medical diagnosis. In the early 1970s, the young MD-PhD student Edward H. Shortliffe started work on his dissertation within Stanford University's Department of Computer Science. His PhD thesis, completed in 1974, involved the development of a computer program called MYCIN, an expert system that provided physicians with advice concerning the diagnosis and treatment of bacterial infections. MYCIN immediately attracted wide attention: it matured into a much larger research enterprise at Stanford and spawned larger conversations about whether and how to apply computers to the problem of medical diagnosis. Chapter 5 recounts this early effort to computerize medical diagnosis and decision-making. It demonstrates that questions about trust and transparency animated the development of, and responses to, the MYCIN project. How could a physician using the system know that its advice was accurate and trustworthy? What did the developers of MYCIN do to make the system's reasoning comprehensible to its human users? The MYCIN team largely pursued technological solutions to the problems of trust and transparency, creating novel technologies, programs, and interfaces that purportedly allowed MYCIN to "explain itself."

As chapter 6 argues, these issues around trust and transparency were entangled with concerns over the physician's authority, identity, and responsibility. To cede important treatment and diagnostic decisions to machines—to allow computers to carry out a fundamental task of medicine—raised questions about what it meant to be a physician as well as questions about the physician's responsibility and their ownership over medical decisions. Despite all that the MYCIN team did to render their system's reasoning transparent, physicians worried about lingering opacities of a computerized system—about the biases that, as one actor put it, may still be "hidden in the code." The technological fixes to issues of transparency thus fell short: they could not cleanly resolve the larger professional, regulatory, moral, and epistemological challenges raised by computerized medicine.

The clinical landscape today is defined by computers. Follow rounds on the inpatient medicine wards and you will witness flocks of residents referencing their smartphones and rolling their mobile computer carts from patient room to patient room. Tag along during some outpatient visits and you may notice physicians oriented not toward the patients before them but toward their computers. In your own conversations with doctors, you may reference your results in your online patient portal and the computer's automated interpretation of those results. Given how deeply the computer is integrated into medical practice today, it is essential to understand how we got here. Yet understanding the origins of computers in medicine first requires returning to a period dominated by pencil and paper. Modern medicine's empire of machines came into being upon an infrastructure of paper.

PART ONE

# PATIENT

CHAPTER ONE

# Indexing the World

Patients who came to the outpatient departments of the New York Hospital through the mid-twentieth century were accustomed to a familiar routine. They would check in at the front desk, be called in from the waiting room, and be seen by an attending physician, perhaps a medical resident. Some walked away, prescription in hand, while others awaited further testing. But patients who happened to come within a certain eighteen-month window—between July 1948 and December 1949—encountered a new and unusual step. These patients were asked to complete a four-page questionnaire. Emblazoned across the top of the questionnaire form were the words "Cornell Medical Index." Each patient spent roughly fifteen minutes answering the index's nearly two hundred questions, which were designed to record the patient's complete medical history. For patients today, having to complete a health questionnaire seems par for the course. To patients in the late 1940s, however, this step was unprecedented: the Cornell Medical Index (CMI) was among the first health questionnaires of its kind.

The driving force behind the CMI was Keeve Brodman, a psychiatrist and professor at Cornell University Medical College. Together with a handful of colleagues, Brodman created the index as a method of improving medical history-taking through standardization. His early interest in standardization soon evolved into an interest in computerization. Beginning in the mid-1950s, Brodman and his collaborators began using data collected from the index to build a mathematical model that could diagnose a range of common diseases from a patient's questionnaire responses. Brodman's team then worked to convert this mathematical model into a program for use on a digital computer.

The method that resulted from this research—the final version of which came to be known as the Medical Data Screen (MDS)—represented one of the earliest attempts to computerize medical diagnosis and decision-making.

Brodman's work was influential in its time. The CMI, among the earliest and most prominent medical history questionnaires, reached hundreds of thousands of physicians and patients around the world, and the MDS represented one of the first attempts to computerize medical diagnosis. His work was published in leading medical journals and covered by the national press. Despite this, Brodman and his initiatives have received little historical attention.[1]

This chapter details the creation of the Cornell Medical Index, and chapter 2 unpacks how this project that started out as a paper-based method of medical history-taking eventually morphed into a computer-based method of making differential diagnoses. Together, the chapters demonstrate the ways in which these two technologies, the CMI and the MDS, created new representations of the patient. The CMI flattened the narratively rich experiences of the patient into a yes-no questionnaire: the patient's identity was transformed into a pattern of answers on a standardized form. The MDS converted patients' answers on these forms into the language of statistics, creating "the statistical patient."

## Brodman's Beginnings

New York City was all young Keeve Brodman knew. Born and raised in the city, Brodman attended the College of the City of New York, earned his medical degree from Cornell University Medical College, and joined Bellevue Hospital's Department of Medicine, where he specialized in psychiatry.[2] Beginning in 1934, he juggled two clinical appointments: one as an Associate Attending Physician at Bellevue, and the other as a physician to outpatients at the New York Hospital. To train at Cornell Medical College and its affiliated hospitals in the 1930s was to train within a vibrant medical ecology at the height of its transformation. During this period, Cornell Medical College not only grew significantly in its own right but also came to be embedded within a much larger network of New York medical facilities. In 1927, Cornell University and the New York Hospital agreed upon the establishment of a joint medical center. The resulting New York Hospital-Cornell Medical Center first opened its doors on September 1, 1932.[3] The twenty-seven-story medical complex, donning a regal alabaster façade, towered over the surrounding Upper

East Side neighborhoods. Behind its impressive physical exterior, Cornell supported clinical and research activities that drew international recognition.

It would take the exigencies of war to unsettle Brodman's New York City roots. In late 1940, as World War II intensified in Western Europe, Brodman wrote to his local US Army Corps area indicating his "desire to co-operate with the armed forces in this national emergency."[4] Less than two years later, Brodman received a notice from the War Department, certifying his military commission as a major in the US Army Medical Corps.[5] On August 18, 1942, Brodman reported for duty at the Station Hospital in Camp Lee, a notable army post in Virginia.[6] There, he quickly climbed the military ladder, starting off as the chief of the hospital's cardiology section before taking on a role as the medical service's assistant chief.

Brodman made his role in the military continuous with his civilian medical role; he treated the medical corps as a new arena to which he could apply his knowledge of psychiatry. Early in his military tenure, Brodman cultivated an interest in psychosomatic medicine, a field that was just beginning to make inroads into the medical mainstream. This interest in psychosomatic medicine temporarily pulled Brodman away from his post in Virginia: in April and May of 1943 he attended a course in psychosomatic medicine with Dr. Helen Flanders Dunbar at Columbia University's College of Physicians and Surgeons.[7] As someone with training in neuropsychiatry, Brodman understood the significance of working with and learning from Dunbar. By the early 1940s, Dunbar had established herself as a leading researcher and clinician in the field of psychosomatic medicine, adopting what one historian has called a "holistic approach" to psychosomatic problems.[8]

Immediately on returning from his six weeks of "detached service" in New York, Brodman began exploring ways of implementing what he had picked up. As early as May 1943, Brodman laid the groundwork for the establishment of a psychotherapeutic clinic in the cardiac section of the 307th Station Hospital at Camp Lee.[9] The clinic offered group psychotherapy to patients whose organic symptoms were determined to be psychogenic; Brodman estimated that such patients comprised 93 percent of all patients seen in the hospital's cardiac section.[10] Through formal talks, Brodman also delivered the tools and tenets of psychosomatic medicine to his fellow medical officers.[11]

At Camp Lee, Brodman's psychosomatic programs and reforms found a receptive audience. Brodman's commanding officer commended his service at Camp Lee's Station Hospital, particularly his work "establishing a psychosomatic clinic, which helped cut down the patient load at the hospital considerably."[12] Despite Brodman's successes locally, his efforts to introduce psychosomatic medicine more widely through the medical corps failed. Upon returning to Camp Lee from detached service in New York, Brodman began drafting a report to be submitted to the Surgeon General's Office (SGO) that proposed a psychosomatic teaching and consultation program for the entire medical corps. By attending to the overlooked psychological and emotional facets of disease—by offering support that could be as simple as a "kindly word, a hopeful attitude, and a sympathetic listening"—such a program, Brodman argued, would address the medical needs of soldiers more effectively and deploy the army's own medical resources more efficiently.[13] The SGO disagreed, explaining to Brodman, "There are not as many cases in the service that need psychosomatic therapy as this article would infer" and that, where such cases did exist, they would "more properly come under the [existing] neuropsychiatric service."[14]

When Brodman received this notice from the SGO, he was in the midst of coming to terms with a more personal setback. Beginning in May 1943, Brodman began experiencing a series of peculiar symptoms. At first, they were slight: a feeling of tenseness in his legs, a sense of instability when climbing and descending stairs. But as the heat and humidity of a Virginian summer settled in over Camp Lee, his symptoms became harder to dismiss. In July, following an hour's worth of vigorous walking, Brodman became unusually fatigued and started noticing a loss of muscle control upon climbing some stairs. His legs grew progressively tired. By November 1943, Brodman was admitted to the Station Hospital of a neighboring army installation, where he was diagnosed with multiple sclerosis, a disease of the central nervous system that variably affects a range of physical and mental functions. By early 1944, Brodman had been reclassified to limited duty at the Walter Reed General Hospital in Washington, DC. Reclassification, Brodman explained in one letter, "is due to the recent development of multiple sclerosis, which for the time being causes considerable difficulty in walking even across the room."[15]

Once reclassified, Brodman lobbied the SGO to be transferred back to New York—to an assignment with "the Cornell Project," a team of Cornell-based researchers working with the National Research Council for the study of psychoneurosis in the army.[16] Brodman viewed the project as a nice fit, blending his interest in psychiatry and psychosomatic medicine with his military background. Harold Wolff, the pioneering neurologist leading the Cornell project, wrote to the SGO supporting Brodman's bid. Wolff detailed Cornell University Medical College's work on "methods for aiding in the screening" of military personnel and "request[ed] that Major Brodman be attached to this project" as a kind of bridge between civilian researchers and the US Army.[17] In particular, Wolff described the group's role in devising "the so-called Cornell Selectee Study which is . . . a brief neuropsychiatric and psychosomatic history having certain quantitative characteristics."[18] According to Wolff, the method allowed for "quick and simple detection" of neuropsychiatric and psychosomatic problems that general medical officers often neglected. By April 1944, Brodman had transitioned to inactive status within the army, and he returned to Cornell to work on the National Research Council project studying psychoneurosis in the military.[19]

## "The Male Pattern of Our Society"

Back at Cornell, Brodman nursed several different academic projects concurrently. One of these projects involved the study of psychiatric health and human relations in industry, which culminated in the 1947 book *Men at Work: The Supervisor and His People*.[20] Although Brodman's research on industrial health proved influential, reaching officials working at high levels in industry, his work on the "Cornell Indices"—the Cornell Selectee Index and the Cornell Service Index—exerted a greater influence over the direction of his later career.[21] The Selectee Index dovetailed with Brodman's own interests and expertise. In line with Brodman's initiatives at Camp Lee, the Selectee Index aimed to deliver a simple, rapid, and accurate means of identifying psychoneuroses and psychosomatic disturbances in troops.[22] The Service Index simply included additional questions tailored for people who had already undergone military training. The motiving purpose of these early indices, then, was to screen and exclude "the neuropsychiatrically unfit" from the military.[23]

Among those targeted for screening and exclusion by the indices were queer, and specifically homosexual, individuals. In creating these new screening tools, the Cornell team included information for the explicit purposes of "drawing conclusions concerning the individual's ability to accept the male pattern of our society."[24] The Cornell Selectee Index, then, participated in broader cultural and federal efforts during this period to enforce sexual norms and penalize homosexuality.[25] Once created, the indices were used to this end. A navy psychiatrist reported using the index to identify "suggestive" and "obvious homosexuality" and concluded that "overt homosexual[s]" like those he had identified "would hardly be suitable material" for "working on ships."[26]

Others further explored and elaborated upon the indices' uses in scrutinizing and policing queer activity and identity. Two clinicians conducted research with the indices (on queer prisoners) to further establish how responses to the questionnaires "revealed certain significant differences among male homosexuals classified in accordance with the degree of homosexual activity and with the predominant role in homosexual activity."[27] These early indices thus incorporated an explicit anti-queer bias into their very structure and content. Even though the items designed expressly for the purposes of identifying homosexuals were not carried forward to the CMI, these origins of the CMI and MDS offer insights into the contingent processes by which computerized systems and medical algorithms may come to incorporate, propagate, and calcify bias (see chapter 3 for greater discussion of algorithmic bias).[28]

Brodman's contributions to these initial indices inspired him to develop a similar instrument except with a broader scope—the Cornell Medical Index. Although the CMI and its immediate ancestors were novel in their particulars, the larger impulse to survey and quantify populations was not. Tools of aggregation have long played important roles in American society—at least since the first US census of 1790.[29] The "quantifying spirit" took a firmer grip on American life through the late nineteenth and early twentieth centuries, as life insurance companies developed elaborate methods for counting, sorting, and measuring people—and for predicting their futures.[30] The logics and practices that animated corporate culture soon flourished in popular culture as well. Beginning in the interwar period, the proliferation of modern surveys, from the Gallup poll to the Kinsey Reports, generated not just large amounts of data on large segments of the population but also new subjectivities.[31] Within medicine, the second half of the twentieth century saw the formation of new and significant links between the fields of medicine and statistics and, as a result of these links, the rising status of epidemiological studies and randomized controlled trials.[32] All the while, the creation and application of standardized tests and questionnaires, particularly within the fields of psychiatry and psychology, followed an upward trajectory through the twentieth century.[33]

It was against this backdrop that Brodman and a number of colleagues (Albert J. Erdmann, Jr., and Irving Lorge chief among them) began work on the CMI in 1947 (Figure 1.1).[34] The CMI differed from the Selectee Index in two primary ways. First, whereas the Selectee Index was designed for use with either members of or applicants to the US Armed Forces (and particularly those deemed "unfit"), the CMI was written to apply to all patients. Second, the CMI aimed to generate a portrait of not just a patient's neuropsychiatric

History Number__________

**(MEN)**

**CORNELL MEDICAL INDEX**

# HEALTH QUESTIONNAIRE

Date________

Print Your Name __________ Your Home Address __________

How Old Are You? ________ Circle If You Are . . . Single, Married, Widowed, Separated, Divorced.

Circle the Highest Year You Reached In School | 1 2 3 4 5 6 7 8 | (Elementary School) | 1 2 3 4 | (High) | 1 2 3 4 | (College)

What is Your Occupation? __________

Directions: This questionnaire is for *MEN ONLY.*
If you can answer **YES** to the question asked, put a circle around the (YES)
If you have to answer **NO** to the question asked, put a circle around the (NO)
Answer all questions. If you are not sure, guess.

**A**

|  | | | |
|---|---|---|---|
| Do you need glasses to read? | Yes | No | 001 |
| Do you need glasses to see things at a distance? | Yes | No | 002 |
| Do your eyes continually blink or water? | Yes | No | 003 |
| Are your eyes often red or inflamed? | Yes | No | 004 |
| Has your eyesight often blacked out completely? | Yes | No | 005 |
| Do you often have severe pains in your eyes? | Yes | No | 006 |
| Have you had cataracts? | Yes | No | 007 |
| Have you ever been told you have glaucoma? | Yes | No | 008 |
| Do you wear contact lenses? | Yes | No | 009 |
| Have you ever had double vision? | Yes | No | 010 |
| Are you hard of hearing? | Yes | No | 011 |
| Have you worn a hearing aid? | Yes | No | 012 |
| Do you notice a ringing in your ear(s)? | Yes | No | 013 |

**B**

|  | | | |
|---|---|---|---|
| Do you have to clear your throat frequently? | Yes | No | 014 |
| Do you often feel a choking lump in your throat? | Yes | No | 015 |
| Is your nose continually stuffed up? | Yes | No | 016 |
| Does your nose run constantly? | Yes | No | 017 |
| Have you ever had a bad nose bleed? | Yes | No | 018 |
| Do you frequently suffer from severe colds? | Yes | No | 019 |
| Do frequent colds keep you miserable all winter? | Yes | No | 020 |
| Do you get hay fever? | Yes | No | 021 |
| Do you suffer from asthma? | Yes | No | 022 |
| Do you have a sinus condition? | Yes | No | 023 |
| Are you troubled by constant coughing? | Yes | No | 024 |
| Have you ever coughed up any blood? | Yes | No | 025 |
| Do you suffer from bronchitis? | Yes | No | 026 |
| Do you sometimes have severe soaking sweats at night? | Yes | No | 027 |
| Have you had a chest X-ray in the last 2 years? | Yes | No | 028 |
| Have you ever had pneumonia? | Yes | No | 029 |
| Are you a smoker? | Yes | No | 030 |

**C**

|  | | | |
|---|---|---|---|
| Do you suffer from angina? | Yes | No | 031 |
| Have you ever had a heart attack? | Yes | No | 032 |
| Does heart trouble run in your family | Yes | No | 033 |
| Have you ever had an electro-cardiogram? | Yes | No | 034 |
| Have you ever had a stress (exercise tolerance) test? | Yes | No | 035 |
| Do you wake up at night short of breath? | Yes | No | 036 |
| Do you get regular (daily) exercise? | Yes | No | 037 |
| Has a doctor ever said your blood pressure was too high or low? | Yes | No | 038 |
| Have you ever been told of high blood cholesterol? | Yes | No | 039 |
| Do you have pains in the heart or chest? | Yes | No | 040 |
| Does your heart often race like mad? | Yes | No | 041 |
| Do you find it hard to breath? | Yes | No | 042 |
| Do you get out of breath long before anyone else? | Yes | No | 043 |
| Have you ever been told to take antibiotics during dental work? | Yes | No | 044 |



Open to next page

*Figure 1.1.* After its original publication in 1949, the Cornell Medical Index (CMI) was updated and revised a number of times. The final version, shown here, largely retains the aesthetic character and content of the original questionnaire. On the recommendation of a committee appointed by Cornell's chairs of medicine, neurology, and psychiatry, the CMI was discontinued beginning in 1990. Courtesy of the Medical Center Archives of NewYork–Presbyterian / Weill Cornell Medicine. The Cornell Medical Index and related historical health questionnaires should only be used for historical reference and not for any research involving human subjects.

well-being (and thus his "fitness" for military service) but his "total medical problem" as well.[35] In short, the CMI widened the Selectee Index's diagnostic parameters to encompass additional medical problems and patient populations.

Arriving at the right questions to include on the questionnaire was a two-year process of iteration and experimentation. The CMI's developers first tried drafting questions as if they were speaking to the patient. To Brodman's surprise, this strategy resulted in patient responses that he found to be "completely inaccurate and unreliable."[36] For example, a first draft of one question seemed simple enough: "Were you ever a patient in a mental hospital?" But after testing the question with a small sample of patients, Brodman noticed that an incredibly large proportion of them responded affirmatively; many patients had apparently overlooked the word "mental." Through multiple rounds of revision, Brodman came to the question's formulation as ultimately included on the CMI: "Were you ever a patient in a *mental* hospital (for your nerves)?"[37]

## The Patient, Indexed

Brodman, Erdmann, Lorge, and their collaborators unveiled the completed CMI to the wider medical community in a seven-part series of articles published between 1949 and 1953.[38] The first of these, published in the *Journal of the American Medical Association (JAMA)*, introduced the questionnaire as "a quick and reliable method of obtaining important facts about a patient's medical history without expenditure of the physician's time."[39] A physician reading any one of these articles would be left with a good sense of the index and how it worked. The index included 195 questions that clustered loosely together into four different categories: questions concerning bodily functions, questions concerning past illnesses, questions concerning family history, and questions concerning behaviors, feelings, or moods. On the questionnaire form itself, these questions were arranged into eighteen sections (A through R) that spanned four pages. The first sections (A through H) mapped onto different organ systems, whereas the later sections concerned disturbances of mood and feeling. In the style of its questions (and in the organization of these questions on the form), the index replicated a common technique in medical history-taking known as a review of systems, whereby a physician systematically asks a patient about subjective symptoms associated with the various organ systems.[40]

Worth noting is the way in which the CMI's standardizing spirit was born out in its very aesthetic form.[41] Each question was assigned an identifying number. To ask "Do you notice ringing in your ear(s)?" was to ask question 013.[42] A patient who reported "frequently feel[ing] faint" had circled "Yes" next to the number 093. Although questions were grouped together according to organ systems, these groupings appeared not under the written name of their respective system but under a simple letter. A physician who wished to examine a patient's visual system needed to consult the responses to questions under the "A" heading. As these letters proceeded alphabetically, the Cornell Medical Index really was, at least visually, a kind of index—an index of, as Brodman described it, "the total patient." Aside from having to write out one's name, address, age, and occupation, completing the questionnaire required virtually no writing and certainly no description or elaboration. Reviewing the CMI was therefore less a matter of interpreting written text than discerning binary markings associated with letters and numbers. In a conventional medical encounter, a patient might vocalize to the doctor their problems of exhaustion and fatigue. But on the CMI they would simply mark as follows:

**I**

. . . (Yes) No 119

In its appearance, then, the index was impersonal, sanitized, anonymous, and universal.

The CMI's formatting, however, was not simply a matter of aesthetics. Questions were designed such that only "Yes" indicated the presence of a symptom that the physician should follow up on. Brodman hoped that CMI users would be able to glean a sense of the patient's "total medical problem" just by scanning the questionnaire and noting the conspicuous pattern of "Yes" answers. A concentration of "Yes" answers within a given section would suggest a medical problem localized to a particular organ system. A smattering of "Yes" answers throughout the entire form might instead point to a medical issue of a more diffuse nature, whether an emotional disturbance or multisystem organic illness. Compared to the question of interpretation, the question of implementation was cake. The second article in the series noted bluntly, "The test is administered simply by handing the form to the patient and asking him to complete it."[43]

The CMI's alphabetical, indexical, and aesthetic character situates it within a much longer lineage of "paper technologies" that have been deployed to help collect, organize, store, sort, communicate, and transmit medical knowledge.[44] Physicians have collected and organized large numbers of patient medical histories (*observationes*) in an indexical fashion since at least the early modern period, as J. Andrew Mendelsohn and Volker Hess have described.[45] The physician Wilhelm Fabry von Hilden (1560–1634), for instance, amassed six hundred patient histories, drawn from several decades of medical practice, and published these histories in a series of six volumes beginning in 1606. These volumes were synthesized into a single edition, the *Opera omnia*, which was published after Fabry's death in 1646. Because few readers could be bothered to read the *Opera omnia*, or even its predecessors, in all their length and detail, the books were alphabetically indexed, directing users to the pages that contained *observationes* of particular interest.

The indexing of texts like the *Opera omnia*, however, differed from the CMI in an important way. In this early modern case, indexing imposed order upon medical knowledge in a post hoc fashion: patient histories that had been collected chronologically over time were retroactively arranged topically or alphabetically.[46] The CMI, by contrast, was prescriptive: order was imposed at the very moment of knowledge collection. All patient histories collected by the CMI contained the same points of data, on the same topics, and in the same format. In its prescriptive and standardized character, the CMI belongs to another lineage of paper technologies that also stretches back hundreds of years. As early as the eighteenth century, hospitals began using "registers," essentially lists of information on a piece of paper, to keep track of the patients entering the hospital, their identifying information, their occupation, the meals they had eaten, and the treatment they had received. Such registers arrived at the hospital largely by way of the broader practices of early modern state administration and accounting. Many physicians soon adopted this "administrative model" of formatting for the purposes of medical history-taking; they recorded patients' medical information not just in a wall of text but in tables, lists, and charts as well. As Hess and Mendelsohn have noted, the proliferation of prescriptive formatting of this kind rendered medical knowledge "comparable and combinable."[47]

In much the same way, the CMI rendered thick, narratively rich patient histories more amenable to aggregation and manipulation, comparison and collation. In Brodman's view, the CMI captured the total patient. But the index transformed and flattened that patient into a four-page standardized survey. It limited the range of answers a patient could give. It translated the patient's history, emotional life, and embodied suffering into a language without words: a pattern of markings on the index. The patient, in other words, had become a kind of data—more amenable to Brodman's research question and, later, his project of computerization.

This new rendering of the patient allowed Brodman and his colleagues to compare how patients with different backgrounds or diagnoses completed the questionnaire. What percentage of patients diagnosed with heart disease answered "Yes" to item 042 ("Do you find it hard to breathe")? To what extent did patients of different genders, occupations, ages, or education levels answer the questionnaire in distinctive ways? Did "neurotic" patients answer more questions on the index affirmatively? In collating CMI data to answer questions of this kind, researchers often conveyed their findings in tables and graphs.[48]

## The Dilemma of Application

The purpose of the series of CMI articles was not simply didactic; in addition to explaining the questionnaire and its clinical uses, these articles worked to build trust in both the specific questions posed by the CMI and the broader project of distilling a patient's medical history into a questionnaire. Brodman and his coauthors first went about establishing the CMI as a legitimate form of history-taking by statistical means. In the 1949 article, the CMI developers examined a sample of 179 patients from the adult general medicine clinic of the New York Hospital Outpatient Department who had both taken the CMI and had their medical history taken by hospital physicians.[49] Comparing the histories obtained by these two methods—one novel, the other routine—the researchers found that the CMI garnered a far more detailed picture of the patient than did the conventional history, recording patient data that the history had missed across every symptom domain. In the case of hypertension, for example, the CMI noted a past history of hypertension in nearly 25 percent of the patients sampled while the conventional history only picked up on a past history of hypertension in 10 percent of the sample.[50]

That the CMI collected a larger quantity of patient data did not mean that these data were of higher, or even comparable, quality. To get at the accuracy of the index's data, Brodman and his colleagues compared the occasions on which the patient data obtained by these methods overlapped. Finding a high degree of correspondence between the methods, the researchers concluded that patients respond to the CMI as honestly and accurately as they respond to existing techniques of history-taking.[51] Brodman and his colleagues expanded on these analyses in subsequent installments to the article series. In a

1951 study, they reported that clinicians examining *only* CMI data made diagnoses that were often more accurate and complete than the diagnoses made through a hospital investigation of the patient's full medical chart.[52] The researchers were not advocating the use of the tool without further medical evaluation, but they presumably felt that evaluating the index as a standalone tool powerfully demonstrated its clinical utility.

To accompany and fill out this statistical evidence, Brodman marshalled narrative evidence, describing cases where the CMI outperformed the examining physician. In one reported case history, the CMI picked up a slate of notable symptoms—chest pain, dyspnea, palpitations, tachycardia, lower extremity edema, cramps, headaches, dizziness, faintness, and muscular twitching—that had apparently evaded the examining physician's scrutiny. Brodman and his colleagues left open the question of "whether the physician did not elicit and record these symptoms because of lack of time, or preknowledge of the diagnosis."[53] In another case history, a woman was admitted to the hospital "complaining of a 'stroke' of three months' duration, with impairment of speech and right-sided weakness."[54] Physicians ultimately identified three conditions—syphilitic aortitis, central nervous system syphilis, and cerebral vascular accident—as the root causes of the patient's affliction, but conventional practices and personnel did not arrive at this conclusion easily: it took five physicians, a laboratory test, and a referral to recognize a crucial piece of medical history (the woman's past history of syphilis) that the CMI had noted immediately.

An official, fifteen-page CMI manual condensed much of this information into an accessible digest and channeled it to the subset of physicians who were considering adopting the index. The manual performed three primary functions: informational, advisory, and political. Although the rise of scientific medicine through the late nineteenth and early twentieth century had embedded the ideal of standardization into many areas of medical thought and practice, there was in the 1940s and 1950s nothing quite like the CMI—at least not on a large scale.[55] As a vehicle for information, the manual conveyed to the uninitiated physician all major aspects of the CMI—its overarching structure, motivating logic, and constituent questions. In its advisory capacity, the manual instructed physicians on the ways in which the index as described could and should be used. The manual, for example, identified the single "most effective method of using the CMI."[56] This involved adopting the index as an adjunct to a more conventional oral interview and having the patient complete, and the physician review, the CMI prior to the interview.

While the manual was prescriptive in the realm of implementation, it was notably deferential in the realm of interpretation: "No rules can be given here on how to interpret symptoms," the manual stated. "Interpretations must be based on the physician's training, knowledge, experiences and insight."[57]

The manual's recommendations and qualifications very likely reflected the honest judgment of its authors, but the document must also be considered in the context of a broader politics of clinical authority. Brodman understood that he had developed an instrument that intervened in an activity—medical history-taking—long considered fundamental both to the practice of medicine and to physicians' sense of autonomy and identity.[58] Statements about the physician's claim to interpretive authority can therefore be read as a way of navigating what some scholars have called the "dilemma of application."[59] In order to demonstrate a need for the questionnaire, the creators of the CMI had to persuade physicians of their own deficiencies in the area of medical history-taking. But doing so also risked antagonizing the very population they needed to accept the tool.

This dilemma also played out in the Cornell group's published articles. In illustrating the CMI's clinical value, Brodman and his collaborators found themselves straddling a fine line between promoting the index and impugning the physician. The developers of the index made measured claims about the CMI's clinical implementation, and they treaded lightly around topics concerning the capabilities and practices of the traditional doctor. The role of the CMI, the authors noted frequently, was that of an adjunct. By their account, the CMI proved most valuable when employed in combination with conventional modes of history-taking: "The most effective technic [*sic*] for use of the CMI as an adjunct to interview has been found to be for the patient to complete the CMI before he sees the physician and for the physician to review the CMI before he interviews the patient. The physician thereby gains a background of knowledge about the patient to orient him in interview."[60] When the researchers inevitably touched on the topic of error in medicine, they privileged exogenous over endogenous explanations. The physician is busy, not inept, they implied: "By calling attention to the patient's symptoms and significant items of past history, it [the index] assures that their investigation will not be overlooked *because the physician lacked time to elicit them*."[61] But despite such assurances, implicit in evidence of the CMI's value and legitimacy were claims about the limitations of physicians and conventional medical methods. A corollary to the statement that the index outperformed the physician was the statement that the physician underperformed the index.

Inevitably words like "overlooked" and "neglected" crept into their discussions of doctors.[62]

Unsurprisingly, then, some physicians objected to the CMI, or at least admonished against its hasty adoption. Critiques of the index found their highest soapbox in a 1952 *British Medical Journal* (*BMJ*) editorial entitled "The Patient Tells His Story." The *BMJ* rehearsed critiques of the index that would become familiar: the editorial mentioned the tool's dehumanizing potential ("It will be remarked that there are other criteria which establish with more certainty and with greater humanism the diagnosis of a neurosis") and its diagnostic blind spots ("It cannot indicate a symptomless early cancer, and the psychological disorders which it clearly reveals are superficial rather than profound, the neuroses rather than the psychoses").[63]

Brodman interpreted the editorial as hostile. In his view the editorial's underlying contention was that "the way to collect a history is not with a printed form but by the physician sitting down with the patient and questioning him."[64] But in fact its tone was more agnostic than antagonistic; the *BMJ* editorial staff ultimately concluded that such critiques missed the index's point: "The CMI is not intended to be the finished portrait: it is but the outline of a rough self-sketch."[65] The worm's-eye perspective of the hurried clinician or medical specialist had something to gain from the bird's-eye perspective offered by the CMI: "If it must be admitted that no general physician sitting in an out-patient clinic addresses 50 questions to the patient's psyche, it will also be agreed that no specialist makes 100 forays beyond his own territory, and no psychiatrist probes the soma 100 times. The CMI does all this with a minimal expenditure of the consultant's time. It tells the hospital doctor almost as much of the patient's complaints and the patient's personality as is known to a good family doctor."[66] During a period with quickening rates of medical specialization, many saw great value in a tool that might capture patients' so-called "total medical status."[67]

The editorial elicited letters from *BMJ* readers holding views across the spectrum. One physician, R. Logan, was so receptive to the idea of medical history questionnaires that their limited uptake at the time left him perplexed: "In fact, it may be asked why such a method is not more widely used by doctors. Perhaps some delay is related to the sanctity of the doctor-patient relationship—about whose emotional aspects some of us are becoming more aware."[68] To Graham Grant and R. A. N. Hitchens, resistance to the CMI's adoption would have made a lot more sense. In a joint letter, these physicians insisted that only a personal interview could effectively build trust between physician and patient, detect important unspoken symptoms, and allay the anxieties of worried patients. Particularly in emotionally charged contexts, they wrote, "the questionary is found wanting."[69]

Occasional squabbles aside, the index was as often ensnared in larger debates about the erosion of medical humanism, the fragmentation of medical knowledge, or the clinical value of questionnaires and mass (multiphasic) screening techniques as it was targeted directly. One such discussion formed around the broader indexical logic of medicine—a logic that one stroke patient suggested in the *New England Journal of Medicine* (*NEJM*) made the physician rigid, the patient unheard, and the relationship between the two adversarial: "A rigid doctor intensifies a rigid patient," this patient lamented.[70] Discussing a medical textbook, he continued, "A certain logic is discernible here, all right, but it is an indexer's logic, and it does chop up the stroke patient . . . into rather small pieces."[71] Mass screening programs, whereby apparently healthy people are examined for disease, had their detractors too. That they yielded too many false negatives and false positives, that they employed faulty tests, and that they left no favorable dent on patient morbidity and mortality were all criticisms that emerged as these screening programs were gaining traction in the 1950s.[72]

Other seeds of criticism were planted in the empirical literature. A 1954 study on medical questionnaires in the journal *Clinical Science* suggested that patients tend to exaggerate the presence of symptoms when those symptoms are mentioned by the questionnaire.[73] This study's findings were discussed widely, occasionally in the context of the CMI. As stated in the leading article for a 1954 issue of the *BMJ*: "It is becoming increasingly popular in the USA for a patient to provide his medical history of filling in a questionary such as the Cornell Medical Index. . . . Galser and Whittow, in light of their findings, issue a warning that the questionaries themselves may produce symptoms."[74] Brodman apparently felt these critiques deeply. In 1965, he confessed to one of his more regular interlocutors, "For the past twenty years I too have devoted myself to a controversial and generally unpopular effort and have endured the loneliness you now experience."[75]

But counterbalancing the criticism and concern among some medical professionals was an interest in and enthusiasm for the index among others. Numerous physicians from around the world wrote to Brodman commending him for his work on the CMI. One physician noted how he was "keen to use the Cornell Medical Index as an important instrument of inquiry" in his own practice of medicine.[76] Other early adopters remarked on the tool's utility, reporting to have "obtained good help" from the CMI.[77] Coverage of the CMI in the lay press also carried a distinctly positive valence. In 1951, the *New York Herald Tribune* ran the story, "Questionnaire Helps Doctors Diagnose Ills," which introduced readers to the index and basic data about its clinical effectiveness. Citing these data, the article concluded, "Since this questionnaire proved so helpful in aiding physicians in the admitting departments to quickly secure a picture of the patient's total medical problem . . . the questionnaire is being introduced in Bellevue Hospital and in numerous private hospital practices."[78] A 1953 article in the Spanish-language magazine *Vision* similarly hailed the index as a remedy to "one of the main headaches plaguing today's busy doctor's [*sic*]."[79]

## Indexing the World

Enthusiasm for the index was backed by its actual clinical use. The distribution and sale of the CMI experienced healthy growth in the decades after its publication. Through the 1950s and 1960s, Cornell Medical College sold and distributed around a quarter of a million copies of the index annually. Thousands more spread through networks of physicians informally. By the 1960s, the CMI was recognized in medical journals as the "most widely used" medical questionnaire.[80] In addition to its broadening influence and visibility as a tool of clinical practice, the index also enjoyed a career as a tool of medical research. From 1949 onward, the number of published articles employing the index in some fashion trended upward. As Brodman and his collaborators pitched it, further research with the CMI would enhance not just medical knowledge but the value of the tool itself. Since the standardized nature of the CMI allowed comparisons across different studies and patient populations, a growing bank of published data derived from the index would incentivize its adoption by other researchers; as the size of the CMI research network grew, so did the expected value of joining that network. Many also speculated that additional CMI research would enrich the index's *clinical* value. As the *BMJ* editorial observed, future research might shed light on yet-undiscovered connections between questionnaire responses and medical conditions.

National and linguistic boundaries hardly inhibited the index's expansion through communities of clinicians and researchers. The CMI gradually became international and multilingual. The first translation of the index—into Spanish—came in the early 1950s, at the behest of officials at Cornell and the New York Hospital. The New York Hospital served a large population of Puerto Rican patients, many of whom came to New York City in the wave of migration to the city following World War II. Brodman therefore commissioned a group of professors at the University of Puerto Rico to make the Spanish translation.[81] Before long, the Cornell Medical Index was not just the *Indice Medico de Cornell* (Spanish); it also became the *Index Médical de Cornell* (French); *Mục-lục Y-khoa Cornell* (Vietnamese), and *Cornell Tıbbi Endeksi* (Turkish).[82] Japanese, German, Arabic, Dutch, Hebrew, Hindu, and Chinese translations also made the index intelligible to patients speaking these languages (Figure 1.2). By and large, these subsequent translations emerged organically—not through the directive of Brodman or Cornell but through the initiative of physicians and researchers working in far-flung regions of the world. One physician who lived and worked in the Lago Colony, a small multinational community located on the east end of the Caribbean island of Aruba, presented Brodman in 1955 with a translation of the index into the island's local language, Papiamento.[83] The physician estimated that this Creole language—influenced by Spanish, Portuguese, Dutch, Arawakan, English, and a number of other languages—was spoken by some 180,000 individuals across the Caribbean islands.

At its core, the CMI was an instrument of standardization. No two physicians confronted with the same patient would take the exact same medical history. Indeed, such variation was, in the early 1950s, emerging as a topic of inquiry—and concern. In 1951, Archibald Cochrane, together with two other British researchers, documented wide variations in the medical histories taken from comparable groups of coal miners, even when the medical observers asked the miners the exact same questions.[84] The authors hypothesized that much of this variation resulted from the "bias" of the medical observers coming into contact with the unstructured nature of the miners' answers. When asked "Have you a cough?" or "Do you spit?" the participants might reply imprecisely, "Only an ordinary cough" or "Only after work."[85] How a physician codes, or follows up on, these responses inevitably turned on factors unique to each individual clinician (i.e., experience, knowledge, background, and personality). Open-ended history-taking, Cochrane and his co-authors implied, left the door open to inconsistency and error. The index, by contrast, imposed sharp boundaries on the possible form a medical history could take. It asked all patients the same questions, in the same order, and in the same fashion; the responses available to patients were binary: "Yes" or "No." The CMI manual, moreover, provided clear instructions concerning the index's clinical implementation, demarcating the "intended" (correct) from the "unintended" (incorrect) ways of using the questionnaire.

Medische Vragenlijst

[illegible]

(FEMMES)

INDEX MÉDICAL DE CORNELL

QUESTIONNAIRE DE SANTE

Date........

DIRECTIONS: Ce questionnaire est pour les FEMMES SEULEMENT.

Si vous pouvez répondre OUI à la question demandée, faites un cercle autour du Oui

Si vous devez répondre NON à la question demandée, faites un cercle autour du Non

Répondez à toutes les questions, si vous n'êtes pas certaine, risquez.

A

1. Avez-vous besoin de lunettes pour lire? ... Oui Non

[illegible]

OUVREZ A LA PAGE SUIVANTE

For Women

CORNELL MEDICAL INDEX

HEALTH QUESTIONNAIRE

Date

Print Your Name

How old are you?

Single, Married, Widowed

DIRECTIONS:

[illegible]

A

1. Do you need glasses to read? Yes No

[illegible]

CORNELL MEDICAL INDEX

健康調査表

[illegible]

(HOMBRES)

INDICE MEDICO DE CORNELL

CUESTIONARIO DE SALUD

Fecha........

Direcciones: Este cuestionario es para HOMBRES SOLAMENTE.

Si puede contestar SÍ a la pregunta, haga un círculo alrededor de (Sí)

Si tiene que contestar NO a la pregunta, haga un círculo alrededor de (No)

Conteste todas las preguntas. Si no está seguro, adivine.

[illegible]

(ERKEK)

CORNELL TIBBİ ENDEKSİ

SAĞLIK SORULARI

DİKKAT

[illegible]

*Figure 1.2.* Various translations of the CMI brought the tool to new populations and parts of the world. *Clockwise from upper left*: Dutch, French, Japanese, Turkish, Spanish, and Hindi translations. Courtesy of the Medical Center Archives of New York–Presbyterian / Weill Cornell Medicine. The Cornell Medical Index and related historical health questionnaires should only be used for historical reference and not for any research involving human subjects.

Despite references in print to a single, universal, and standard CMI, in practice there existed a multiplicity of CMIs. As the index pushed through geographic and linguistic barriers, the tool sometimes changed along the way, adapting to its various local contexts. Even within the United States, some physicians who integrated the CMI into their private practices tailored the questionnaire to the needs of their practices and patients. One internist wrote to Brodman in 1966, "I have used the old Cornell Medical Index beginning about 1951 and a *personal modification* since 1961. I find these extremely useful in my practice of Internal Medicine."[86] But not all changes to the index were intentional: meaning was also lost—and gained—in translation. The creators of the index were very deliberate about the wording of the 195 items on the questionnaire. The slightest modification of word choice, Brodman discovered in the process of creating the CMI, could significantly alter patients' responses. "We found," Brodman wrote in 1949, "that every word had to be chosen with the greatest care, and that every question had to be rigorously tested after it was put together."[87]

The chief criterion for choosing between different formulations of a given question was clarity; the CMI's developers wanted to design a questionnaire that could be answered by people with "no more than three or four years of elementary school education."[88] For Brodman, making the index linguistically accessible meant making it conversational and idiomatic—incorporating common expressions and dressing many questions up in a colloquial style. For example, item 145 on the index read, "Does your work fall to pieces when the boss or a supervisor is watching you?" Idioms, like "fall to pieces," vary across languages, so maintaining the spirit of such questions sometimes proved difficult.[89] Once translated into another language, the questionnaire was never equally befitting of all dialects within that language. The Cornell-sponsored Spanish translation, customized for speakers of Puerto Rican Spanish, was, to speakers of certain other dialects, intelligible but imperfect. A Venezuelan doctor raised these issues to Brodman in a 1962 letter: " 'Eyeglasses' are called 'espejuelos' in Cuba. In Venezuela we called them 'lentes' which would be more widely understood. 'Anteojos' used in Colombia is also more clear than 'espejuelos.' "[90]

Dwarfing the challenge of translating across languages was the challenge of translating across societies and cultures. Built into the CMI were certain theories of illness along with certain assumptions about the population's health behaviors, views on medical disclosure, and distribution of disease. Researchers found that these assumptions did not hold in all contexts. In the early 1950s, the psychiatrist Ludwig Laufer used the CMI among people native to the Okinawa Islands located to the south of Japan. From the outset, Laufer identified what he believed to be a mismatch between the index and the local culture: Okinawan society (in his view) was more group-oriented than the individualistic milieu from which the CMI developed. As Laufer saw it, a local Okinawan was more inclined to answer the index's questions as part of a family unit. Laufer therefore administered the index not to individuals but to "cooperative family group[s]" that discussed and responded collectively to each questionnaire item.[91] Compounding issues with the CMI that were more structural in nature, individual items on the questionnaire were often incongruous with local norms and distributions of disease. In a culture with a different family and social structure, what was the meaning of a question like, "Do you wish that you always had someone at your side to advise you"? Or, more materially: given the higher prevalence of endamebiasis and intestinal parasites, what was Laufer to make of questions about respondents' bowel movements?

About a decade later, an anthropologist-physician team from Harvard faced similar problems in applying the index to Zulu communities in Southern Africa.[92] The team created a modified version of the CMI, (modestly) adapted to the linguistic and cultural characteristics of the population studied. These slight modifications did little to rescue a number of questions from cultural opacity. According to the study's authors, it was a common practice in Zulu communities to look upon strangers with a healthy degree of suspicion. As a result, an affirmative answer to the question "Do strange people or places make you afraid?" was indicative not of any paranoid or neurotic mentality but of a perfectly normal cultural attitude. Beyond problems with individual items, the entire structure of the questionnaire came under strain. The index's organization, based on Western ideas about disease causation and the human body, came into conflict with other theories of illness and systems of nosology. Zulu indigenous culture, the researchers reasoned, "provides a competing and highly organized system of classifications of disease and concepts of disease etiology, so that the classification of CMI questions into organ-systems or by disease areas may seem, to them, to present symptoms in a meaningless or confusing context."[93] It was not the conclusion of these researchers that the CMI had buckled under the weight of these cultural forces; rather, the team suggested that the index proved useful in unintended ways. They proposed that the index and culture had a bidirectional relationship: the CMI must be interpreted with adequate knowledge of the participating population's culture, but they came to believe that, when interpreted as such, the CMI "yields clues" not just to the respondents' health status but to their "cultural and social situation."[94]

The CMI's national and international spread highlights the role of the instrument's users in driving its clinical expansion and shaping its clinical use.[95] Brodman himself recognized the possibility that, once developed, the tool might mature in unexpected, even regrettable, ways. As he wrote in a draft of a 1949 magazine article, "An[d] now, we're wondering about the future. Will the Health Questionnaire be used properly? Will it be recognized for what it is, simply a large collection of medical data for the doctor to study and combine with other information? Or will it be used like a radio tube tester, and all by itself, in an attempt to make automatic diagnoses?"[96]

To discuss the role of the index's consumers is not to diminish from the work of its producers in promoting and legitimating the tool.[97] Brodman and his collaborators had grand ambitions for the CMI, and they chased these ambitions through a variety of means. To publicize the index, these researchers reported on the tool in leading medical journals; to facilitate its clinical implementation, they created a user manual that addressed logistical issues surrounding its clinical use. The first wave of publications on the index relied on a single patient population: outpatients at the New York Hospital. This limited subject pool satisfied these early studies' primary aim of illuminating the index's basic value in more structured and conventional clinical settings. But how would the index fare among rural people? Or people who did not seek outpatient medical care? These questions were hanging in the minds of Brodman and his colleagues.

## Oneonta, New York, as Laboratory

By the early 1950s, Brodman and others had initiated a research venture to demonstrate the CMI's utility in far different, sometimes even nonclinical, environments. One of these studies, the Oneonta Health Survey, was ambitious. The study, conducted in November 1951, surveyed 1,800 adult residents from six hundred randomly selected families in Oneonta, a town in central New York State.[98] The study was a logistically complex operation, and the Cornell researchers enlisted the Bureau of Applied Social Research at Columbia University to assist in coordinating and undertaking the study's fieldwork.[99] The Bureau's staff instructed and supervised twelve fieldworkers, drawn from the local Oneonta population, who distributed copies of the CMI to each of the study's adult participants and gathered additional medical, social, personal, and economic information about the participants from the head of each household. The fieldworkers directed participants to return the completed index by mail and personally revisited participants who, after two weeks, failed to do so. By the end of the study, 85 percent of the study participants had responded.[100]

The American public was not always well acquainted with surveys, questionnaires, and population statistics, as Sarah Igo has shown.[101] Brodman and his collaborator Irving Lorge made no assumptions about the Oneonta public's familiarity with—or their warmness toward—either the CMI specifically or health questionnaires in general. Cornell researchers orchestrated an information campaign not only to raise awareness about the health survey but also to put the survey under a positive light. The campaign, as Harold Wolff related in a 1952 letter, began ten days prior to the fieldwork and recruited the cooperation of "local physicians, Public Health Service personnel, civic leaders, school authorities, newspapers, and radio stations."[102] The campaign's various organs worked together under a common slogan: "To help the doctor help you." The "you," one team member explained in the month leading up to the study, "is both singular, referring to the individual completing the form, and plural, the community."[103]

To convincingly claim that the study would help the local community, the study's architects ironically needed the local community's help. "We were always going to accent that this is a community affair," the team member wrote, "that the civic organizations, schools, churches, physicians, health officers, newspaper, and community leaders were backing the project."[104] Brodman and his colleagues recognized that the campaign's message would be amplified if channeled through the voice of local officials, institutions, and community members: "The publicity should mention the fact that the community can take pride in being selected for this survey. Statements to this effect from local leaders are probably the most effective method of making this point."[105]

The formal objective of the Oneonta Health Survey was, as stated in some July 1951 notes on the project, "to determine the health status of the population of Oneonta N.Y. and the contiguous rural area."[106] But behind this primary research objective lay a grander secondary objective. In effectively appraising the health status of Oneonta, the developers of the CMI hoped that the study would prove the questionnaire's suitability for larger scale, even national, health surveys. Researchers selected Oneonta over alternative locations largely because the city, with its mix of urban and rural areas, seemed nationally representative; success in surveying the health of Oneonta, these researchers figured, would augur well for the index's successful application at a national level. Oneonta was the perfect laboratory, they believed. In December 1951, just months after the survey had wrapped up, Harold Wolff saw an opportunity to introduce the index into discussions about national health initiatives. That month, President Harry S. Truman signed an executive order establishing the President's Commission on the Health Needs of the Nation. The president left the commission with a broad directive: "During this crucial period in our country's history it [the commission] will make a critical study of our total health requirements, both immediate and long-range, and will recommend courses of action to meet these needs."[107]

Part of estimating the nation's total health requirements involved estimating its total health status. How many Americans had heart disease? What percentage complained of vision problems? This is where Brodman, Wolff, and their associates thought that the CMI could be of use. In January 1952, Wolff wrote to commission member Joseph Hinsey in an effort to bring the questionnaire to the commission's attention. Wolff singled out the group's work in Oneonta as a point of particular interest. He opened the letter, writing, "As a member of the commission . . . you may be interested in our experiences with the Cornell Medical Index-Health Questionnaire, especially those in making a health survey of an upper New York State community."[108] He closed on a similar note: "Our experiences in this local [Oneonta] survey have convinced us that the Cornell Medical Index-Health Questionnaire may be useful in conducting a national health survey."

Wolff's suggestion indeed piqued the commission's curiosity. Commission chair Paul B. Magnuson followed up with Wolff in a series of letters, all of which homed in on certain administrative aspects of collecting health data with the index. Magnuson was eager to know how many people were surveyed in Oneonta, how long it took to conduct the survey, how long it took to analyze the information collected, and how much money conducting a health survey of this nature cost. "These questions," Magnuson explained, "are important to us in determining whether or not this Commission should sponsor such an undertaking on a larger scale."[109] The commission ultimately decided against using the index, curbing hopes that the CMI might be adopted as a government-backed, nationwide survey. To be sure this was a disappointment, but not one that stopped Brodman from pushing the CMI in new directions.

CHAPTER TWO

# The Statistical Patient

In January 1955, J. Robert Oppenheimer, the former scientific head of the Manhattan Project's Los Alamos Laboratory, appeared on Edward R. Murrow's popular television series *See It Now* to discuss his new, civilian role.[1] Since 1947, Oppenheimer had taken over as director of the Institute for Advanced Study, a research center in Princeton, New Jersey, that served as the intellectual home for luminaries like Albert Einstein, Kurt Gödel, and John von Neumann.[2] Brodman happened to watch the program and was immediately struck by two things: first, Oppenheimer's commitment to "interdisciplinary thought in science," and second, Oppenheimer's personal connections to the world's most prominent scientists and mathematicians.[3] Brodman therefore wrote to Oppenheimer asking if he might recommend a mathematician "with competence and interest" in a particular problem.[4]

Brodman's problem was this. The fact that the Cornell Medical Index (1) aided physicians (and even unskilled personnel) in making comprehensive diagnostic decisions, (2) quickly collected large amounts of data on large numbers of patients, and (3) collected these data in a binary form suggested to Brodman that it was possible "to derive a mathematical model of the operation of making diagnoses from the data, as an analogue to human thinking."[5] Although Brodman believed that he had identified an auspicious problem area, he recognized his own limitations in navigating it solo: "My own inadequacy as [a] mathematician has permitted the construction of only a crude model, but even this Simple Simon gives promise that further study may be fruitful."[6]

This chapter follows Brodman's project as it evolved from a paper-based technology that sought to assist with medical history-taking to a digital technology that aimed to automate diagnosis. This evolution was driven by a confluence of factors, including Brodman's own personal interest in cybernetic thought as well as a broader societal interest in applying new computing technologies to all kinds of medical, social, and distributional problems of the day. Ultimately, the chapter demonstrates that the final product of Brodman's work—the Medical Data Screen (MDS)—created statistical and aggregative representations of patients and their disease states.

## The Cybernetic Psychiatrist

For Brodman, the hope of developing a diagnostic model from CMI data was inextricably linked to the hope of shedding light on the nature of human reasoning. From the beginning, the idea that a mathematical model could both incorporate and illuminate human cognitive processes consumed him. As he noted to Oppenheimer, "Study of such a model may have not only value in pure science but may also give information about the mechanisms of higher brain functions such as memory, concept formation, and judgement."[7] By way of response, Oppenheimer advised Brodman to contact Julian Bigelow, a cyberneticist, engineer, and computing pioneer based at the Institute for Advanced Study.[8] Brodman dutifully did just that. In a letter to Bigelow, Brodman highlighted his team's finding that nonphysicians and trainees—medical interns, nurses, and technicians—made diagnostic deductions from CMI data nearly as effectively as full physicians did. Even a layman, Brodman elaborated, "with not as much pertinent information as a physician, can usually make partial diagnoses."[9] To Brodman this hinted that (contrary to the CMI manual's insistence otherwise) the secret ingredient to interpreting patient data was not to be found exclusively in the physician; perhaps a mathematical model, based on human reasoning generally, would suffice. Brodman posed this question to Bigelow: "Since a human being with this information in binary form can make correct diagnostic decisions, is it not possible to derive a mathematical model of the operation of making these decisions?"[10]

Brodman offered a rough sketch of how, by his estimation, humans reason in a clinical context: "Some of the methods a person uses in reaching decisions for diagnoses are known . . . For example, in determining which organ system is likely to be associated with a complaint on the questionnaire, the diagnostician unconsciously scans his memory. He estimates the frequency with which the complaint occurs with disorders in each organ system, and selects the one with which the complaint is most frequently associated."[11]

Bigelow, having spent much of his career thinking about the application of computing and mathematics to practical domains of this sort, was stimulated by these ideas. He agreed that the proposal warranted further serious study, but he gently implied that Brodman was not fully appreciating the complexity of human cognitive processes: "This is not at all easy to do in a valid way, as the scarcity of genuine successes reported in the literature may indicate."[12] Like Brodman, Bigelow believed that there existed a mechanism by which humans make decisions from observational data, but in his view this mechanism was "of the most complicated and obscure type."[13]

In Brodman's mind, the complexity of human cognitive functions depended on the scale of analysis. At lower, more basic levels of cognition, Brodman insisted on simplicity. Either a neuron fires or it doesn't: "The unit mechanism is almost certainly simple, a yes discharge or a no discharge. The next level for some functions may still be simple neurones arranged in configurations permitting such operations as 'and,' 'or' and 'not.' Then I stop."[14] Beyond this stopping point, Brodman conceded that speculating about the mechanism of higher-level thought processes was difficult, noting "the immense and bewildering complexities of interrelated functions." But this complexity spurred Brodman. He saw the proposed study as a possible entry into a "vast unknown field of knowledge."

Brodman's view of human thought processes was refracted through the lens of his own experience with multiple sclerosis. Once Brodman returned to New York from his military service, his condition worsened. From 1948 onward, he was conducting all of his work from home due to his physical mobility challenges; when he met with correspondents and collaborators like Bigelow, it was always at his residence. In 1954, Brodman more fully elaborated on the nature and progression of his symptoms: "For the past dozen years I have developed increasing disabilities due to multiple sclerosis. Their marked progression during the past six months has made it extremely difficult for me to keep up with my work or, for that matter, to carry out the daily routine of living."[15]

But Brodman's disability informed as much as it distracted from his work: it was his experience with multiple sclerosis that first convinced him that human reasoning could be formalized, mathematized, and computerized. Brodman began deriving ideas about human cognition from his neurologic disease as early as 1953. In a 1953 letter to Norbert Wiener, Brodman described his own experience with multiple sclerosis in terms that Wiener, as the leading voice of cybernetics, would have understood well—Brodman revealed how central nervous system tracts degenerate "as if small groups of wires in a communication system were cut." He continued, "This suggests that a study of functions disordered by the disease may give useful leads to the understanding of central nervous system mechanisms. I am thinking not only about spinal and cerebellar functions but more particularly about the unknown mechanisms of such activities as memory, association, judgement, intellegence [*sic*], and behavior."[16] Two years later, in a letter to Bigelow, Brodman invoked this same cybernetic metaphor, comparing neurodegeneration to communication system wires being "cut at random." Brodman went on to explicitly trace out the causal pathway linking his experience of multiple sclerosis to his interest in formalizing human reasoning: "It was my observation of the subtle progressive changes in my higher functions that led me to believe the basic unit of these functions to be simple, similar in many areas, and describable in mathematical terms."[17]

Brodman's letters to Wiener and Bigelow point to the pathway by which Brodman, a clinician trained in psychiatry and psychosomatic medicine, came to work on computing projects. Wiener and Bigelow were founders of the field of cybernetics.[18] In 1948, a year before Brodman and his colleagues released the CMI, Wiener published his influential book *Cybernetics*.[19] The book defined the field of cybernetics, the study of "control and communication in the animal and the machine," and helped establish some of its guiding tools (mathematical models) and metaphors (mind as machine). Though peppered with complex equations and technical language, *Cybernetics* aroused considerable interest among both academic and lay audiences. The book's content (and title) struck most of its readers as utterly new, but the book popularized, synthesized, and elaborated upon a line of thinking that had been in the making for a few years. In 1943, the neurophysiologist Warren McCulloch, together with the twenty-year-old logician Walter Pitts, published a landmark paper that described the first mathematical model of a neural network (Figure 2.1).[20] The paper, demonstrating that neural nets could perform the logical operations of a Turing machine (a mathematical model of computation), invigorated ideas that mind and machine were fundamentally analogous.[21]

These early cybernetic ideas appealed to scholars with a wide range of disciplinary backgrounds—from the anthropologist Margaret Mead to the mathematician and engineer Claude Shannon. Between 1946 and 1953, this diverse network of researchers came together for a series of cybernetics conferences organized by the Josiah Macy Jr. Foundation.[22] The conferences served as a venue for thinking through cybernetics in its many different instantiations: as

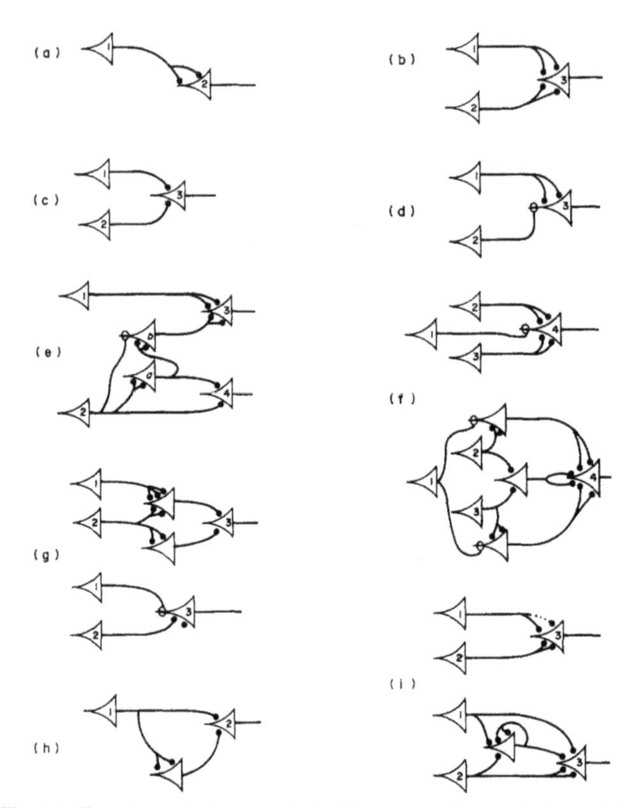


Figure 1. The neuron $c_i$ is always marked with the numeral $i$ upon the body of the cell, and the corresponding action is denoted by "$N$" with $i$ s subscript, as in the text:

(a) $N_2(t) . \equiv . N_1(t-1);$

(b) $N_3(t) . \equiv . N_1(t-1) \vee N_2(t-1);$

(c) $N_3(t) . \equiv . N_1(t-1) . N_2(t-1);$

(d) $N_3(t) . \equiv N_1(t-1) . \sim N_2(t-1);$

(e) $N_3(t) : \equiv : N_1(t-1) . \vee . N_2(t-3) . \sim N_2(t-2);$
$N_4(t) . \equiv . N_2(t-2) . N_2(t-1);$

(f) $N_4(t) : \equiv : \sim N_1(t-1) . N_2(t-1) \vee N_3(t-1) . \vee . N_1(t-1) .$
$N_2(t-1) . N_3(t-1)$
$N_4(t) : \equiv : \sim N_1(t-2) . N_2(t-2) \vee N_3(t-2) . \vee . N_1(t-2) .$
$N_2(t-2) . N_3(t-2);$

(g) $N_3(t) . \equiv . N_2(t-2) . \sim N_1(t-3);$

(h) $N_2(t) . \equiv . N_1(t-1) . N_1(t-2);$

(i) $N_3(t) : \equiv : N_2(t-1) . \vee . N_1(t-1) . (Ex)t-1 . N_1(x) . N_2(x).$

*Figure 2.1.* The McCulloch-Pitts artificial neuron. Each neuron can either fire or not. The neural arrangements represent different Boolean functions or logical propositions, such as "AND," "OR," "NOT," etc. In this figure, part (b) represents "OR" (i.e., neuron 3 will fire if neuron 1 fires OR if neuron 2 fires at a given time), part (c) represents "AND" (i.e., neuron 3 will fire if neuron 1 AND neuron 2 fire at a given time), and part (d) represents "NOT" (i.e., neuron 3 will fire if neuron 1 fires but NOT if neuron 2 fires at a given time). Brodman's intellectual debt to this work is apparent in his 1955 letter to Bigelow: "The unit mechanism is almost certainly simple, a yes discharge or a no discharge. The next level for some functions may still be simple neurones [*sic*] arranged in configurations permitting such operations as 'and,' 'or' and 'not.'" Warren S. McCulloch and Walter Pitts, "A Logical Calculus of the Ideas Immanent in Nervous Activity," *Bulletin of Mathematical Biophysics* 5 (1943): 115–133. Courtesy of the Society for Mathematical Biology.

a mathematical theory of communication and control, as a transdisciplinary study of the analogies between minds and computers, as an engineering enterprise concerning the construction of automata, and even as a more philosophical inquiry into what it means to be human.[23] Though heterogeneous, cybernetics animated widespread hopes that the behaviors of both inanimate and living systems could be modeled mathematically.

If the Macy Conferences served as an early platform for the field of cybernetics, the Dartmouth Summer Research Project on Artificial Intelligence, a 1956 workshop organized by mathematician John McCarthy, helped to introduce artificial intelligence as a field.[24] The aim of the Dartmouth workshop was described in a proposal written for the conference in 1955: "The study is to proceed on the basis of the conjecture that every aspect of learning or any other feature of intelligence can in principle be so precisely described that a machine can be made to simulate it."[25] McCarthy, together with colleagues (and competitors) at institutions like MIT, Carnegie Institute of Technology (now Carnegie Mellon University), and Stanford University, defined a new approach that came to be known as symbolic artificial intelligence.[26] Through the 1960s and 1970s, "symbolic," "expert systems," and "pattern recognition" approaches moved to the mainstream while overtly "cybernetic" approaches migrated increasingly to the fringes.[27]

While cybernetics is often conceived of as a militaristic science, the sociologist Andrew Pickering has helped elevate the role of psychiatry in the field's development. As Pickering describes it, psychiatry was a "surface of emergence" for the field of cybernetics—a disciplinary arena in which cyberneticists thought through ideas about feedback, control, and communication.[28] These intellectual exchanges between psychiatry and cybernetics arose out of a shared interest in the human nervous system. A central aim of cybernetics was, as Wiener noted in a 1948 essay, to study "the common elements in the functioning of automatic machines and of the human nervous system."[29] And the hallmark approach within cybernetics for probing these "common elements" between minds and machines was the development of mathematical models of the nervous system. Brodman's early musings about how to formalize clinical cognition therefore carry a distinctively cybernetic flavor. Like Wiener, Bigelow, and other early cyberneticists, Brodman exhibited not only an intense fascination with the analogies between the human mind and automatic systems but also an inclination to pursue these analogies through mathematical modeling. Beyond showing *that* Brodman was attracted to cybernetic approaches, these exchanges with Wiener and Bigelow also suggest *why*

Brodman was so drawn: the letters showcase his embodied sensitivity to cybernetic principles of communication and control. What primed Brodman to the possibility of applying mathematical models and computers to the problem of medical diagnosis and decision-making was his own experience of illness—an alertness to the sensations of his own body.

Citing the weight of other commitments, Bigelow backed out of their collaboration a few months after it began.[30] But around the time of Bigelow's departure, in the summer of 1955, Brodman received a serendipitous letter introducing him to someone who might be able to fill Bigelow's shoes: Adrianus van Woerkom.[31] A Dutchman, Van Woerkom trained in astronomy at Leiden University, earning his doctorate in 1948. That same year, Van Woerkom began serving as an assistant professor of astronomy at Yale University, where he also directed the nascent Computing Laboratory. Van Woerkom wore many hats as an academic: he was introduced to Brodman as "Adrianus J. J. van Woerkom, astronomer, mathematician, and master of the IBM machine."[32] One of Van Woerkom's interests was the application of mathematics to psychology—particularly areas of psychology where there existed large amounts of high-quality data.[33] This was precisely the kind of area in which Brodman believed himself to be working. Human psychology was Brodman's chief intrigue, and he was working with large quantities of patient data procured from the CMI beginning in 1948. Brodman therefore followed up with Van Woerkom by presenting his research "problem" as he had presented it to Oppenheimer some seven months earlier.[34] Within a month, the two began a collaboration that would become the most important of Brodman's career.

In his collaboration with Van Woerkom, Brodman continued his cybernetically inflected quest to develop a model of human cognition, one that might serve as the basis for his computerized diagnostic system. Contemplating the implications of such a model often left Brodman palpably excited. In 1960, as he was brainstorming a new model, he wrote to Van Woerkom, "I have so many thoughts about the new model that I feel like Handel when he said after he finished an oratorio that it was as if all heaven was opened before him. I feel as if all truth wer[e] opened before me."[35] At this early stage of development, Brodman's ideas were both vague and grandiose, and they centered on one primary topic: pattern recognition. Diagnosing disease, Brodman ventured, was fundamentally an exercise in discerning patterns. As he expounded to Van Woerkom, "A physician certainly does not make computations when he makes a decision, nor does a person consciously use statistical techniques when he makes any decision. People recognize and manipulate patterns, gestalt. The model will do likewise."[36]

In the context of medical diagnosis, Brodman ventured that a pattern might consist of a "configuration of symptoms." It was the whole collection of symptoms that served as the meaningful unit of analysis in diagnostic reasoning. As Brodman described it, a physician, after "recogniz[ing] some elements of a disease concept" would "search for other elements [of the pattern] to convince himself that the disease concept exists in reality."[37] According to Brodman, that diagnosing disease involved pattern recognition was simply a consequence of the fact that pattern recognition underlay all human (even animal) cognitive processes:

> The principles of the model are by no means limited in application to the making of a diagnostic decision. What I like most about the model is that we use a single simple principle, that the CNS [central nervous system] recognizes reality by its pattern, to explain decision function, psychiatric phenomena, thinking, animal behavior, and many other living activities that heretofore have required complicated and unrelated formulations to explain each independently. It is not a large step to extend this principle to explain how the CNS recognizes abstract phenomena such as mathematical concepts, beauty, concept formation, creativity, and language, and how the CNS creates.[38]

Brodman wasn't just computerizing diagnosis; by his estimation, he was modeling a unified theory of cognition.

These reflections on pattern recognition bear the mark of contemporaneous research in the fields of cybernetics and artificial intelligence. Pattern recognition emerged as a favorite topic within cybernetics owing in large part to Warren McCulloch and Walter Pitts's 1947 article "How We Know Universals: The Perception of Visual and Auditory Forms." Aiming to shed light on the neural basis of "the *Gestalten* of Wertheimer and Köhler," the article outlined two neural mechanisms "which exhibit recognition of forms."[39] That is, the article was an effort to understand (and describe mathematically) how humans could, for example, perceive a given object as the same (as "invariant") even when viewing it from different sides and angles. Related discussions of gestalt perception also figured prominently in Wiener's *Cybernetics*.[40] By the late 1950s, the intellectual seeds of pattern recognition research that had been planted within the field of cybernetics began to germinate within the field of artificial intelligence.[41]

Pattern recognition offered one important cybernetic analogy between digital computers and human minds; psychiatric disorder offered another. Various cyberneticists drew parallels between psychiatric problems and problems in the operation of a computer. Humans develop psychoses and neuroses; machines crash, stall, and run amiss. Even psychiatric treatments had their digital correlates: Wiener believed, for instance, that electroshock therapy was akin to the wiping of a computer's memory.[42] Here again, Brodman's views are remarkably consonant with those of early cyberneticists. Brodman mused that an ideal model would be one that failed in the same way that human minds tend to fail. He wanted the model to be a little bit "neurotic": "In general," Brodman wrote in some notes in 1955, "the math model should have the possibility of doing what humans do, even of developing the same defects in judgement and behavior as a human with a neurosis or psychosis."[43]

It would be a mistake to claim that Brodman was a full-fledged cyberneticist; he wasn't. Brodman never cited any key cybernetic works in his writings, nor did he identify his views as being cybernetically inspired.[44] But considering his unsolicited letter to Norbert Wiener, his engagements with Julian Bigelow, and the parallels between cybernetic thought and his own, Brodman was certainly interested and invested in cybernetic thought. It was this interest that catalyzed the evolution of a project of medical history-taking into one of computerizing diagnosis.

## Digitizing Data

Brodman's work traversed the heady and the mundane. At the same time that Brodman was engaged in airy philosophical meditations concerning various models, he was also consumed by the labor and monotony of more earthy data practices. The CMI data collected from New York Hospital patients between 1948 and 1949 provided Brodman, Van Woerkom, and their collaborators with three basic kinds of information about some five thousand patients: their diagnosis as determined by New York Hospital clinical staff, their responses to the CMI, and their demographic characteristics.

Originally, this "raw" data took the form of thousands of paper questionnaires. The data, in this form, exhibited a lot of what the historian Paul Edwards has called "data friction"—the questionnaires were bulky, they took up physical space, they demanded great labor to sort through, and they could be (and were) physically lost and misplaced.[45] At some point, by the mid-1950s, this information had been abstracted and coded onto punched cards, and later magnetic tape, for computer processing. Although difficult to know with certainty, these data may have also existed in an intermediate, abstracted paper "database" as well. Brodman hinted at this possibility in a 1970 letter, when he noted that the "original volume" of 1948–1949 data had been lost: "All data derived from the Cornell Medical Index of course remains in the public domain, but by this time all except published material have been lost. The original volume of data was enormous with over 23 thousand entries for one table alone."[46]

By the mid-1950s, Brodman's team had articulated an overarching strategy for building a diagnostic model from this information. Their model would permit making diagnoses from CMI data "on the basis of the frequency of each complaint in different diseases."[47] In other words, they hoped to exploit the fact that patients with a given disease responded to questionnaire items in a generally distinctive way. With this framework in place, Brodman and his collaborators turned to questions of mathematics. Although building a mathematical model was necessarily technical, Brodman believed that his clinical intuition would effectively guide their early work. He wrote to Van Woerkom, "My clinical experience suggests that the complexities of the problem will make many pitfalls and booby traps, and we must be alert and careful in planning if they are to be avoided. Fortunately, clinical experience can not [*sic*] only help avoid these traps but can also yield the intuitive approach to successful planning that is so important in studying a new area of knowledge."[48]

The fruit of all this labor—a working statistical model suitable for computer implementation—was announced in a series of articles published between 1959 and 1961.[49] These articles described a four-step statistical method. First, using the 1948–1949 CMI data, it assigned each questionnaire item a significance value for each of the sixty most common diseases according to the following formula:

$$P_{ij} = \frac{R_{ij} - R_i}{2(\sqrt{R_i})} \pm 1,$$

where $P_{ij}$ is the significance value, $R_i$ is the frequency of a given complaint ($i$) in the entire patient population, and $R_{ij}$ is the frequency of the complaint in the subset of patients with disease $j$.[50] The logic behind this formula was this: a given complaint (or symptom) is diagnostically valuable when its frequency in the overall patient population is very different from its frequency in the subset of patients with the disease in question. Second, for a particular patient, and in a given disease, the significance values of the separate questionnaire items were combined using the formula:

$$N_p = \sum P_{ij}^2.$$

Third, this total value, $N_p$, was corrected for the patient's age—a statistical nod to the fact that physicians expect diseases to present differently in differently aged populations. Finally, the corrected total score for the particular patient was converted into a "likelihood score," $L$, by relating it to the mean corrected total score for all patients known to have the disease, $N_m$:

$$L = \frac{N_p}{N_m} \times 50.$$

The patient in question was diagnosed with the disease if $L$ surpassed a given threshold. Brodman and Van Woerkom developed a program to run these computations on an IBM 704 computer, which was capable of making these computations at a rate of one patient per second (Figure 2.2).[51]

In presenting the model, Brodman speculated about the ways in which it might "simulate" clinical cognition.[52] He and Van Woerkom tested various formulas for calculating the total score ($N_p$) for each disease. Besides the formula that was eventually adopted—summing the *squares* of the significance values—one of the alternative formulas that they favorably considered involved simply adding together the significance values of all the pertinent symptoms. A number of these formulas seemed to work satisfactorily. But Brodman was drawn to the formula that squared the significance values because it captured what he believed to be an important aspect of clinical reasoning. Specifically, Brodman believed that physicians weigh symptoms that are hallmarks of different diseases especially strongly. According to Brodman, the formula simulated this clinical tradition by squaring the diagnostic value assigned to each item, which inflated the diagnostic weight of items with large significance values (consider: $1^2 = 1$; $3^2 = 9$).[53]

Brodman's engagement with the CMI, mathematical modeling, large quantities of data, and computers prompted him to generate new ideas about how doctors think. The MDS method would in turn come to contain—in its code—these very ideas. The computerization of diagnosis was clearly a generative space for thinking about, and encoding, the medical mind and its inner workings. As Lucy Suchman has noted, and as Stephanie Dick has reiterated in the context of mathematical proof, computers can be "powerful disclosing agents"—prompting humans to look inward and articulate certain views of

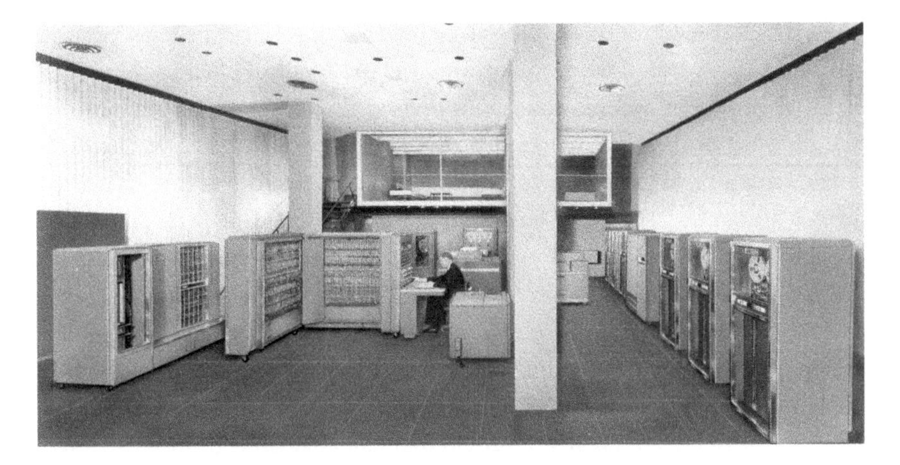

*Figure 2.2.* The IBM 704. *IBM 704 Electronic Data Processing Machine: Manual of Operation* (New York: IBM Corp., 1955), 4. Reprint courtesy of IBM Corporation © 1955. IBM, the IBM logo, and ibm.com are trademarks or registered trademarks of International Business Machines Corporation, registered in many jurisdictions worldwide. Other product and service names might be trademarks of IBM or other companies. A current list of IBM trademarks is available on the Web at "IBM Copyright and trademark information" at www.ibm.com/legal /copytrade.shtml.

themselves.[54] Brodman's case illustrates that this is not just a process of disclosure. It is also one of inscription and propagation: views articulated by humans can come to be encoded in computer programs and the mathematics underlying them.

For all that Brodman said about the possible analogies between the model and the human mind, he was the first to admit that the model as published fell short of his earlier, roaming speculations. "The machine cannot yet do as well as a physician," he admitted to Van Woerkom in 1958. "It doesn't have the background of a physician's information, and we don't know how to program a method of analysis a human being uses."[55] He struck similar notes of moderation in his article describing the model, noting that the human mind remained a "black box," shut off from perfect analysis.[56] Due to setbacks, combined with the mounting pressure to produce something concrete from all this work, Brodman's focus increasingly moved away from the model's form—the extent to which it accurately mimicked human cognition—and toward its function—the extent to which it generated correct diagnoses.[57]

## Finding a Market

The "machine method" as described between 1959 and 1961 served as the basis for what would become the Medical Data Screen.[58] Only two features differentiated the MDS from these earliest descriptions of the method. First, the MDS screened for one hundred, rather than just sixty, diseases. Second, the MDS made use of a new questionnaire: the Medical Data Index (MDI). Even as Brodman and his colleagues revised the original questionnaire for the purpose of the computerized method, the revised version retained the logic, structure, form, and many of the individual questions that characterized Brodman's earlier paper-based work. Like the CMI, the MDI favored informal over technical language and grouped questions on the questionnaire form according to sections of the body. Although the MDI contained fewer questions than the CMI (Brodman omitted the questions that did not help differentiate among the one hundred diseases), many of the MDI's 150 questions were taken from its ancestor questionnaire with minimal changes.[59]

The research team created an MDS manual, analogous to the CMI manual, that outlined the intended operation of the method. The patient would complete the self-administered, paper-based MDI questionnaire, the results of which would be mailed to those with access to a digital computer for analysis. After human workers coded and input the MDI data, the computer would generate a paper output, which would be sent back to the physician. Finally—and most importantly in Brodman's eyes—the physician would interpret this output in light of their "own training, knowledge, experiences and insights" (Figure 2.3).[60]

By the mid-1960s, Brodman had "become convinced . . . that there is an urgent need to have our method in operation and for sale as quickly as possible."[61] To help bring the MDS into wider clinical use, Brodman created the Medical Data Corporation, a small company staffed by Brodman, his research associates, and a few additional personnel to handle business and administrative affairs. Though established in 1961, the Medical Data Corporation ramped up its activities in 1966, after the MDS method was finalized and reported in the medical literature. The Medical Data Corporation saw large companies as the MDS's most promising market. This focus on industrial health was somewhat circumstantial, driven by Brodman's personal interest and expertise in the field. But Brodman and his associates also had good reason to believe that industry was particularly well suited for such a tool. Large companies had strong incentives to maintain and monitor the health of their employees, and they often lacked well-developed or well-equipped medical departments to do so.

The Medical Data Corporation initiated discussions about the MDS method with a handful of large corporations, many with tens of thousands of employees: General Electric, General Motors, Olin Mathieson, Mobile Oil, Owens-

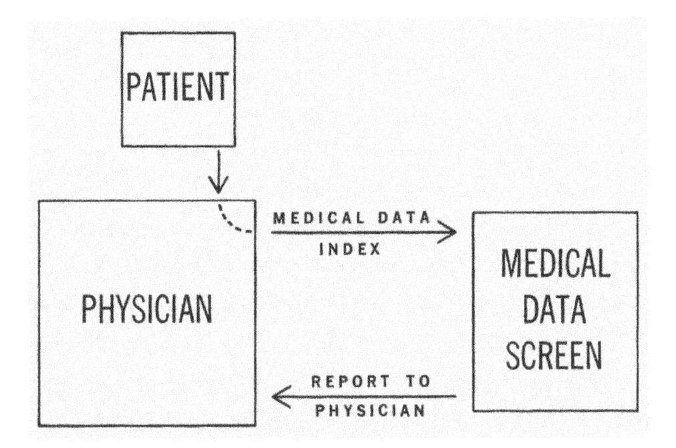


*Figure 2.3.* A schematic of the Medical Data Screen's imagined implementation. Note the size of the patient's icon relative to those of the physician and the computer. Courtesy of the Medical Center Archives of New York–Presbyterian / Weill Cornell Medicine. The Cornell Medical Index and related historical health questionnaires should only be used for historical reference and not for any research involving human subjects.

Illinois, New York Telephone Company, Prudential Life Insurance Company, Mountain States Telephone Company, and Tennessee Eastman Company—among others. As the Medical Data Corporation pitched it, companies would use the MDS method as follows: First, the Medical Data Corporation would provide the company with the needed quantity of MDI questionnaires at a cost of $4.00 per fifty questionnaires. After having employees complete the MDI, companies would send the completed questionnaires to the Medical Data Corporation for servicing. The Medical Data Corporation would then use a computer program to screen the questionnaires for the one hundred common diseases, sending the resultant computer output back to the company at a cost of $1.00 per report.[62]

As soon as he began developing and marketing the MDS, Brodman experienced something with which he was becoming all too familiar: pushback. The reactions provoked by the MDS echoed those provoked by the CMI some two decades earlier—only now they were amplified. This intensified response resulted from two key differences between the MDS and the CMI. First, the MDS made use of a technology, the computer, about which many physicians and lay people had negative or uneasy preconceptions.[63] Second, the MDS method, by its very nature, contradicted Brodman's earlier assurances in the CMI manual about the physician's interpretive monopoly over medical data. In the late 1940s, Brodman was reassuring the medical community that the interpretation of symptoms belonged to the physician and the physician alone;

some ten years later he was developing "a machine method of making diagnostic interpretations" and publishing articles with titles like "Interpretation of Symptoms with a Data-Processing Machine."[64]

The headwind came the moment Brodman and his collaborators began seeking out research funding. In 1962, after hearing rumors about the availability of "substantial sums of money to spend for medical research," Brodman wrote to a research branch of the US Army Medical Research and Development Command to inquire about funding for his work.[65] The response to Brodman's inquiry was polite but blunt: "[S]ome of us are rather vigorously opposed to this sort of thing. I am sure you must have experienced this yourself from other members of the medical profession."[66] Brodman and his colleagues faced similar opposition once they started submitting their work to medical journals. In 1960, an anonymous reviewer for *Biometrics* tentatively recommended Brodman and Van Woerkom's article for publication, in part as a way of recognizing "the courage to undertake such a difficult study" and in part as a way of "stimulat[ing] interest and controversy." But this recommendation came with a caveat: "I tremble at the thought that someone might be persuaded to use this procedure for practical purposes."[67]

It did not take long for Brodman to appreciate what he called "the expressed and unconscious antagonism" of many physicians to a machine method of diagnosis.[68] A deeper understanding of the specific concerns underlying this antagonism came after the Medical Data Corporation started exploring the potential market for their new technology. Perhaps the most common refrain the Medical Data Corporation heard was this: "[d]octor feels [that the] program may jeopardize his position or job." To these physicians, the MDS was no mere adjunct; it was "a threat."[69] If the computer didn't take their job, many physicians thought the method risked changing it in detrimental ways. The medical director of Mobile Oil related to the Medical Data Corporation the sentiment among some physicians "that the computer would replace his personal contact with the patient."[70] A magazine article on the MDS method gave voice to this same concern, reporting the fear among some physicians "that increased mechanization of the diagnostic phase of medical practice will dehumanize the doctor-patient relationship."[71] General practitioners at Owens-Illinois, a large glass company, similarly bristled at the thought of the MDS—a reaction that the company's medical director attributed to the fact that general practitioners were "not statistically minded" enough "to accept the MDS as a feasible approach."[72]

Brodman believed that much of the opposition to the method was unfounded, fueled more by emotion and ignorance than reason. But many critiques of his method were in fact quite practical. One repeatedly voiced concern was that the time lag between (1) sending the questionnaire responses to the Medical Data Corporation for computer analysis and (2) receiving the results of that analysis would be too great for the service to be effective and practicable.[73] There was also a healthy degree of skepticism around the claim that the MDS would save companies, hospitals, and physicians large sums of money. The cost of the MDS, some industrial physicians noted, was not just the cost of leasing the program itself. They also worried privately about the added cost of having to pursue medical problems that had otherwise gone unrecognized. Critics today might draw comparisons to the cost of pursuing one "incidentaloma" after another.[74] Failing to follow up on the many problems identified by the MDS, moreover, might put the physician in legal jeopardy. The MDS sales manager Arnold Wander summarized such concerns from his discussions with a half-dozen industry physicians: "Confidentially their attitude was, why look for trouble?"[75]

As he did with the CMI, Brodman issued assurances designed to defang the MDS method as it existed in many physicians' minds. For example, he labored over the wording of one paragraph in the MDS Manual, a paragraph he included for the sole purpose of appeasing uneasy physicians. As Brodman explained in a 1972 letter, "I want this paragraph to be as clear as possible because it is being entered to allay the fears of those physicians who may feel that an automated method of identifying symptom complexes threatens to replace them."[76] This paragraph cast the computer as subservient to the physician, stressing that by using the MDS physicians were merely "delegat[ing] to a computer the rote task of matching symptoms while reserving for himself the clinical evaluation of data which the MDS develops." The passage also enumerated the computer's limitations, a device "totally incapable" of making sense out of uncertain or inconsistent data. This strategy of confining the computer's role to only "rote," mindless, and unsavory medical work is one that many other boosters of computerized medicine would also adopt—and one that would shape the identities of physicians and the value of their work, as later chapters outline.

Whatever their effect on computerphobes, computerphiles saw straight through such assurances. In a 1966 manuscript submitted to the *Journal of the American Medical Association* (*JAMA*), Brodman and his coauthors assured that computers would not partake in value judgments anytime in the near future. One of the manuscript's anonymous reviewers found this statement indefensible: "The comments . . . to the effect that value judgment will not be made by the computer in the forseeable [*sic*] future will be balm to the ears of many an MD in the US. The fact is that such an opinion can only be held (1) for the purpose of soothing the obvious fears, (2) out of ignorance, or (3) by an intellectual Luddite. Clearly, in the future, the computer will in many cases be making better value judgments than the average M.D."[77]

This reviewer's response brings out the degree of variability in attitudes toward the MDS and computers more broadly. After Brodman published his first article on the MDS method in 1966, letters poured in from around the country with reactions that ranged from curious intrigue to outright enthusiasm. Some physicians happily imbibed Brodman's vision of the MDS as an invaluable adjunct to the busy physician. Some countered that technologies like the MDS would, in fact, replace physicians but reasoned that such an outcome wasn't necessarily bad. The steady advance of technology would not be kind to the sentimental, they warned. Some hoped that the MDS might one day stand in for doctors but only in "underdeveloped" areas without an adequate supply of medical personnel.[78] Physicians committed to various medical projects—telemedicine, regional medicine, preventative medicine—also envisioned a productive place for the MDS in their respective undertakings.

The MDS method appealed to many companies as well. But despite many wet toes, no one would take the plunge. By 1967, members of the group reported the feeling of "spin[ning] ones [*sic*] wheels," disappointed by the unfulfilled potential of what they hoped would be a "million dollar enterprise."[79] Success evaded the Medical Data Corporation for manifold reasons; among them were poor coordination among Brodman's associates, reluctance among industry physicians, the company's limited capital, and lingering imperfections in the operation of the MDS method.

In spite of the Medical Data Corporation's troubled efforts to sell and distribute the MDS, the computerized method enjoyed some positive media coverage. *Medical World News*, a magazine for the medical profession with a circulation of nearly 250,000, published an article on the MDS in its February 16, 1968, issue.[80] The article opened in a distinctively journalistic vein: "The electronic brain is now being readied for a move into the vital core of a doctor's practice—the diagnosis of his patients' diseases."[81] While Brodman found nits to pick with the article, his business-minded colleagues at the Medical Data Corporation were giddy. "[T]his exposure," one member noted, "is extremely valuable."[82]

Even better news came a few months later, in the form of a letter from

Marvin L. Miller, the director of Roche Psychiatric Service Institute, an arm of the multinational health care company Hoffmann–La Roche. Hoffmann–La Roche had recently been involved in creating and distributing an automated version of the Minnesota Multiphasic Personality Inventory (MMPI), and Miller indicated that the company might be interested in doing something similar with the MDS.[83] Managers at the company, Miller noted, were "extremely interested in exploring the possibility of making such an automated service available nationally."[84] Brodman jumped at this opportunity—and understandably so. In light of the Medical Data Corporation's limited, disorganized, and largely ineffectual efforts to distribute the MDS, the prospect of a large health care company orchestrating a national rollout of the program surely appealed to Brodman and his colleagues. By late spring, representatives of the two organizations had hammered out a formal agreement; the Medical Data Corporation terminated its independent efforts to lease the MDS and granted Hoffmann–La Roche exclusive rights to pilot test the program.

## The Medical Data Screen in the Johnson Era

What value did Miller see in the MDS? What led Brodman and his people to conclude, in the mid-1960s, that there was "an urgent need to have our method in operation and for sale as quickly as possible?"[85] Optimism about the MDS was buoyed by a number of medical reform efforts underway during this time period. On February 10, 1964, President Lyndon B. Johnson delivered his "Special Message to the Congress on the Nation's Health," which set forth his administration's health care agenda for the coming year. The address drew popular attention primarily for what it said with respect to the establishment of a national insurance program for aged Americans—Medicare. Although Medicare may have occupied the top of the president's agenda, Johnson also packed into the address other significant policy proposals that together were to "comprise a vigorous and many-sided attack on our most serious health problems."[86]

The largest targets of Johnson's "many-sided attack" were three diseases: heart disease, cancer, and stroke. These diseases, Johnson pointed out, afflicted 15 million Americans and had long remained the leading causes of death in the United States. Johnson believed that the health challenges posed by these diseases, and their possible policy remedies, demanded further study. To this end, Johnson announced the creation of a Commission on Heart Disease, Cancer, and Stroke "to recommend steps to reduce the incidence of these diseases through new knowledge and more complete utilization of the medical knowledge we already have."[87] A few months after giving his health message to Congress, Johnson tapped Michael DeBakey, an internationally renowned cardiac surgeon at Baylor College of Medicine, to head the commission. In December 1964, the twenty-eight-member body published its findings and recommendations in an expansive two-volume report, *A National Program to Conquer Heart Disease, Cancer, and Stroke*, which Johnson received at a ceremony in the Cabinet Room of the White House.[88]

The DeBakey Report recommended what would become known as the Regional Medical Program (RMP).[89] The RMP's primary goal was to better integrate academic research centers with the medical needs of regional communities.[90] In proposing this kind of institutional regime, the report espoused a logic that had guided health policy and reform throughout the twentieth century. This logic was one of "hierarchical regionalism," whereby the knowledge, practices, and technologies developed in academic laboratories and teaching hospitals would spread to regional locales through the hierarchies of schools, hospitals, clinics, and private practices.[91] As the DeBakey Report framed it, the proposed national network would "link every private doctor and every community hospital to a national—and indeed worldwide—network transmitting the newest and best in health service."[92]

The RMP bill that Johnson signed into law in many ways represented only a bare tendril of the program originally envisioned by the DeBakey Commission—a consequence of the vigorous lobbying against the law by the powerful and conservative American Medical Association.[93] Though watered down, the bill was far from trivial. Indeed, the RMP funded a host of early projects in the computerization of medicine and medical diagnosis, believing that such efforts could advance the RMP's larger "circulatory" aims: computerized systems might help move the knowledge and expertise generated at the "heart" of the medical system (medical schools and teaching hospitals) out to the system's regional "extremities" (patients and clinics in rural America). Among the more colorful of such RMP-funded initiatives was the Automated Physician's Assistant (APA). Designed to "bring modern medicine out to the rural areas in Missouri," the APA equipped a small-town Missouri physician named Billy Jack Bass with automated medical history-taking systems and other information acquisition devices.[94]

Although the MDS did not receive any RMP funds directly, many viewed the method within the context of these larger efforts. Brodman surely did: he urged Roche personnel to "consider the opportunities in other important areas as, for example . . . in government-supported efforts, such as the Regional Medical Program or Welfare Program."[95] Brodman's interest in the RMP was reciprocated by RMP personnel's interest in the MDS: certain members of various RMP initiatives looked on the computerized method with great interest. In 1968, a leader of the Missouri Regional Medical Program wrote to Brodman, asking about the MDS and its possible incorporation with their efforts in computerized medicine: "I have just discovered your article on the Medical Data Screen and am very interested in it. Here in the Missouri Regional Medical Program, we are working on an Automated Patient History Acquisition System (project APHAS) [part of the APA project] and some of the data you allude to would be very helpful in designing our program."[96]

RMP initiatives, like the APA project, were but single instantiations of a broader ethos. Owing to the rapid pace of technological change, many began to imagine the computer as an antidote to many of medicine's steepest social and economic challenges. Such perspectives were voiced prominently in the 1966 report of the National Commission on Technology, Automation, and Economic Progress. Traveling under the title *Technology and the American Economy*, the congressionally commissioned report aimed to define areas of "unmet community and human needs" and recommend ways of deploying new technologies to meet said needs.[97]

Against the backdrop of such national discussions, an anonymous reviewer of one of Brodman's manuscripts picked up on the MDS's broader timeliness: "I find this paper informative, interesting, and timely—particularly in the light of (1) the increasing strain that will shortly be placed on medical manpower by Medicare and the Regional Medical Programs, (2) the Adult Health Protection Act of 1966 currently being proposed by Congressman Fogarty and Senator Williams, and (3) the burgeoning interest in the possibility of Regional Health Computer Systems as indicated in the February 1966 report of the President's Commission on Technology, Automation, and Economic Progress."[98] Indeed, the report identified four main recommendations to improve health care in the United States, two of which were very closely aligned with the CMI and the MDS: (1) "broader and bolder use of the computer and other new health technologies" and (2) "increased spread and use of health statistics, information, and indexes."[99]

Besides the MDS's alignment with ongoing national reform efforts, Brodman viewed the computerized method—and its paper ancestor—as well positioned to solve some of the most pressing medical problems of the time. For Brodman, the primary trouble with the medical system was a lack of resources—human resources, in particular. There were too few doctors with too little time. According to Brodman, the numerical imbalance between the provider and consumer sides of health care manifested in the form of rushed doctors and hurried clinics. Under the pressure of time, physicians tended to examine patients narrowly, taking into account only their most immediate concerns and problems. Any foray a physician hoped to make into additional areas of health risked further draining already scarce resources. As Brodman explained to one correspondent in 1969, "Heavy patient loads prevent physicians or clinics from obtaining and interpreting comprehensive medical history on any but a few patients. Physicians thus must treat patients for their chief complaints and without reference to their total medical problems."[100]

This concern about a national shortage of medical personnel was shared by many during the 1950s and 1960s. The country's perceived shortfall of doctors was a dominant theme of the 1952 report by the President's Commission on the Health Needs of the Nation. The issue surged again onto the national agenda a few years later, in 1959, with the publication of a report by the Surgeon General's Consultant Group on Medical Education. Named after the consultant group's chairman, Frank Bane, the "Bane report" projected that the country would face a deficit of 40,000 doctors by 1975.[101] The report attributed medicine's workforce problem to two principal causes. The first was numerical: there were simply too few doctors in the field and too few trainees in the pipeline. This numerical problem was further compounded by a distributional problem: on top of the fact that there were too few doctors overall, the distribution of this limited supply of personnel was not optimized to meet the nation's health needs. Unacceptably large shares of physicians pursued some kind of specialty training over general practice.[102]

Brodman fashioned the CMI and the MDS as partial solutions to this problem. Neither the CMI nor the MDS deployed any more boots on the ground, of course. But they did aim to assist, extend, and optimize the manpower that was already in place. These tools allowed the busy physician to gain a wider perspective on the patient "with no expenditure of the short supply of physicians' time."[103] "The Medical Data Screen," Brodman elaborated in 1967, "is unique in bringing comprehensive information to the physician about a person's total medical status, and in doing so rapidly, inexpensively, and with little burden to physician or patient."[104] The patient as revealed by the CMI and the MDS was not the "diabetic patient" or the "cancer patient" but, as Brodman put it, "the total patient."[105] Elsewhere, Brodman broadened "the total patient" even further—to "the whole person."[106] Much has been said about the tendency of modern medicine to reduce the patient into their disease or collection of medical signs and symptoms. Brodman hinted that the CMI and the MDS corrected this tendency, redirecting the physician's attention from "a particular symptom" to "the total patient," perhaps even "the whole person." In the frantic, and increasingly compartmentalized, world of medicine, the MDS conferred both speed *and* completeness.

As strongly as Brodman emphasized the importance of seeing "the total patient," he characterized his initiatives as a species of laboratory test. The MDS "essentially is a laboratory technique," he noted frequently.[107] Brodman pointed out, however, the MDS was a laboratory test of a distinctive kind. Existing laboratory tests were typically limited in scope. To obtain even a reasonably comprehensive picture of the patient, the physician had to order multiple costly tests.[108] Brodman and his associates maintained that the MDS "avoid[ed] [this] 'shotgun' approach," garnering information on multiple diverse common diseases and conditions with a single "test."[109]

Framing the MDS as a laboratory test was a rhetorical strategy: Brodman's way of making something innovative and strange look banal and familiar. This was a tool, Brodman suggested, that would improve medical decisions and diagnoses by developing upon—rather than disrupting—conventional modes of medical practice. In terms of the physician's daily practice, the MDS would not change a thing. It was just like the other lab tests they had been ordering day-in and day-out. The likening of the MDS to a laboratory test therefore represented the familiar impulse to anticipate and allay the fears of wary physicians. In fact, the Medical Data Corporation's sales manager confessed as much in a 1967 correspondence: "Dr. Brodman suggests that the advertising program . . . emphasize that our MDS is a program of laboratory technique designed to alert the physician to disease present and in no way diagnosis [*sic*] or treats and in no way endangers doctors [*sic*] position as the final factor in the determination of disease present or treatment."[110]

Comparisons between the MDS and laboratory tests provided arrows in the quiver as Brodman and his colleagues defended their computerized method against common critiques. In August 1968, the head of the Regional Medical Program in Texas voiced an objection to the MDS that was later characterized during a conference between Roche and Brodman's team: "He said that the one objection he has to the Medical Data Screen is that it may lead physicians to give up the practice of thinking and let the computer make diagnoses."[111] The computerization of medicine, some worried, might slowly blunt physicians' clinical skill and acumen. Brodman and his colleagues countered this line of thinking by invoking the now-accepted reliance on laboratory tests. The mainstream medical community had long accepted laboratory tests as central components of care—occasional bouts of overreliance notwithstanding. Why should the computer, Brodman's team wondered, be held to a different standard? "This comment," they wrote, "could be made about any effective laboratory. Indeed, physician[s] now too often rely on laboratory tests instead of making an extensive investigation of each patient and interpreting the data collected. . . . We have always emphasized that the MDS is no more than a laboratory test and should be treated as such even though the results are reported in terms of named disease[s]."[112]

## The Statistical Patient

Critics of the CMI and the MDS sometimes invoked the humanistic dimensions of medicine. To some, the CMI and MDS harbingered a deadening of the clinical encounter—a reduction of the patient into binary variables and a distancing of doctors from their patients. Yet Brodman, having been trained in psychiatry and psychosomatic medicine, was not only sensitive to the goals of holistic medicine but also convinced that the MDS was consistent with them. If one facet of the total patient was particularly overlooked by modern medicine, it was the emotional facet. In Brodman's eyes, this oversight was significant, for he "strongly suspect[ed]" that patients' suffering and illness lie "in large measure with the emotions as well as with organic disorders."[113] He found the medical system's uneven response to different kinds of illness and suffering troubling. "It is sadly true," Brodman wrote in 1965, "that whereas a person in our civilized society can usually get help for his bodily disorders he can rarely find help for disorders of the spirit and feelings."[114]

Brodman evidently felt that the CMI and the MDS, with their capacity to elucidate patients' psychiatric and emotional status, could bring such people into the medical fold. These instruments, he argued, would allow physicians to engage these patients on a deeper level. By liberating physicians from the monotonous task of conducting a full review of systems, tools like the MDS promised to free up time for physicians to better understand the rich emotional and psychological life of each patient. These sentiments demonstrate that even as Brodman blazed forward on projects of computerization and standardization, he continued to hold onto many ideas about medicine that he had developed earlier, through his training in psychiatry and psychosomatics.[115]

As much as Brodman and others contemplated medical holism and the individuality of each patient, the MDS method in fact subordinated the eccentric, the individual, and the particular to the aggregate, the average, and the statistical. Brodman believed that the MDS's object of study was "the total patient." A better description of its object of study, however, would be "the statistical patient": the MDS method generated statistical characterizations of patients and the disease categories to which they belonged. Brodman described these statistical renderings of diseases as symptom complexes—the groupings of questionnaire complaints found in specific diseases. For each disease, Brodman could list its associated complex of symptoms. For instance, the symptom complex for disease F572 (chronic enteritis or ulcerative colitis) with respect to male patients included three items with a significance value of three, 047 (intestinal trouble), 051 (bloody bowel movements), and 052 (pain on moving the bowels); three items with a significance value of two, 044 (indigestion), 049 (diarrhea), and 050 (mucus in stools); and an additional six MDI items with a significance value of one.[116]

The specific content of each symptom complex, importantly, was derived from population health data as collected by the CMI (and later the MDI). By collecting questionnaire data on thousands of patients, by synthesizing and categorizing these data according to different variables, and by creating an algorithm for comparing an individual patient's questionnaire responses to population data, Brodman and his colleagues had created a new way of defining and diagnosing disease—one that was statistical and aggregative. The CMI and the MDS therefore did not just standardize medical history-taking or discipline clinical observation, they also facilitated new disease concepts and new ways of thinking about patients and patient populations in relation to these concepts. As much as these methods reconfigured the act of clinical observation, they also reconfigured the object of that observation: patients and their diseases. Ulcerative colitis was now F572.

Who decided the contours of the symptom complex? Who chose which symptoms mattered, and how much? To these questions Brodman gave a provocative answer: the computer. "Our study shows," he asserted in a 1961 draft grant proposal, "that with proper programming, a machine can develop *for itself* a hierarchy of diagnostic significance for symptoms in specific diseases . . . that proves to be effective in the screening of patients for these diseases."[117] This was a claim that Brodman had been making since 1959. In his first publication on the machine method published that year, Brodman referred to the "syndromes [of symptoms] 'discovered' independently by the machine."[118] Of course, the computer was not actually determining diagnostic weights "on its own": it simply applied a formula (that Brodman and Van

Woerkom had worked out) to an existing set of data. But the computer did create new possibilities by allowing researchers to engage with and manipulate large amounts of data in ways that would have otherwise been immensely, if not prohibitively, time-consuming and labor-intensive.[119]

Such language separated Brodman's views from those of other leaders in early biomedical computing. In a widely distributed 1960 report on medical electronics, for example, the biomedical computing pioneer Robert Ledley stipulated that "rigorous diagnostic criteria for the various diseases must be established by medical investigations before computer programming can be meaningful."[120] Brodman dissented. "This attitude," he wrote in some notes, "is contrary to mine. I believe that the computer should be programmed to establish its own criteria. Our research shows that it is indeed possible to do so and that the machine criteria transcend in usefulness for the machine operation those extablished [*sic*] by the accumulated experience of the medical profession."[121] By Brodman's rendering, the computer was almost an agentic participant in the knowledge-making process, "discovering" on its own the symptom complexes for each of the one hundred diseases. The mathematics and materiality of digital computing facilitated twin redefinitions: patients as numerical representations of their questionnaire responses and diseases as averages and aggregates of those numerical representations.

Brodman and his colleagues were not the only actors interested in how the CMI and the MDS constructed disease categories. Others who encountered this work also speculated about the relationship between "symptom complex" and "disease." Was the symptom complex equivalent to, indicative of, or subsumed by its associated disease? In 1966, a reviewer of one of Brodman's first MDS manuscripts asked for clarification on the nature of the symptom complex: "What is the definition of disease? Did all the physicians in the study agree that the symptom complexes detected by the medical data screen were really indicative of disease that should have been detected by the physician? Or did some physicians feel that those symptom complexes were really detected by the physicians but the physician did not feel they constituted disease and were therefore not reported?"[122]

Brodman grappled with similar questions himself. He frequently pointed out that "there is no one-to-one relation between disease and symptom."[123] If Brodman could easily articulate what the relationship between the MDS's symptom complex and the physician's disease was *not*, he had a harder time offering a positive articulation of what, exactly, their relationship *was*. The MDS manual included a Venn diagram to illustrate the overlap between disease and symptom complex.[124] Yet Brodman wavered when it came time to decide on the degree of overlap as well as the best labels for the two respective circles. Were these diseases identified by two different methods, or different conceptual entities entirely? As time went on, he increasingly emphasized the differences between the thing physicians diagnosed and the thing his computer system identified. The MDS computer printouts included warnings about the difference between disease and symptom complex. One such warning read, "the Medical Data Screen (MDS) has matched this patient's symptoms on the MDI questionnaire with complexes of symptoms found in 100 diseases. The MDS identified symptom complexes that occur in the diseases named below. These identifications become proven diagnoses when confirmed by examination of the patient."[125]

Here, Brodman suggests that what distinguishes diseases and "proven diagnoses" from symptom complexes is the physician's proverbial "touch": a symptom complex only becomes a real disease when the physician says so. Although symptom complexes as operationalized by the MDS were quite different from conventional definitions of disease, the crucial difference, for Brodman, had less to do with any properties internal to these concepts and more to do with their source—with *who* (or *what*) was doing the diagnosing. A machine diagnosed symptom complexes; a human diagnosed diseases. Brodman's efforts to drive a conceptual wedge between "disease" and "symptom complex" therefore represented a way of signaling that, even with the introduction of computers into diagnosis, the real work of medicine remained the province of human physicians.

The MDS put the symptom front and center. This privileging of symptoms ran counter to trends in mid-twentieth-century medicine. Due to the growing reach of laboratory medicine, symptoms were losing ground to signs. "Subjective" measures of health—markers of disease that only the patient could discern—were increasingly relegated to a secondary role in comparison to "objective" measures of health—markers of disease that a physician could discern independent of the patient's experience.[126] Consider diabetes. Once made entirely on the basis of symptoms like polyuria (increased urination), polydipsia (increased fluid intake), and polyphagia (increased appetite), the diagnosis of diabetes was increasingly made on the basis of hemoglobin A1C tests, urine tests, blood glucose tests, and glucose tolerance tests.[127] Whereas the patient's symptomology represented the surface expression of disease, many hailed these kinds of laboratory tests as windows into its etiological mechanism.

In defending his method's reliance on symptoms over signs, Brodman invoked the accumulated wisdom of centuries of medical practice. The diagnostic significance of symptoms seemed self-evident to Brodman; even in the age of laboratory medicine, physicians attended to patients' symptoms, just as they had for centuries. Brodman concluded in one grant application, "Physicians recognize the diagnostic value of symptoms," drawing upon the authority of the 1952 text *Signs and Symptoms*: "It is widely recognized by experienced clinicians that a carefully taken history . . . will more frequently than not indicate the probable diagnosis, even before a physical examination is made or any laboratory tests performed."[128] The defense of symptoms did not come with the derision of signs. Brodman saw the two as mutually supportive and brainstormed ways of eventually incorporating laboratory data into the MDS method.[129]

By conventional accounts, defining disease in relation to symptoms and defining disease in relation to numerical thresholds sit in opposition. Glucose levels, breathing rates, blood pressures, pulses—these were easy to quantify. But a patient's description of their own condition? Not so much. The MDS method, however, bound these two ways of defining disease together—its definitions were both symptomological *and* numerical. The MDS method turned a given patient's questionnaire responses (their symptomology) into different numerical scores. To calculate these scores, the MDS used significance values derived from the patterns in the symptomology of the larger populace. The computer's representation of the patient—including even their subjective symptomatology—as these numeric scores is the process of creating "the statistical patient."

To convert these diagnostic scores into an estimation of diagnostic likelihood, the MDS compared the score of a particular patient against the mean score of all patients who were confirmed as having the disease in question (Figure 2.4). The MDS method thus made the larger population (or at least a supposedly representative sample of the population) the ultimate reference point for health and disease. This was the second "statistical patient" created by the MDS: in addition to the scores derived for the patient being diagnosed, also stored in the computer were the averaged and aggregated numerical scores of a population of patients with a given disease. By attaching a numerical score to patterns of symptoms, the MDS functioned as what Steven Shapin has called an "objectivity engine": it transformed subjective experiences (symptoms) into a form that could be readily measured, quantified, manipulated, compared, and communicated.[130]

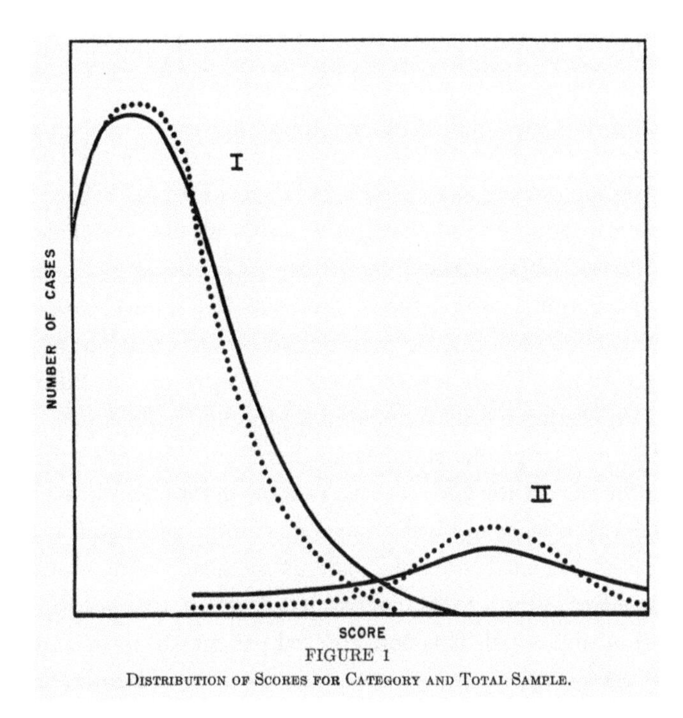


*Figure 2.4.* The translation of symptoms into the language of numbers meant that individual patient scores could be compared against a normal distribution of scores in the population. Population statistics thus became the reference point for determining health and disease. As part of the Medical Data Screen method, Brodman and Van Woerkom compared the distribution of calculated Cornell Medical Index scores among patients with a given disease (II) to the distribution of scores among the larger population (I). The dotted line indicates the distributions of scores after adjusting for patient age. Adrianus van Woerkom and Keeve Brodman, "Statistics for a Diagnostic Model," *Biometrics* 17 no. 2 (1961): 299–318, p. 307. Copyright International Biometrics Society. Courtesy of John Wiley & Sons.

The aspirations that Brodman had for the MDS remained just that—aspirations. In December 1972, Miller wrote to Brodman alerting him to Roche's most recent market survey results: "We find that the most recent survey findings challenge the successful marketability of MDS. Further, it appears that the market may be smaller than was originally anticipated."[131] Because Roche's primary interest in the MDS was financial, these new insights into the limited profitability of the program sounded the death knell: "Regrettably, as a matter of reasonable business judgment, we find it necessary to terminate both agreements between Roche and yourself."[132] The news came as "a shocking surprise" to Brodman.[133] It apparently also surprised Roche personnel, who were actively working on edits to the MDS as late as one week before Miller's notice.

The revelation came as Brodman's career was already in its eclipse. Brodman had been retired from Cornell since 1971, and since the late 1960s he found his multiple sclerosis to be almost "incapacitating."[134] The intellectual environment around him was changing as well, with the cybernetic ideas that spawned his work in sharp decline. By the end of the 1960s, the movement to establish cybernetics within the United States had unraveled (though it remained a dynamic field in select international contexts, including Chile and the Soviet Union).[135] Roche's withdrawal from work on the MDS therefore wrested from Brodman his last remaining academic engagement.

The MDS is of far greater significance than its ultimate fate might suggest. Above all, the case of the CMI and MDS show that the rendering of patient and disease identities is not just a social or cultural process. It is a material process as well. The CMI converted patients' medical history—long rendered as rich narratives—into a form that was pared-down, stripped of interpretation, emotion, and detail. This new indexed patient was more amendable to statistical analysis and computerization. The rise of "the statistical patient" was facilitated by the use of computers and the digitization of questionnaire data. Patients' questionnaire responses allowed them to be represented as a set of numerical scores pertaining to different disease categories. Diseases, in turn, were defined statistically, by the patterns of questionnaire responses among the larger patient population.

PART TWO

# DISEASE

CHAPTER THREE

# The Disease Concept Incarnate

At 11 a.m. on December 10, 1957, an interdisciplinary group of researchers in Camden, New Jersey—comprised of physicians and engineers and headed by the television pioneer Vladimir Zworykin—gathered at the laboratories of Radio Corporation of America (RCA) to witness a demonstration of one of the first instances of a computer diagnosing disease in US history.[1] They watched as RCA's Bizmac computer rendered, from inputs of patient data, diagnoses of hematologic diseases (Figure 3.1). Recognizing the significance of this moment, the researchers organized around the demonstration a series of speeches, discussions, and panels, and they invited a select group of leading physicians and engineers with an interest in the emerging field of medical electronics to participate. Others registered the significance of this effort too. In 1965, the *New York Times* ran the headline "Computer Now Can Diagnose Ills," announcing that Zworykin's group had "invented an automatic system for diagnosing disease" and had recently filed for a related patent.[2] The demonstration in Camden was only the beginning: the hematology program carried on for nearly three decades, evolving in its aims, methodologies, and group membership.

The hematology program offers a window into the role of the computer as an agent of disease definition. Part II argues that physicians and engineers, in creating computer systems that screen for and diagnose disease, simultaneously shaped the meanings and definitions of disease themselves. This process of disease redefinition was a material one—the result of having converted medical knowledge into different material forms. As Zworykin described it, this was the process of "translat[ing]" medical knowledge and patient information "into the standardized language of the machine."[3]

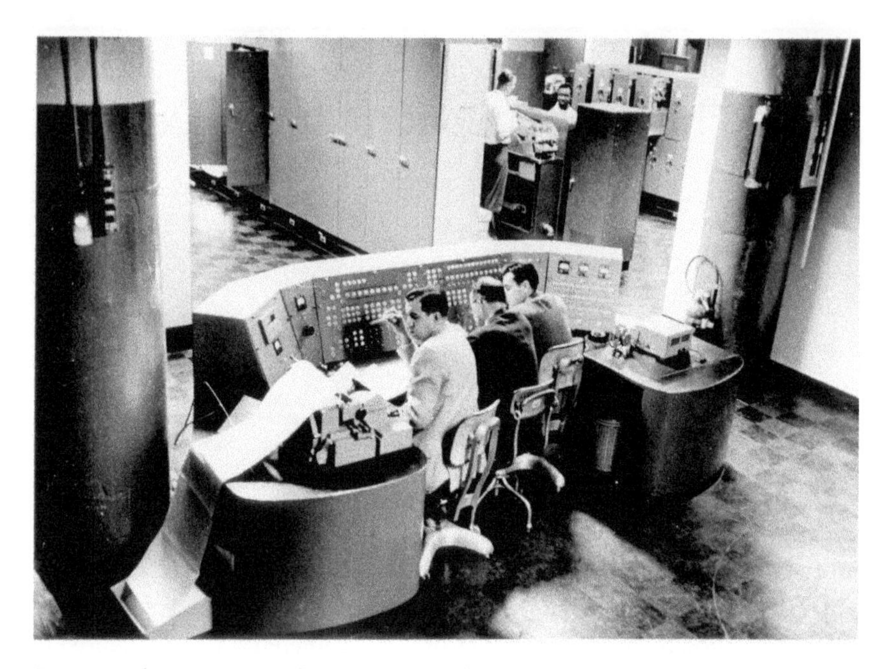

*Figure 3.1.* The Bizmac at Radio Corporation of America's Camden, New Jersey, facility. Courtesy of the Computer History Museum.

Existing scholarship on the definitions of disease foregrounds the social, intellectual, and cultural factors that give rise to different disease concepts. From venereal disease in the nineteenth century to diabetes in the twentieth, much has been said about how historically contingent moral attitudes, intellectual tools, social arrangements, clinical behaviors, and marketing practices have shaped our understandings and definitions of disease. But the process of disease (re)definition is not just a social or intellectual process. It is a material process as well, shaped profoundly by the material media with which physicians work. Charles Rosenberg has noted that "concepts of disease . . . always exist in both social and intellectual space."[4] As this section seeks to make clear, our ideas about and definitions of disease exist in material space as well. Disease concepts are corporeal: they cohere, come apart, and reconfigure in and through material bodies, whether paper notebooks or magnetic tape.

## Recoding Disease

The demonstration in Camden was the culmination of some five years of work. Toward the middle of September 1954, a lavish event was held to honor Zworykin in the wake of his retirement from the RCA.[5] Then sixty-five years old, Zworykin was a towering figure not just in the world of engineering but in American intellectual and cultural life more generally, having invented the iconoscope and the cathode ray tube that made modern electronic television possible.[6] Attendees who knew Zworykin well predicted that retirement, in his case, wasn't so much an end as it was a new beginning. As RCA president David Sarnoff declared at the event, "I see no relationship whatever between retirement and Vladimir Zworykin . . . he will continue to do whatever work interests him most."[7] Sarnoff was right, and what began to interest Zworykin most was the nascent field of medical electronics. He started imagining and inventing all kinds of medical devices and designs: a "radio pill" to visualize the gastrointestinal tract, an electronic patient "passport" to organize medical information, a television system with medical applications, and of course, a computerized diagnostic system.[8]

Around the time of his retirement, Zworykin grew interested in the work of two physicians, Martin Lipkin and James Hardy. Since 1952, Lipkin and Hardy had been studying medical decision-making and developing a mechanical method of using edge-notched cards (also called McBee punch cards) to aid in the differential diagnosis of hematologic disease (Figure 3.2). The device they proposed was ingenious in its simplicity.[9] For each disease considered, the researchers prepared a single "master card." Punched onto the periphery of every master card were holes, each of which corresponded to a different piece of clinical information. For a given master card, triangular wedges were then punched into a unique set of marginal holes, marking the clinical data that were characteristic of that particular disease. Once prepared, the master cards for each disease were collected and arranged into a deck. Diagnosing a given hospital case involved inserting a rod through the punched hole corresponding to a clinical finding present in that case. After the rod was inserted and raised, only disease cards without triangular wedges at that specific punched hole (i.e., diseases for which that clinical finding was *not* characteristic) were raised and removed from the deck. By repeating this process for additional clinical findings in the hospital case, a physician could continually reduce the number of disease cards that matched the patient's clinical picture. Eventually, the physician would arrive at just a few cards. Among these cards, Lipkin and Hardy hoped, would be the patient's most probable diagnosis.

Zworykin saw in Lipkin and Hardy's work an opportunity. He reached out to them and pointed out that their mechanical strategy of matching patient data with disease descriptions was amenable not just to paper methods but to

FIG. 5-1 Card selection with an edge-notched card system.

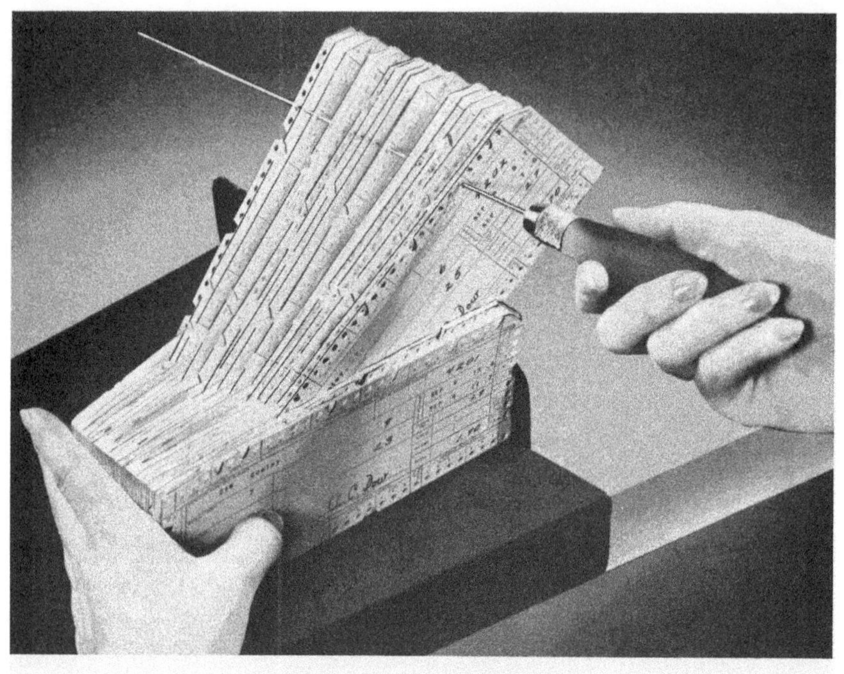

*Figure 3.2.* Lipkin and Hardy developed a mechanical method of diagnosing hematologic disease using edge-notched cards, similar to those depicted here. After a rod is inserted through one of the holes associated with a given clinical finding, only the cards with the edged "notched" at that location remain in the deck; cards without a notch are removed by the rod. Repeating this process with additional clinical findings allowed the user to narrow their differential diagnosis, with fewer and fewer cards (diseases) remaining in the deck after each round. Courtesy of Computer History Museum.

electronic computing procedures as well.[10] The same year that he retired from RCA, Zworykin had secured a new perch from which to explore this possibility. As the director of the Medical Electronics Center at the Rockefeller Institute, he oversaw various research projects in the area of medical electronics. Working at the Rockefeller Institute proved highly conducive to the pursuit of exploratory, novel, and ambitious research projects of the kind that interested Zworykin. The Rockefeller Institute stood apart from other academic institutions in its decentralized arrangement. Organized around individual researchers rather than departments, the institute provided researchers like Zworykin with more latitude to pursue research in any area, irrespective of how this research might breach conventional disciplinary and departmental boundaries.[11] For Zworykin's part, this freedom was particularly important;

Zworykin stressed that the field of medical electronics was nothing if not interdisciplinary. "In the new interdisciplinary field of medical electronics," he explained in a 1961 speech, "we hope to break down these walls and restore the unity of science in at least one sector of vital importance for human welfare."[12]

True to this ideal, Zworykin forged an interdisciplinary team of researchers to explore the question of how to computerize medical diagnosis. The team brought together engineers (Zworykin and his associate Carl Berkley), computing experts from the RCA Bizmac Computer Processing Center (Russell Ebald, Robert Lane, and Marvin Sendrow), and physicians (Lipkin, a gastroenterologist, along with B. J. Davis and Ralph Engle, Jr., both hematologists). This original nucleus of researchers was soon joined by a statistician (Max Woodbury), a sociologist (Louis Gerstman), and another hematologist (M. A. Atamer).[13] The group convened at the Rockefeller Institute for monthly seminars, during which they discussed virtually all aspects of computer aids to diagnosis. At some meetings their discussions were technical and mathematical. But on other days, they ventured into more philosophical territory, discussing how—and how much—physicians can know.

Wandering into uncharted territory, the research group recognized that they would need to set certain parameters and select a narrow subfield of medicine with which to work and test their ideas. For a number of reasons, hematology quickly emerged as the team's field of choice. One reason was path dependence: hematology was the field that had been selected by Lipkin and Hardy in their earlier work using marginal-punched cards. More significantly, though, the researchers believed hematology to be a field of medicine that was uniquely objective, well understood, and quantitative. Whereas some medical specialists worked with messy concepts like human behavior and emotion, hematologists worked with clear and quantitative measures: theirs was a world of blood cell counts, red cell distribution widths, sedimentation rates, clotting times, and numerical fragility measurements. As the group explained in 1957, "Hematology has been chosen for the initial study . . . because many of the findings in hematology are from clinical laboratory data which are relatively independent of subjective findings of either the patient or doctor."[14]

As the team ventured into the weeds of clinical hematology, Lipkin realized that it would be prudent to recruit additional hematologists to join the group. In 1955, he reached out to Ralph Engle, a hematologist at Cornell, inviting him "to join a group of computer specialists and physicians meeting at

Rockefeller Institute to discuss and develop ways in which electronic computers could be used to help physicians."[15] As one of the team's resident hematologists, Engle later quipped that views about the "objective" nature of hematology reflected less the reality of hematology and more Martin Lipkin's status as a gastroenterologist: "The other fellow's specialty always seems more straightforward and less complex!"[16] Without the separation of time, Engle's emotions on the matter seemed a little more raw, less playful; in 1960, he registered being "upset to learn that others thought hematology was so clear-cut and so definite, without any diagnostic problems, that everything could be handled by computer."[17]

With many boasting about the promises of a diagnostic machine, the clinically oriented Engle often found himself as the tempering voice. As early as 1960, he was pushing back against the idea that the program could be viewed as an autonomous diagnostic entity: "There has been some criticism of the program—in particular, that it is developing a diagnosis machine. I think we have to do everything possible to discourage this concept. It really represents a giant textbook of medicine, which stores not only a clear picture of a particular disease, but also such things as bibliographic data and all types of medical information which the physician can then use to improve his practice and to help him with diagnosis; but this is not a diagnosis machine."[18]

The team's first computer program functioned analogously to the mechanical, punched card method that had been outlined by Lipkin and Hardy: a given patient's findings were compared to "characteristic" descriptions of each hematologic disease. These definitions of each disease were arrived at through a fairly straightforward process. The group's hematologists assigned weights to different clinical items (i.e., symptoms, physical findings, and laboratory findings) depending on how—and how strongly—the item was associated with the disease. A weight of 0 indicated that the item was typically present in the disease ("relevant"); 1 indicated that the item was necessary but not necessarily sufficient ("critical"); and 2 indicated that the item was either unconnected to, or not typically present in, the disease ("irrelevant").[19] Mechanistic, organic, or pathophysiological conceptions of disease held little purchase in the computer's diagnostic process. The definition of each disease, as far as the computer program was concerned, was a collection of numerical representations of the association between the disease and given clinical variables.

In her work on the history of automated mathematical proof, historian Stephanie Dick demonstrates how epistemologically interesting things can happen in the process of implementation.[20] The material affordances of computers and machines, Dick argues, can affect how knowledge is organized and structured. Mathematicians, engineers, and computer scientists—in the process of moving mathematical proofs from analog media dominated by pencil and paper and to new electronic and digital media—were forced to alter their approaches and epistemologies to suit new materialities. For example, Dick shows how Allen Newell, John Clifford Shaw, and Herbert Simon, in their work automating theorem proving on the JOHNNIAC computer, introduced new ways of formulating logical propositions (i.e., linked lists) as a way of navigating the JOHNNIAC's material requirements (i.e., limited memory availability). These linked lists rendered logical propositions in a very different form than their pen-and-paper instantiations (a "concatenated series of symbols").[21]

What Dick observes in the context of automating mathematical proof also applies, at least in some cases, in the context of automating diagnosis. The hematology research team was forced to reckon with the material constraints of the computer from the outset. Among these constraints were the computer's memory and processing speed. Even with their first program, which considered only twenty-one hematologic diseases, the researchers found that the computer would take too much time if it went about individually checking the degree of correspondence between the patient data and each of the twenty-one disease descriptions. "One of the problems in computer diagnosis," the team expounded in a 1962 report, "is to reduce the number of diseases under consideration by the diagnostician and the computer at any one time."[22]

The group found a taxonomic solution to this material problem: they grouped the twenty-one diseases into nine classes. By clustering diseases into larger disease classes, the computer could perform a preliminary matching between the patient's findings and the smaller number of disease classes. Only diseases within the subset of classes found to meet some level of correspondence would be investigated further. These groupings, importantly, were brand new: they did not, the team noted in one grant application, "conform completely to any recognized medical classification."[23] Their concepts of disease were incarnate in the material world of the Bizmac, and as a result, the contours of these disease categories were redrawn.

With descriptions of both disease classes and individual diseases stored in the computer, the last piece of information that needed to be fed into the computer was the clinical data from the patient under consideration. To facilitate this process, the researchers devised standardized case history forms, or what they called an "Information Code" (Figure 3.3).[24] These forms performed two primary functions. First, they prompted physicians to collect medical information that was useful to the operation of the computer program. More importantly, these rigidly standardized forms helped translate the patient's medical picture into information that could be input into the computer. The forms were created, then, to serve as a conduit between two different kinds of media: the material world of pen and paper that physicians had been accustomed to for centuries, and the new digital medium of the computer that the Rockefeller team was venturing into for the first time. As Zworykin and Berkley elaborated in an unpublished paper, these forms represented part of the team's larger effort "to arrive at some standardization from which data could be more readily entered into a machine storage."[25]

"For a computer to accept data," Zworykin reiterated elsewhere, "it is essential that all of the data supplied to it must be consistent."[26] Traditional case histories and patient records, heterogeneous and discursively rich, would not suffice. Medical information in such a traditional format, they believed, was ill fit for transcription onto magnetic tape.

As a longer-term goal, the team imagined that the computer program would be dynamic, updating disease descriptions on the basis of new and increasing amounts of input data. Jordan Baruch of Bolt, Beranek, and Newman broached this point following a presentation by Lipkin at the Rockefeller Institute's 1959 conference on "Diagnostic Data Processing."[27] Baruch raised "the possibility of introducing a feedback system whereby the machine improves its performance as time goes on."[28] Lipkin responded affirmatively: "We believe a long-term study involving feedback mechanisms should be undertaken. For example, in describing diseases, instead of using the various opinions regarding the significance of the data, or even literature, case hospital data themselves might be used as a basis of the information."[29] Lipkin thus saw a clear path toward a future where computers were beginning to define disease descriptions "for themselves"—not unlike how Brodman viewed symptom complexes as defined by the Medical Data Screen (MDS).

One member of the hematology group, B. J. Davis, worked with IBM's Taffe Tanimoto to create a computerized program that could tackle "the taxonomy problem" in medicine.[30] Tanimoto developed a computer program that, through application of a mathematical model, could classify cases into disease-like categories. Essentially, the program defined certain "centroid" points of naturally occurring clusters, which purportedly represented the case that is most prototypical of all other cases in that cluster. The centroid points, in other words, may define discrete disease representations out of an

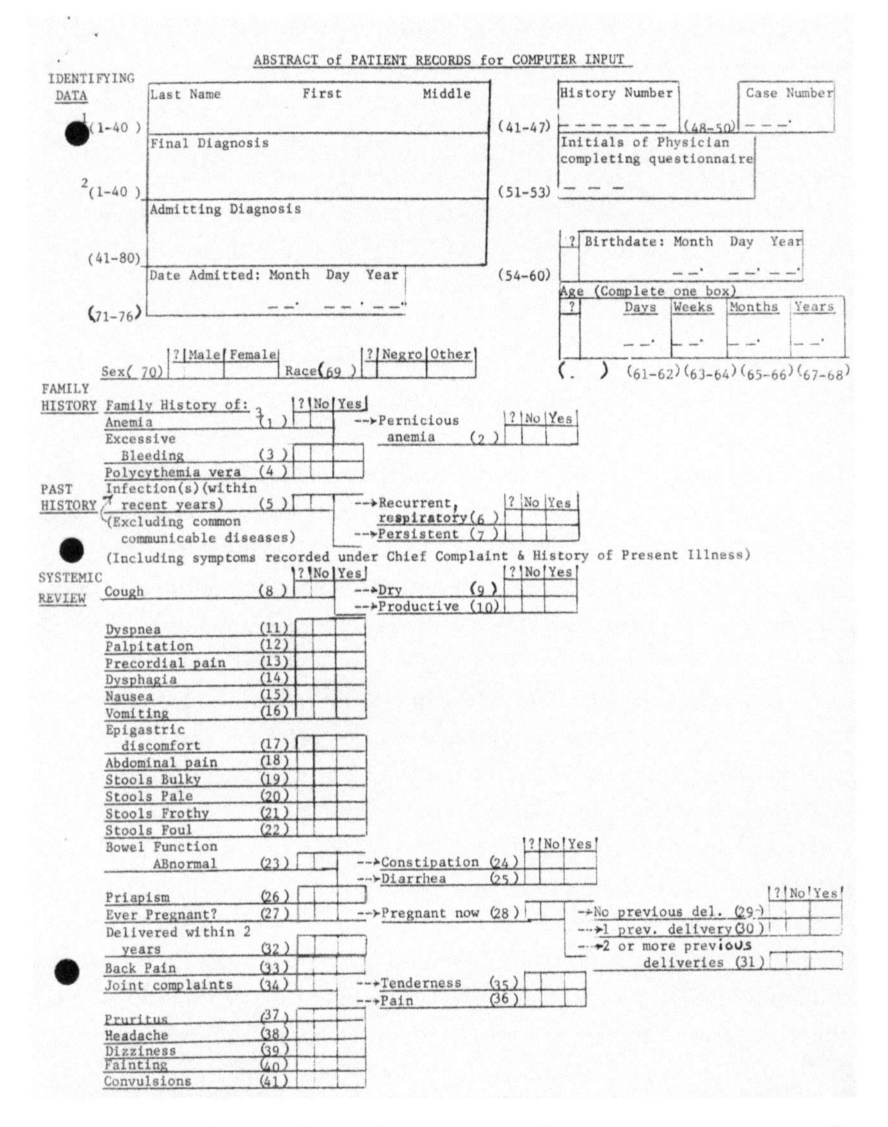

ABSTRACT of PATIENT RECORDS for COMPUTER INPUT

IDENTIFYING DATA

(1-40) Last Name First Middle
(41-47) History Number (48-50) Case Number

Final Diagnosis
Initials of Physician completing questionnaire
(1-40)
(51-53)

Admitting Diagnosis
(41-80)

? Birthdate: Month Day Year
(54-60)

Date Admitted: Month Day Year
(71-76)

Age (Complete one box)
? Days Weeks Months Years
( ) (61-62) (63-64) (65-66) (67-68)

Sex (70) ? Male Female
Race (69) ? Negro Other

FAMILY HISTORY
Family History of: ? No Yes
Anemia (1) --> Pernicious anemia (2) ? No Yes
Excessive Bleeding (3)
Polycythemia vera (4)

PAST HISTORY
Infection(s) (within recent years) (5) --> Recurrent, respiratory (6) ? No Yes
(Excluding common communicable diseases) --> Persistent (7)

(Including symptoms recorded under Chief Complaint & History of Present Illness)

SYSTEMIC REVIEW ? No Yes
Cough (8) --> Dry (9) ? No Yes
--> Productive (10)

Dyspnea (11)
Palpitation (12)
Precordial pain (13)
Dysphagia (14)
Nausea (15)
Vomiting (16)
Epigastric discomfort (17)
Abdominal pain (18)
Stools Bulky (19)
Stools Pale (20)
Stools Frothy (21)
Stools Foul (22)
Bowel Function ABnormal (23) --> Constipation (24) ? No Yes
--> Diarrhea (25)
Priapism (26)
Ever Pregnant? (27) --> Pregnant now (28) --> No previous del. (29) ? No Yes
--> 1 prev. delivery (30)
--> 2 or more previous deliveries (31)
Delivered within 2 years (32)
Back Pain (33)
Joint complaints (34) --> Tenderness (35)
--> Pain (36)
Pruritus (37)
Headache (38)
Dizziness (39)
Fainting (40)
Convulsions (41)

*Figure 3.3.* Standardized case history forms were created to impose structure upon medical information for the purposes of computer input. Courtesy of Hagley Museum and Library.

otherwise mess of data. The method, when presented at the 1959 Rockefeller conference, stirred considerable discussion. Ledley, while speculating that the method "would probably be the basis of a good method for finding new diseases which have not been previously defined," also probed, "Why should the centroid point be the diagnosis? That is not clear in my mind."[31] Carl Berkley, another member of the hematology group, responded on Tanimoto's behalf, noting that the clusters should be thought of not as narrow diagnoses but broader classes of illness (e.g., arteriosclerosis versus diffuse degenerative-circulatory disease). Not all attendees were so optimistic about this program's promise. One physician questioned whether the method would really work in medicine, a domain where clinical pictures frequently overlap and blur together. "I don't have quite as much faith in medicine's being so well ordered as some here have shown," he warned.[32]

## The Hydraulics of Clinical Judgment

For a first attempt, the hematology program performed reasonably well. After examining forty-nine hospital cases, the program identified the correct disease (as diagnosed by hospital staff)—either as the definitive "positive diagnosis" or among the shortlist of possible pathologies—in all but two of the cases.[33] Although the program seemed to demonstrate the feasibility of computerized diagnosis, the researchers conceded that it was limited in important ways: the program considered only a sliver of all hematologic diseases, it omitted complex cases, and it incorporated rough human estimates. This original program, Carl Berkley wrote to Louis Gerstman in 1966, "reflected the experience of physicians in a relatively cursory way."[34] In updating the program, the team's primary aim was twofold. One, they wanted to include additional hematologic diseases and patient findings. And two, they wanted to determine the symptom weights through objective data rather than through the subjective clinical judgment of a panel of hematologists. Lacking access to enough clinical data to determine these symptom weights, the researchers took to systematically reviewing the medical literature. By extracting and combining the data from enough studies and published case histories, they hoped to garner empirically robust information about the incidence of each clinical finding in each hematologic disease of interest.

Led by M. A. Atamer, one of the group's hematologists, this process of culling data from the medical literature to produce a database proved to be "a tremendous undertaking."[35] When Atamer and others turned to clinical data and the medical literature, they encountered a state of information anarchy, with physicians collecting and reporting clinical data according to their own preferences, particularities, and proclivities. A lawless environment bred various problems. The team found, for example, that different physicians referred to different diseases by different names. Von Willebrand disease, a bleeding disorder, went by fifteen different names at the time, and myeloid metaplasia had twenty-five different possibilities in the existing terminology.[36] Atamer also ran into problems arising from a marked degree of variation in how physicians and researchers reported clinical data. For example, if a study didn't report information about a given clinical finding, did that mean that the finding was found to be absent, or simply that it wasn't tested for? On top of this, the Rockefeller team had to grapple with vague and imprecise phrases strewn throughout the medical literature. What did it mean, numerically, when a study stated that a certain symptom or clinical finding was "infrequent" or "uncommon" in a given patient population?

As a result of the indeterminacy and heterogeneity of clinical data, the process of collecting and collating data from multiple sources—that is, the process of amassing a database—was not an objective one. It was shot through with subjective judgments.[37] Members of the Rockefeller team had to judge for themselves which studies to include in their review, what to make of studies with anomalous findings, and how to quantify ambiguous descriptors like "few" and "many." Subjective judgment, they discovered, was hydraulic; like water, it could not be easily controlled or done away with.[38] Attempts to levee clinical judgment at one location in the diagnostic process often just shifted human judgment into new and different channels and outlets. The need for clinical judgment remained.

The researchers were internally cognizant of this challenge. In a 1962 letter to Zworykin, Berkley described how contemporaneous researchers who were attempting to make sense of data reported from drug tests faced "the same kind of bottleneck that we have had on the hematologic diagnosis, that is, it requires experts in Biochemistry and Pharmacology to translate from the drug report to the computer format."[39] An internal progress report on the project, produced in 1967, echoed these sentiments. Pulling data from the world literature, it noted, "necessitated employing some subjective judgment since different investigators differed in their definitions of certain symptoms as well as in the thoroughness of their reports. One author, for example, might cite 100% incidence of a particular symptom where another author did not cite the symptom at all."[40]

The persistence of human judgment in increasingly "rationalized" domains of medicine is a dynamic that runs through the history of medicine. As Harry Marks has shown, the advent and rise of the randomized controlled trial (RCT)—the "gold standard" of medical research—sometimes failed to permanently settle open questions of therapeutic efficacy and clinical decision-making.[41] In fact, RCTs could introduce new forms of judgment and decision-making into the equation. Was the trial adequately designed? Is the study population generalizable? Did researchers adequately adhere to study protocol during the process of implementation? Even after a given RCT produced some result about comparative efficacy, the matter was sometimes far from settled: clinicians continued to debate—and make human judgments about—the quality of the study, the validity of the result, and the extent to which the study's findings applied to their particular patients. Clean statistical designs do not always supplant the messy political and professional debates around therapeutic choices and "best practices."

The University Group Diabetes Program (UGDP) study offers a case in point.[42] After longstanding controversies about the clinical management of diabetes, the UGDP was intended to settle these affairs through state-of-the-art clinical trial design. Contrary to expectations, however, the results of the trial fueled, rather than squelched, debates about the use of long-term hypoglycemic drugs in the treatment of diabetes. When the study produced unexpected findings (that the popular hypoglycemic drug tolbutamide actually increased cardiovascular complications), many physicians were forced to decide whether the force of the clinical trial evidence warranted an overriding of what Yale University's Alvan Feinstein called the clinician's "biologic logic" and "clinical judgment."[43]

In a similar vein, ceding the task of diagnosis to database or machine introduced forms of judgment at both the development end and the implementation end. Developers like Atamer had to employ subjective judgments in the process of creating the database, and clinician-users would have to make subjective judgments about the database's accuracy and fidelity.

## Algorithmic Bias

Databases, because they were judgment-laden, could also be biased.[44] They could reflect systematic errors, lapses, assumptions, and oversights that affected the functioning of a computerized diagnostic system. This possibility did not escape actors at the time. Many framed this problem as one of "garbage in, garbage out": computer-generated results are only as sound as the information entered into them. Biased inputs begot biased outputs.[45] A 1967 article in *Medical World News*, for example, pointed out that computers could only be as rational as their creators: "Diagnosis requires judgment, and a computer must rely on its human programmers to supply that judgment. The 'electronic brain' is no brain at all. It has been called 'an idiot machine, capable of generating errors at the same fabulous rate at which it generates correct answers.' Program it wrongly and it spews out nonsense. In cybernetic jargon, this awkward situation is called GIGO—'Garbage In, Garbage Out'—meaning that a computer is no better than the people who run it."[46] A computer program, some at the time realized, did not necessarily transcend the human faults of its makers. It could incorporate, and even amplify, these faults.

Keeve Brodman, too, considered the possibility of biased data. Like the early hematology project, the MDS was seen as being "data-driven." Brodman and his colleagues did not decide, a priori, how symptoms were weighted, or how symptom complexes were defined. Rather, these weightings and complexes emerged from patterns in the Cornell Medical Index (CMI) and Medical Data Index (MDI) data. Introduction of bias and error into the data—whether during their creation, processing, or application—could thus translate into inaccurate results.

In his 1960 paper "Diagnostic Decisions by Machine," Brodman considered the analogy between "the machine method" and the human mind. He noted that "the machine method was devised to simulate what is postulated to be the operation of a mind free from any intellectual or emotional bias, and because every mind has many such biases the machine at best can operate analogously only to any isolated human function."[47] Brodman was careful to note, however, that despite the computer's absent emotionalism, biases could also be introduced into the machine method. "Biases similar to those associated with decision function can be introduced in a machine system," he warned. This bias entered the system through the back door: through its "reference data":

> We now have under study machine systems which have been biased in a systematic manner by being supplied with invalid reference data. (This is similar to what is found in people who use invalid information because of ignorance or an emotional disturbance.) Decisions made by these systems are often incorrect in a predictable manner, not because the data are processed illogically but because the logical operations make use of reference data different from those which yield correct decisions. Other systems which have been biased in a random manner (as are individuals with certain central nervous system disorders, such as disseminated atherosclerosis) yield incorrect but logical diagnostic decisions that are unpredictable.[48]

The processing of biased data—no matter how logical or unbiased—generated bad and biased decisions.

The CMI's very structure as a written, paper technology almost ensured some degree of bias within its sample of patients. The tool made a critical assumption of its users: literacy. Many patients in the 1950s could not read or write in any language, and many more were subliterate.[49] The challenges of illiteracy were not shared equally among all members of society. Large racial and socioeconomic disparities in literacy rates reflected long histories of discrimination and dispossession. Even if the CMI's user was literate, there was no guarantee they could read English (the index's most prevalent version). This was especially true in a place like New York City, where more than 20 percent of the population at midcentury was born outside the United States.[50] Technologies like the CMI and MDS thus overlooked and erased certain kinds of people. The patients and diseases that tools like these constructed were far from universal, only representing particular strata of society. Given the index's lineage from the Cornell Selectee Index, more overt forms of bias could have also infiltrated the MDS. This computerized method evolved directly from tools that were explicitly designed for the purposes of discriminating neuropsychiatrically "unfit" queer people from their straight counterparts.

Among the most prominent voices arguing against uncritical reliance on data during this period was Alvan Feinstein—the same Feinstein who warned against naïve adoption of clinical trial results.[51] A leading epidemiologist, Feinstein's critiques did not come from a place of nostalgia or mysticism about clinical reasoning.[52] Indeed, in his 1967 book *Clinical Judgment*, called "revolutionary" by reviewers at the time, Feinstein urged clinicians to adopt "improved scientific methods for observing and analyzing the intact body, mind, existence, and clinical treatment" of patients—to make the act of clinical judgment, despite its unavoidable subjective elements, into a kind of "basic science" of its own.[53] But it was important, Feinstein believed, that physicians bring this clinical judgment—which could be learned, dissected, studied, communicated, and cultivated—to bear in their engagements with clinical data and computers. Feinstein therefore worried about computerized systems based on faulty data—about the consequences of clinically-oriented physicians ceding the realm of diagnosis to professionals with little clinical grounding. As he explained in 1966, "The right kinds of clinical data and numbers must go into the computer. The big danger is that clinical physicians will stand off and let the mathematicians, PhDs and laboratory-oriented MDs take charge."[54]

Despite glimmers of self-awareness about the problems of bias, judgment, and error, many of Zworykin's contemporaries viewed the computer as relatively immune to the biases that commonly befell human physicians. Humans tire, forget, and get emotionally invested in their work. Computers, by contrast, have no emotions; they don't have bad days. Each case is treated the same as the last. These views were expressed by Edmund McTernan and Dean Crocker in a 1969 issue of *Hospital Physician*. "No matter how many physicians and related personnel we train, we can't keep up with the demand for health services," they wrote.[55] "One big reason is that we are *too* human. Our receptors of information are subject to error: Hearing cannot be perfectly trained; vision may fail by degrees, unnoticed; touch is imperfect; personal worries, prejudices, or mind-sets may distort our perception."[56] They concluded, "Thus, our ability to gather all the data we need is limited by our humanity, affected by our need to eat, sleep, love, and eventually die." Their point was simple: to err is human. But their point also had an important corollary: if error is human, accuracy is mechanical.

Such views about the limits of the physician's mind were buoyed by mounting awareness of human-generated medical error through the mid-twentieth century. By the 1960s, and increasingly through the 1970s, numerous studies began to cast aspersions upon the credibility of physicians and the soundness of their decisions. Certain studies, for example, started to reveal a marked degree of regional variation in medical care. One 1969 study showed that, within a single US state and under a single insurance scheme, certain surgical procedures were performed in some regions at a rate three to four times that of other regions.[57] Another study, published four years later in the journal *Science*, documented "wide variations" in health care expenditure, utilization, and provision even among neighboring cities.[58] Viewed from a global perspective, these variations were often starker. In 1968, an international team of researchers from the United States, the United Kingdom, and Sweden found up to fourfold variations in hospital discharge rates and surgical operation rates across the three locales.[59] That a given patient might go under the knife in one zip code but not in a neighboring zip code seemed arbitrary. The existence of regional discrepancies therefore eroded the credibility of physicians and medical institutions. As one commentator would later write, such findings cast "doubt on [physicians'] knowledge base, on their competence to interpret it, or both."[60]

Proponents of computerization seized on such findings. A duo of physicians wrote an article in 1966 addressing the question, "Why use computers as an aid to diagnosis?" The first answer they offered: to reduce errors. Human physicians, they observed, sometimes dropped the ball, whether due to oversight or misdirection:

> Whenever there is a *decision* to be made on diagnosis, prognosis, or choice of therapy, the physician faces the possibility of making the "wrong decision" in relation to the future course of his patient. A number of investigators have reported the intrapersonal and interpersonal *inconsistency* of medical observation and diagnosis. Though inconsistency may not necessarily imply error, physicians would generally agree that significant errors do occur in the practice of medicine. Important errors of decision may be due to *errors of omission*—failing to observe certain facts or failing to consider certain implications—or may be due to *errors of commission*—choosing the wrong course of action, possibly because of a mistaken diagnosis and/or prognosis, or possibly because of error in judgement.[61]

Incorporating computers into the decision-making process represented to many one promising way of rooting out medical error.

The growing concern about clinical error and irrationality recapitulated broader intellectual trends across the cognitive and economic sciences.[62] In the early postwar period, a number of fields—psychology, cognitive science, political science, sociology—saw the flourishing of rational choice theory, a perspective that underscored the rationality, autonomy, and flexibility of human reasoning processes. Canonical views about human rationality during this period found a platform in *Theory of Games and Economic Behavior*, written during the 1940s by the mathematician John von Neumann and the economist Oskar Morgenstern, and subsequently in Leonard "Jimmie" Savage's *Foundations of Statistics*. These works in the field of decision theory represented attempts to standardize ways of weighing possible choices under conditions of uncertainty.[63] Von Neumann and Morgenstern, for example, described a set of assumptions, or "axioms," that underlie rational decision-making; when decision-makers satisfy these axioms, they will assess uncertain prospects according to their expected utility, or satisfaction. Rational choice theory therefore relied on the idea that humans function primarily as rational agents—that decision-makers possess a full understanding of the actions and events that make up their environment, have clear and consistent objectives, judge probabilities in a reliable way, and logically weigh values and uncertainties.

By the 1960s, and increasingly through the 1970s and 1980s, a different cohort of psychologists, economists, and computer scientists started to poke holes in the rational model of human cognition that had been constructed by their own fields.[64] Irrationality, not rationality, these scholars argued, was a defining characteristic of human reasoning. At the Carnegie Institute of Technology, Herbert Simon was among the first to revise this assumption that people are rational entities.[65] In 1957, Simon coined the term "bounded rationality" to capture how the human mind's ability to reason through problems and process information is inherently limited.[66]

A pioneer in artificial intelligence research, Simon, together with his colleagues at the RAND Corporation, Allen Newell and Cliff Shaw, created the Logic Theorist, a computer program designed to solve logic problems as humans do: by using "rules of thumb," or "heuristics."[67] His engagement with computing and dominant theories of neoclassical economics informed his understanding of bounded rationality; that is, Simon associated bounded rationality with what was human and unbounded rationality with what was economic and algorithmic (*homo economicus*). As Simon wrote in a 1991 letter, "To say that [people's] rationality is bounded is simply to acknowledge their (our) humanity."[68] Simon continued, "I coined the phrase many years ago as a contrast with the (unboundedly) rational person of classical economics who goes about godlike, choosing optimal behaviors with no concern for the superhuman feats of computation required to select them."[69] Even as some recognized the vulnerabilities of computerized diagnostic systems, many others believed them capable of effortlessly carrying out these "superhuman feats."

## Numbers over Narrative

Even as the hematology team recognized the subjectivities and biases attached to the data collection process, they nevertheless pushed forward in their efforts to collect more "objective" data for their program. After two years of work, Atamer had compiled data from some 18,000 cases reported in the published literature. He arranged these data into a matrix with 76 columns and 538 rows—each column representing a hematologic disease and each row representing a given patient finding.[70] Each cell in the matrix reported the incidence of the particular patient finding in the particular disease. In 1963, Atamer published the information contained within this matrix in the form of a book titled *Blood Diseases*.[71] Even before the team began to produce computerized disease descriptions from these data, the process of methodically reviewing the world literature generated new ideas about different disease categories in the hematologic field: "In doing this [creating a database]," the team observed in an annual report, "it has been found possible to reduce the number of presently recognized disease entities and to combine results from a number of diagnostic tests."[72]

The information contained in Atamer's matrix formed the basis for the disease descriptions that were input into the computer's memory. As with the original program, the representation of disease in this updated version looked nothing like conventional conceptions of disease. Instead, disease here was essentially a constellation of statistical averages, derived from the population data that Atamer had culled from the literature. Consider the condition of iron deficiency anemia. In the computer's memory, this form of anemia was defined as a collection of some twenty-nine clinical variables that were found to be associated, whether positively or negatively, with the disease designation (Figure 3.4). The strength of the association was expressed in the form of incidence data. Such numerical definitions of disease were viewed as a solution to the problem of getting disease concepts into the digital medium of the computer. Their project, Zworykin wrote, "demonstrated that it is possible to reduce the symptoms of a particular disease into numerical data which can be stored in the memory of a computer."[73] The hematology team hoped that by creating numerical definitions of diseases outside of the hematologic field, the program could be easily applied to other fields of medicine.[74]

That their project in computerized diagnosis resulted in numerical definitions of disease was a point of pride among some members of the team. When asked, in 1963, to identify the primary achievements of their work, Zworykin, Engle, Woodbury, and Berkley responded in a joint letter that one of their two chief accomplishments had been "the numerical specification of the characteristics of diseases to a greater extent and more quantitatively than has previously been attempted."[75] Zworykin believed that these numerical disease descriptions existed in stark contrast to the discursive descriptions that had dominated much of clinical practice and the medical literature.[76] In a 1961 speech, he derided some disease descriptions from Byrd S. Leavell and Oscar A. Thorup's 1960 textbook *Fundamentals of Clinical Hematology* as "grossly non-numerical." To illustrate with a specific example, Zworykin invoked the book's description of agranulocytosis. In a typed draft of the speech, he underlined the portions of the disease description that he believed to be lamentably "vague": "Prodromal symptoms such as fatigue, headache, weakness, insomnia, and restlessness usually occur. The majority of patients complain of a sore throat. This often progresses rapidly as chills, increasing fever, and dysphagia develop."[77] Many physicians may not have found fault with such a

```
    126600000      78      7    BM,  HYPOCELLULAR
    128200000      87      6    BM,  M/F RATIO DECREASED

                        NO. OF SYMPTOMS
WEIGHT ONLY                  10
INCIDENCE AND WEIGHT         36
TOTAL-----------------       46


                           FE DEF A

       200000      20      3    MALE
       400000      80      7    FEMALE
       600000     999      2    AGE OF PT. L.T. ONE WEEK
      2200000     999      6    MULTIPARAF
     11000000       6      5    ANOREXIA
     12000000      18      5    BRITTLENESS OF NAILS
     13800500      43      5         DYSPNEA - ON EXERTION
     19200000      50      7    PALLOR (ANEMIA OR RECURRENT ANEMIA)
     21400000       1      5    TONGUE, SORE
     61800000      36      5    CONG HEART DIS/CHR LUNG DIS/A-V ANEURYSM, EVIDENCE OF
     65400000       5      5    HEPATOMEGALY
     69000000      22      7    MASS IN THE ABDOMEN
     70201000       0      5         NEUROLOGICAL ABNORMALITIES - PARAESTHESIA
     71800000      61      7    PERICARDIAL RUB
     77400000      14      5    SPLENOMEGALY
     79000000     999      7    THROMBOSIS, EVIDENCE OF
     79200000      25      5    TONGUE,ATROPHIC OR SMOOTH
    100200000     100      8    A,HGB LTE 12.5 GM. PCT,PCV 35 PCT,RBC 4.10(6) PER CU.MM.
    100200500      98      7    A-HYPOCHROMIC ,MCHC LT 32 PCT/MORPHOLOGICALLY HYPOCHROMIC
    100201500      71      7         ANEMIA - MICROCYTIC (MCV L.T.E. 80 C.U)
    100203000      30      6    A-SEVERE,RBC LTE 2.5X10(6) PER CU.MM.,HGB 7 GM.,PCV 22 PCT
    100800000      70      6    ANISOCYTOSIS, POIKILOCYTOSIS
    101700000     999      6    ERTHROCYTES HYPOCHROMIC
    103400000     999      0    ERYTHSIS,HGB GT 16 GM. PCT,RBC MTE 6X10(6) HEMATCT MT 55
    105400000     999      6    NUCLEATED ERYTHROID CELLS IN PB
    105800000      81      7    PROTOPHORPHYRINS IN ERYTHROCYTES,  INCREASED
    106200000     999      6    RETICULOCYTE COUNT,NORMAL
    112600000      11      5    LEUKOPENIA (L.T. 5,000 PER CU.MM.)
    126400000      87      7    BM,  HYPERCELLULAR (NORMOBLASTIC)
    127200000     100     10    BM,  IRON DECREASED
    155200000      54      6    ACHLORHYDRIA
    158200000      81      7    COPPER (PLASMA),INCREASED
    159200000     100      8    IRON ABSORPTION,INCREASED
    159600000     100     10    IRON BINDING CAPACITY (SERUM),INCREASED
    160200000      93      7    IRON (SERUM),DECREASED
    201400000     100     10    IRON.  GOOD RESPONSE

                        NO. OF SYMPTOMS
WEIGHT ONLY                   7
INCIDENCE AND WEIGHT         29
TOTAL-----------------       36
```

*Figure 3.4.* The definition of iron deficiency anemia, as stored in the computer. The fourth column represents the collection of items associated with the disease. The third column represents the degree of association between each item and the disease—according to clinical judgment. The second column represents the degree of association between each item and the disease—according to prevalence data. Courtesy of the Medical Center Archives of New York–Presbyterian / Weill Cornell Medicine. The Cornell Medical Index and related historical health questionnaires should only be used for historical reference and not for any research involving human subjects.

description. But compared to disease definitions based on numerical weights or statistical averages, individual case histories and discursive descriptions such as these looked nebulous and imprecise. For the hematology team, the project of computerizing diagnosis was inextricably linked to the project of "obtain[ing] accurate probabilistic statements to replace vague disease descriptions."[78]

To be sure, computers did not spawn numerical representations of disease, nor did they create the standardized patient chart. Computerization followed in the wake of existing processes of standardization, as the arc from paper CMI to digital MDS outlines. Paper data practices and epistemologies enabled the computer's introduction into medicine. By the mid-nineteenth century, hospital-based physicians in Great Britain and France began to produce numerical, rather than narrative, disease descriptions of rheumatism.[79] The paper chart took on an increasingly standardized form over the first quarter of the twentieth century, its "crisp typography" evoking "the clear, manufactured, metallic lines of engineering science."[80] This hospital standardization movement emerged from a confluence of factors, from the growing scientific ethos of medicine to the desire among hospital administrators to gain control over an increasingly complex hospital structure.[81] Standardized patient charts had therefore been facilitating communication among physicians and supporting the clinical research enterprise at many hospitals decades before the advent of the digital computer. In this busy and increasingly bureaucratic clinical environment, some lamented the "meager and often inadequate" social histories being recorded in patients' medical records.[82]

Nevertheless, the hematology program demonstrates the potential role of the computer as a driver behind the evolution from clinical descriptions that were discursive to clinical descriptions that were numerical and aggregative. The latter was seen as more suitable for the material conditions of the computer. Even following the standardization of patient charts in the early twentieth century, the landscape of medical information looked chaotic to many creators of early computerized diagnostic systems. In many ways, the spreading use of computers created a new cognitive model about what it meant for medical knowledge to be truly standardized.[83] While the content of Leavell and Thorup's text surely looked structured by comparison to the discursively rich case studies of the nineteenth century, early pioneers in biomedical computing instead saw chaos and anarchy. They were working with a new and different cognitive model.

## The Bayesian Bandwagon

At the same time Zworykin was launching his work on the hematology project, another team—the duo of Robert Ledley and Lee Lusted—were just beginning a fruitful intellectual collaboration. This collaboration ultimately elaborated a strategy of automating diagnosis that attracted an exceptional level of attention.[84] The strategy revolved around Bayes's theorem. In 1959, this pair of researchers published their groundbreaking article "Reasoning Foundations of Medical Diagnosis" in the journal *Science*.[85] Although the article gestured to the use of digital electronic computers in medical diagnosis, its immediate aim was more abstract: to outline different methods of rendering diagnostic reasoning in mathematical terms. The article addressed many intellectually delicate questions. What is the optimal way of representing, with symbolic logic, the relationship between combinations of symptoms (symptom complexes) and combinations of diseases (disease complexes)? How can one mathematically analyze treatment decisions given that a patient's choice of treatment "not only depends on the established diagnosis but also on therapeutic, moral, ethical, social, and economic considerations"?[86]

The article's most enduring intervention, however, was its application of the well-known Bayes's theorem to medical diagnosis. Ledley and Lusted proposed that a physician, provided with a large enough set of patient data, could calculate the probability of an event (i.e., the diagnosis) based on prior knowledge about conditions that might be related to that event (i.e., symptoms, demographic factors, etc.).

Ledley and Lusted's interest in Bayes's theorem was very much a reflection of their times. The theorem's origin dated back to the mathematical work of the eighteenth-century English minister Thomas Bayes.[87] After enjoying an early period of critical engagement, Bayes's theorem lapsed in and out of relative obscurity over the ensuing centuries. By the early twentieth century, many statisticians believed that Bayesian methods fizzled out essentially from a lack of oxygen: few scholars gave the theorem the thought and attention necessary for its survival and acceptance. But World War II, and the Cold War that followed, changed the landscape of statistics and gave the theorem new life. Alan Turing used Bayes's theorem while working as a code breaker at Bletchley Park, and across the pond, US institutions deployed the theorem for its own military matters, whether locating missing vessels or estimating the probability of a potential nuclear event.[88]

Within the academy, a group of scholars based predominantly at the University of Chicago and Harvard University promoted Bayesian methods as part of what some scholars have called the "neo-Bayesian revival" of the 1950s and 1960s.[89] The leaders of this revival, including Leonard J. Savage, Dennis Lindley, and I. J. "Jack" Good (who worked as a cryptologist with Turing), argued for an approach to statistical inference in which decision-makers use Bayes's theorem to update an initial state of knowledge as more information and evidence becomes available. Soon, this interest in Bayesian statistics within the military and the academy spilled over into a number of applied domains. Medicine was no exception.

Ledley and Lusted's professional trajectories mirrored the life course of Bayes's theorem. As Bayesian methods migrated from military to medical contexts, so Ledley and Lusted arrived at the topic of computers in medical reasoning by way of their military backgrounds. Ledley's foray into the computerization of medical reasoning came during his time at the Operations Research (OR) Office at Johns Hopkins University, where he was working on applications of formalized mathematical logic to complex problems of military strategy and biomedicine.[90]

When Ledley was in Chevy Chase, Maryland, investigating OR applications to biomedicine, Lusted was on active duty just down the street at the National Institutes of Health (NIH). For someone interested in electronics, the mid-1950s was a stimulating time to be in Bethesda. During this period, the NIH initiated, in partnership with outside companies, a range of projects geared toward developing new medical electronic devices.[91] Lusted, though stimulated by many of these projects, was left a little longing; what the field still lacked, he felt, was a broader understanding of how computational techniques might assist the more fundamental processes of medical diagnosis and reasoning. It was while in this frame of mind that Lusted first made contact with Ledley.[92] They began a series of conversations about the computer's uses in biomedicine and medical diagnosis, conversations that would culminate in their paper "Reasoning Foundations of Medical Diagnosis."

Much to their surprise, this 1959 paper (despite its quiet and circumstantial origins) attracted an enormous audience, one that included groups as various as computer specialists, medical practitioners, mathematicians, logicians, and enlightened lay people. Their article quickly circulated among biomedical researchers, physicians, and computer scientists, through both personal correspondence and professional journals.[93] As Ledley later recalled, the paper "stimulated a tremendous amount of work in these areas [medical informatics] and has been called the seminal paper starting a lot of this work. It's very hard to believe, looking back, but there's no way I could have visualized at that time how influential that paper would turn out to be."[94] Media outlets further amplified the article's reach. The *New York Times*, *New York World Telegram*, and *New York Post* all used Ledley and Lusted's work as a springboard into speculative discussions about the future of computers in medicine.[95]

A few research centers translated the theoretical sketch offered by Ledley and Lusted into functioning diagnostic systems.[96] The most prominent of these was based out of the University of Utah and the Latter-day Saints (LDS) Hospital in Salt Lake City.[97] There, Homer Warner, together with his colleagues Allan Pryor and Reed Gardner, began building what would arguably become the most successful health information infrastructure in the country.[98] The project started small. Inspired by Ledley and Lusted's mathematical formalizations, Warner and his colleagues grew interested in the possibility of applying ideas about Bayes's theorem and conditional probabilities to actual clinical data.[99] They quickly settled on congenital heart disease as their test domain.[100] Their reasons for selecting this domain were twofold: data quality and data quantity. Quality-wise, the accuracy of diagnoses made on the basis of clinical findings could be verified against the gold standard of cardiac catheterization and findings at surgery. Quantity-wise, the team believed that "relatively objective clinical findings" could be easily obtained.[101] The team thus assembled a database: a matrix that included incidence information on about fifty-seven symptoms and thirty-five diseases.

Warner translated this mathematical approach for implementation on a digital electronic computer.[102] The computer's performance impressed Warner—and many others. The group found that, in a sample of seventy-four patients with congenital heart disease, the diagnostic performance of the computer was on par with that of physicians who had seen the same patients. The results grabbed national attention. "Computer Is Found Useful in Heart Disease," the *New York Times* reported. "A computer has been programmed so that it can diagnose congenital heart defects as accurately as can an experienced heart specialist. In fact, it was reported, physicians working alongside the computer improved their own diagnostic skill while the computer improved its own ability to pinpoint heart defects."[103] Excitement around the findings roused familiar speculation about the technological deskilling of the profession, with "computers . . . tak[ing] the place of highly skilled specialists, and more physicians . . . becoming well-trained data-collectors."[104] The findings also put wind in the sails of Warner's larger research enterprise at Utah. Before long, Warner's narrow focus on cardiac diagnosis broadened. The project that started in the Cardiovascular Laboratory soon spread outward, evolving into a larger health information system called Health Evaluation through Logical Processing (HELP). By the late 1960s, HELP had been adopted widely across the LDS Hospital.[105]

Yet, the growing excitement around Bayes's theorem was tempered by growing realizations about its limitations. Members of the hematology team were highly tuned into these limitations and were among the loudest in pointing them out. Carl Berkley described the team's abnegation of Bayes's theorem in a 1966 letter: "In the evaluation of various problems of diagnosis we have been led to a detailed examination of diagnostic processes and to a realization of the inherent pitfalls in total reliance on Bayesian methods."[106] Max Woodbury, a statistician at New York University who would come to lead the hematology project for a period of time following Zworykin's retirement in 1961, unpacked some of the "inherent pitfalls" to which Berkley was referring.[107]

In a 1963 talk delivered at the Fifth International Conference on Medical Electronics, Woodbury discussed the mathematical and logical basis behind what he saw as the "Inapplicabilities of Bayes' Theorem to Diagnosis."[108] Woodbury emphasized the assumptions that were required by Bayesian models of diagnosis yet violated by medicine. "The primary difficulty in the application of the theorem," Woodbury explained, "is that it has been assumed that diseases are mutually exclusive and that diseases outside of the list assumed do not produce symptoms considered in conjunction with the diagnosing of diseases in the group."[109] Such assumptions ran afoul of medical reality—almost to a laughable degree. Of course patients can have multiple diseases at once; of course certain clusters of symptoms run together; of course the diseases considered by a diagnostic system are not exhaustive of all diseases that patients could possibly have. Indeed, such Bayesian violations may have been the rule, not the exception, for many patient populations.

Besides faulty assumptions, the hematology team also worried about the data requirements of Bayes's theorem. The theorem depended upon the existence of accurate conditional probabilities. But apart from places like Utah and diseases like congenital heart disease, few areas of medicine were sufficiently data rich to derive these probabilities from population data. For a computerized diagnostic system to have any generalizability, the hematology team believed, a different approach was needed. It was a decision, however, the team would come to revisit.

# The Medical Mind

"The coming of high speed computers has been the wind of change for many of the sciences and their applied technologies."[1] So John A. Jacquez opened a conference on "The Diagnostic Process" held at the University of Michigan in 1963. In his opening remarks, the dean of University of Michigan's School of Medicine, William N. Hubbard, Jr., further clarified the circumstances leading up to the conference and identified some of its goals:

> We are aware of the interest that has developed in the last few years in the use of mathematical models and electronic equipment in the diagnostic process. We have not been confident, however, that we understood the intrinsic nature of the diagnostic process well enough so that we could proceed with the kind of transitional research that would carry us effectively into use of mathematical models and machine data processing. We have had some concern that one might adapt the diagnostician to the device rather than vice versa, if one did not have clearly in mind the role that the mathematical model and the machines can appropriately play.[2]

With computers entering the diagnostician's domain, the conference organizers saw the meeting as an "opportune time to re-examine some of the features of the diagnostic process"—to corral together a group of experts to discuss and define how diagnostic decisions might be made.[3]

The hematology team was well-represented at the conference. Ralph Engle delivered the opening paper, "Medical Diagnosis," where he proposed a philosophical framework for thinking about how physicians reason and classify diseases. Martin Lipkin's paper, though more technical, also touched upon the question of how physicians think—and whether the computerized system approximated such human reasoning. As interdisciplinary teams worked to automate medical diagnosis, they repeatedly bumped up against fundamental epistemological questions. How do doctors think? What is the nature of human reasoning? Are human modes of reasoning amenable to computerization? If they are, *should* computers aim to mimic them? In what ways do physicians come to define and classify disease categories? Are these categories even necessary? While carrying the hematology program into its final decades, this chapter explores how computers both generated and incorporated ideas about the medical mind and its inner workings.

## Informational Medicine

The hematology team's engagements with computing technologies gave them a new repertoire of metaphors with which to frame and understand medicine more broadly. As people like Vladimir Zworykin began working on computerized approaches to diagnosis, they began to see medicine differently. Physicians were computers; patients, repositories of data. Zworykin wanted to create a future "in which a physician will extract the proper information from the patient and dial this information in a central computing agency."[4] The patient, in Zworykin's mind, was above all a site of data extraction. The role of the physician was one of managing and manipulating such data. After a talk delivered by Engle on computing and clinical reasoning, an audience member concluded, "The diagnostic process really is a kind of information retrieval problem."[5]

Members of the hematology team weren't the only ones who started describing the practice of medicine in the language of information and computing. Some of Zworykin's contemporaries rethought the entire medical system along these lines. Starting in 1964, IBM undertook the development of the Clinical Decision Support System (CDSS) "to aid in the acquisition of patient data, and to suggest appropriate decisions on the basis of the data thus acquired."[6] The CDSS broke down the decision-making process into micro-decisions and used threshold logic to generate decisions.[7] Overseeing this effort was the physician-turned-engineer Frederick J. Moore.[8]

In June 1968, Moore published a report on the effort, analyzing the medical system's defining challenges and arguing for the computerized decision support system as a fitting solution. The way Moore argued for this fit was through a reframing of the medical system as an information system. This reframing, Moore claimed, was less of an interpretation than a concrete "finding" of the report: "In this report we examine medical care as a system, find that it is primarily an information system in which the decision element is crucial."[9] The report reformulated nearly every aspect of medicine—from the tectonics of the system to the granular details of the clinical encounter—as matters of information processing:

> The function elements of health maintenance . . . are summarized as follows:
>
> 1. The acquisition of data to establish health status,
> 2. The comparison of these data with stored knowledge,
> 3. The decision as to
>    a. what added data are needed
>    b. what treatment is indicated,
> 4. The administration of the treatment and the acquisition of follow-up data, and
> 5. The addition of all this experience to stored knowledge.[10]

By Moore's rendering, examining a patient boils down to the "acquisition of data," and diagnosing a patient involves the process of comparing these patient data to the "stored" preexisting "data" in the physician's mind. Having outlined the medical system's core elements, Moore felt comfortable concluding that medicine's defining processes, opportunities, and challenges were informational in nature: "Thus, it appears that the medical care system is predominantly *informational*—i.e., it depends largely on the acquisition, storage, and interpretation of information by both the patient and the doctor—and that the decision process is the pivotal element in the system, toward which all data acquisition is directed and upon which the action taken by the patient or by the doctor depends."[11] Such a view recast the role of patients and physicians as sources and consumers of data: "The doctor, as well as the patient, stores, retrieves, and processes data regarding the patient's present disorder and data from relevant clinical experience."[12] Viewed as an information processor, the doctor's shortcomings came to the fore. The doctor, Moore claimed, relies upon "two forms of information storage: human memory and records."[13] The former, however, is notoriously error-prone: "it is subject to bias, false drops, and failures, a major factor governing retrieval being the area of interest or attention at the moment."[14] If medicine was all about data—their creation, storage, management, processing, and distribution—the computer held great promise.

This informational view of medicine gave a perennial crisis in medicine—the perception of "information overload"—sharper outlines and greater urgency. Many physicians worried that the medical field was facing a threat that was almost Malthusian in nature: whereas human cognitive abilities remained relatively fixed over time, the quantity of medical knowledge available to the clinician seemed to be growing exponentially. The result? Too much information for even the academic medical specialist, let alone the general practitioner, to know.[15] If medicine was, fundamentally, about the accumulation, management, and application of "information," as many increasingly believed, then information chaos and overload loomed as outsized threats. The hematology team, like so many others at the time, isolated this as a driving motivation of their program. To Zworykin, the dynamics of information overload and its implications for the human physician were unmistakable: "The need for such an undertaking is obvious; medical knowledge advances at much too rapid a rate for assimilation by the medical practitioner."[16]

Most medical and scientific commentators spoke of this phenomenon in rather general terms, gesturing to "the exponential explosion of knowledge" unfolding around them.[17] But one researcher, David Durack of Duke University, adopted a more quantitative, if peculiar, approach. In his classic (and jocular) 1978 article "The Weight of Medical Knowledge," Durack sought to "take some objective measure" of perceptions among physicians concerning the impossibility of keeping abreast of the current literature.[18] Durack's "objective measure" of choice was the *Index Medicus*, a comprehensive bibliographic index of all journal articles published in the medical sciences. Durack found that the *Index*, as measured by weight, was indeed undergoing exponential growth: between 1879 and 1945 the *Index* hovered steadily around two kilograms, before doubling in weight between 1946 and 1955, and increasing another sevenfold, to reach nearly thirty kilograms, between 1955 and 1978. It therefore comes as no surprise, Durack quipped, that "most of us feel weighed down by the heavy and increasing burden of medical reading."[19] Despite its playful tenor, the article gave voice to real and pervasive anxieties about the challenge of providing quality, up-to-date medical care in an era of information overload.

The informational metaphors adopted by those like Moore populated not just the realm of language but also the realm of images. A 1968 issue of *The Sciences* featured an anatomical drawing of the human body on a punched card, recasting the patient's body as "data"—as the material input ready for computer processing (Figure 4.1).[20] Other images portrayed the physician as a consumer of data, whether a computer or some other machine. One such image presented the physician as a mosaic, constructed out of wires, gears,

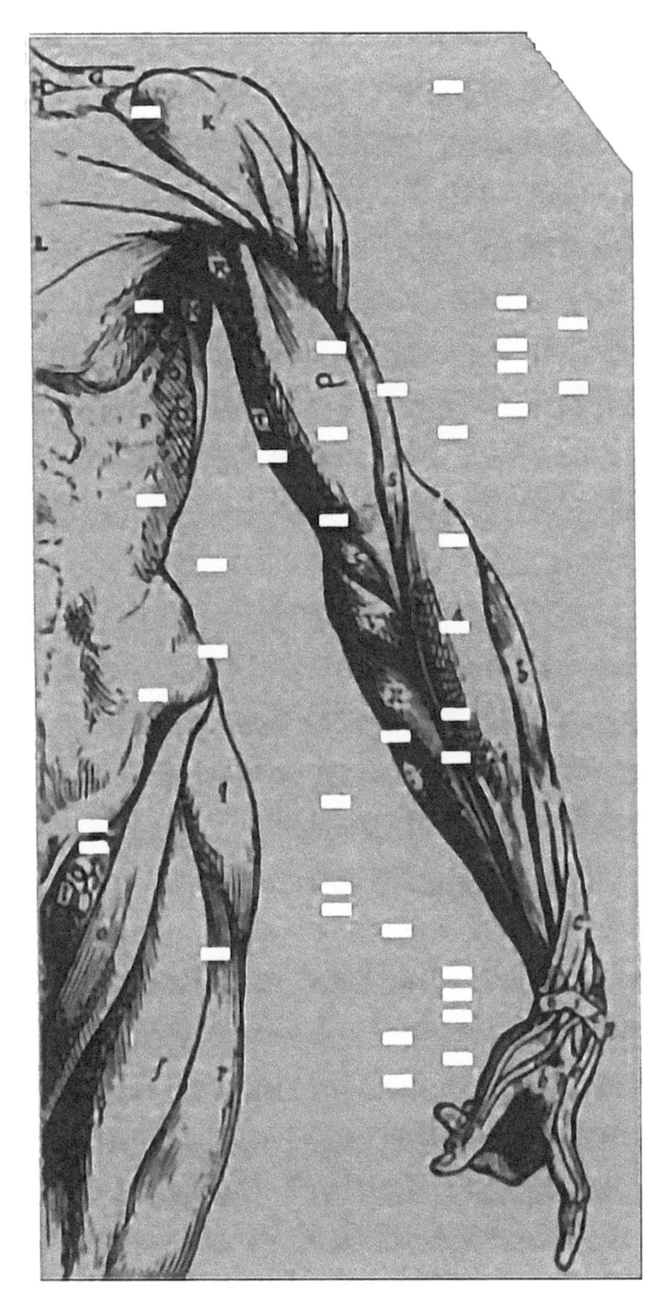

*Figure 4.1.* Patient as punched card. "Computers and Clinical Medicine," *The Sciences* 8, no. 3 (1968): 32–38. Copyright New York Academy of Sciences. Courtesy of John Wiley & Sons.

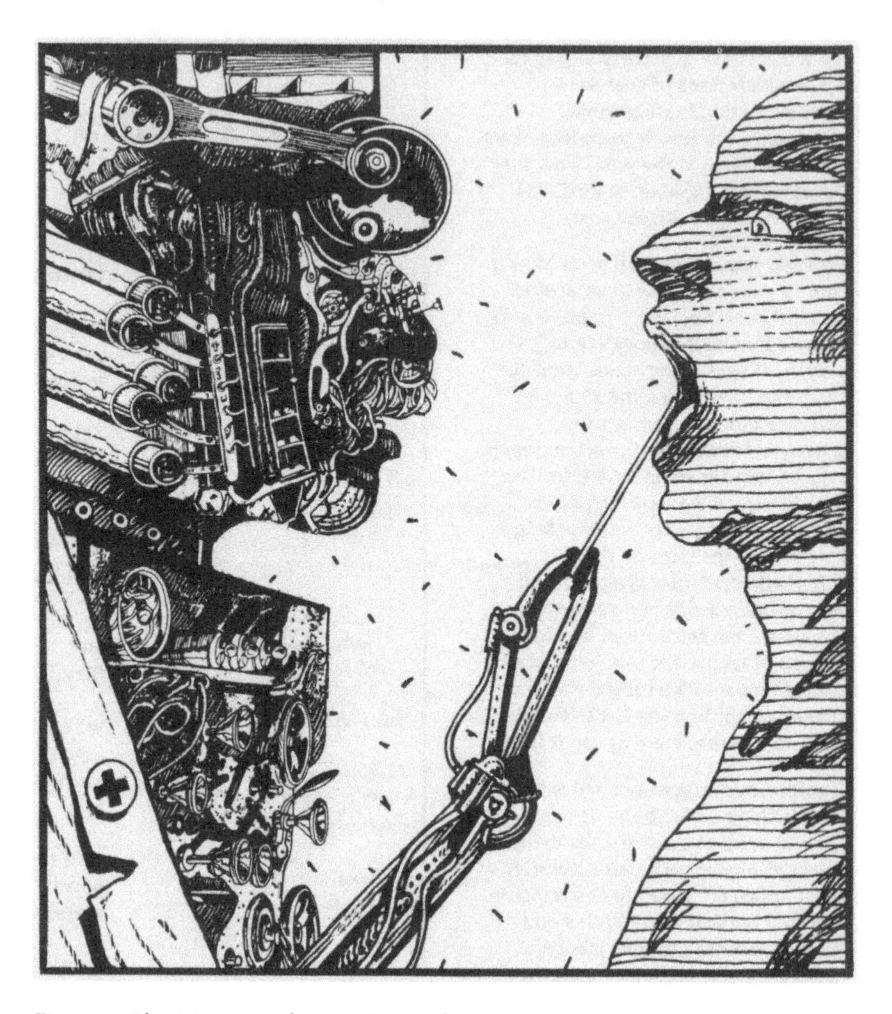

*Figure 4.2.* Physician as machine; patient as data. Richard Friedman, "Myths about Computers and Medicine," *Cornell University Medical College Alumni Quarterly* 47 no. 2 (1984). Courtesy of Weill Cornell Medicine.

nuts, and bolts (Figure 4.2).[21] These visual metaphors swarmed press and popular accounts of computerized diagnosis.

The power of medicine's metaphors to shape patient experience and drive therapeutic decision-making has been richly described by historians and social critics alike.[22] Historian David Jones, for example, has demonstrated how understandings of the heart and cardiovascular system as a system of "pipes" and "plumbing" affected intuitions about which cardiac therapeutics might work—and why. The metaphor that heart attack and angina were little more than problems of clogged pipes (i.e., obstructive atherosclerotic plaques) generated a powerful intuitive logic that surgical approaches of undoing or bypassing the clog would surely remediate, if not cure, the condition. Jones explains, "The plumbing analogy makes a powerful claim: since angioplasty or surgery can relieve the obstruction or bypass it altogether, they must work. The pairing of theory and therapy is so persuasive that excellent outcomes seem inevitable."[23]

Like certain cardiac interventions, computers and protocols have ridden on the coattails of certain metaphorical and rhetorical constructions.[24] Science and technology studies scholar Marc Berg, for example, has charted the emergence of a "cognitivist" discourse in the second half of the twentieth century that "locates the scientific status of medical practice in the mind, and also likens the physician's mind to a computer."[25] Under this discourse, the threats to a rational medicine come not from any forces external to medicine but from *within* the physician—from the human biases and errors that can get in the way of a mechanical, rote application and interpretation of medical information. This rhetorical, discursive, and metaphorical shift allowed for the proliferation of decision support tools throughout medical practice: "Once the diagnostic task is seen as an exercise in statistics," Berg reasons, "physicians' performance is seen as second-rate."[26]

The causal arrow also went in the opposite direction: the introduction of computers into medicine indeed benefited from, but also created, ideas about medicine's computational and informational underpinnings.[27] The creep of computational tools into medicine gave researchers and practitioners a new vocabulary for understanding and framing the fundamental tasks of medicine. Increasingly through the 1960s and 1970s, developers of computerized diagnostic systems began to see medicine through the lens of computational metaphors. To them, medicine seemed to be little more than an information-processing discipline. Their immediate material world—the world of punch cards, magnetic tape, processing units, and even yes-no surveys—shaped their cognitive world, their way of understanding medical work. These new cognitive outlooks about the fundamentally informational nature of medicine in turn circled back to fortify and justify their material practices and research efforts.

## Computerization as Valuation

Renderings of the physician as an information processing machine tapped into a familiar set of fears. Analogies between mind and machine suggested to many that physicians could be replaced. Some, like Utah's Homer Warner, ventured that computers would one day turn physicians into mere "well-trained data-collectors."[28] Many physicians saw such a future as both unattainable and unacceptable. In pushing back, these physicians emphasized the fundamental aspects of clinical work that seemed to defy formalization and computerization. The former president of the American Medical Association (AMA) held such a stance, one that surely pleased many members of the organization. While discussing the potential benefits of automation to practicing physicians, the AMA official at the same time reassured them that "there is no danger of practices being taken over by computers. Some patients and disorders just do not respond to impersonal treatment either from a doctor or from a machine. The human need for personal contact is what makes the practice of medicine an art as well as a science."[29]

In defending medicine against the threat of automation, many physicians espoused what historian Christopher Lawrence has called an epistemology of "incommunicable knowledge."[30] In his study of the British medical profession from the mid-nineteenth to early twentieth century, Lawrence identifies a rhetorical tradition whereby traditional physicians invoked an "epistemology of individual experience" to "defend the autonomy of clinical practice."[31] By describing clinical practice as an art that eluded analysis, these physicians cordoned off clinical medicine from encroachment by new technologies like the sphygmomanometer and new "scientific" modes of analysis.[32] Although physicians in the mid-twentieth century faced the specter of new digital technologies, they drew upon these long-standing rhetorical strategies. They cast the practice of medicine, and the work of diagnosis, as artful, intuitive, tacit. Excellence in these realms, they argued, derived more from years of irreducible experience than from pages of book-bound knowledge. Many at the time understood the stakes behind these varied descriptions of the diagnostic process. For some, to concede that medicine was communicable was to relinquish the realm of diagnosis to the machine. One physician reasoned during the 1963 conference on the diagnostic process: "I would submit that if clinical diagnosis is a science then a computer can do the job better than a clinician. If it is scientific, it is communicable and if it is communicable then a computer obviously can do it more quickly and more reliably."[33]

Questions about how to describe and represent computers nagged at the hematology team as well. Ralph Engle's perspective on the nature of the computer—and its relationship to the human—was rather more nuanced than that of many of his contemporaries. Pioneers in biomedical computing frequently lamented that physicians seemed to suffer from the computer allergy more severely than did any other professional group. The unreceptive attitude of many traditional practitioners was widely recognized as a, if not *the*, central barrier to getting computing technologies out of the research laboratory and into the clinic.[34] In 1966, Stephen Yarnall and Richard Kronmal characterized the "psychological resistance" among physicians to computers in diagnosis. In their view, this resistance had three primary facets: "First, physicians have traditionally approached diagnosis in their own individual manner, and attempts at systematization are generally unwelcome; second, many of the systems introduced to-date have required more, rather than less, work by the physician with no immediate gain apparent to him or his patient; third, physicians, and many laymen, fear computers as strange and impersonal machines which may destroy meaningful doctor-patient relationships and even displace physicians to some extent."[35]

Engle shared these concerns about an unreceptive, even antagonistic, clinical audience. But it was actually the opposite attitude—uncritical acceptance—that came to trouble Engle more deeply. Physicians, he believed, needed a deep understanding of how a computer program worked; only then would they be able to effectively evaluate its clinical value and, more crucially, its limitations: "It concerns me that some physicians are only too anxious to let a laboratory test or a computer make their decision. These tools should only be one input into the decision-making process. The physician must add his own perspective."[36] The output of a computer program, Engle warned, can convey a false decisiveness that physicians may be all too eager to accept uncritically. "The aura of finality and correctness of the computer," Engle predicted, "will be difficult for some physicians to overcome."[37] The single computer output did little to convey the messy, contingent, partial, and uncertain choices that the developers made in creating the program. The computer's rigid outputs might convey a false impression of certitude.

Engle feared that the language surrounding computerized diagnosis, with phrasing like "thinking machines" and "artificial intelligence," may undercut any measured understanding of a computer program's limitations. Specifically, Engle seems to have feared that a "living" metaphor about the computer risked gradually shading into a "dead" one; that is, he worried that metaphors may lose their status as mere figures of speech and begin to be interpreted as real or literal. Artificial intelligence may come to be taken as intelligence, full stop. As a result, when Engle did invoke metaphors, he was careful to point out their status as such. His views on this subject were heavily informed by the work of the German philosopher Hans Vaihinger.

In his book *The Philosophy of "As if,"* Vaihinger argues that much human knowledge is a mere assemblage of "fictions" but that there is often value in acting "as if" these fictions were true for pragmatic reasons.[38] In much the same way, Engle believed it a "fiction" to speak of a computer's "intelligence," but he nevertheless granted that such language could be justified pragmatically. He reasoned, "Great benefits can result from acting 'as if' models of artificial intelligence were real life human intelligence especially if it may lead to an effective coupling of the computer with the human brain."[39]

Other members of the hematology team also often acted and spoke "as if" the computer was a kind of human—although surely with less of a philosophically inflected self-awareness about what they were doing. The storage of incidence data in the computer's memory, the team wrote in one progress report, represented a kind of "experience" not unlike the physician's own experience: "This type of information stored in the 'permanent' computer memory will eventually constitute a body of 'computer experience' which will exceed human capability."[40] In a 1963 letter, members of the team similarly discussed the value of "the cumulative experience of a computer."[41] Many others took these metaphors further, assigning computer systems varying degrees of educational attainment—"medical students," "residents," "attendings"—based on the quantity and quality of information stored within them.

Decisions about where computers ought to go—what parts of medicine they were well suited to automate—were not just technical decisions. Behind these decisions were implicit valuations of different kinds of medical work. Historians of computing have described how new digital technologies create "new economies of intelligence" that dictate "whose cognitive labor is valued and devalued, displaced or replaced."[42] To carve out certain aspects of medicine for computerization was to partition medical work into tiered categories: from work that was human, cognitive, and artful (high value) to work that was mechanical, mindless, and rote (low value). Many developers of early computerized diagnostic systems insisted that computers would only take over the "rote" aspects of medicine, leaving physicians able to dedicate more of their time toward the human, and humanistic, dimensions of medicine.[43] Delegate to the computer the rote and the routine; leave to the physician the complex and contradictory. The two, mind and machine, were different but complementary. As the pioneer in the computerization of electrocardiograms, Cesar

Caceres wrote in 1968, "Proper use of both the machine's tireless ability for routine analysis and the physician's inimitable ability to put together sensed or intuitive impressions is the key to improvements in tomorrow's diagnostic practice."[44] Computers, these physicians and engineers suggested, would take over only the subset of the physician's work that was *beneath* them. In doing so, the physician would be "free" to pursue the aspects of medicine that they found more interesting and rewarding.

Members of the hematology team thought along similar lines. Engle believed that the diagnostic process was not just one thing but represented a collection of heterogeneous activities. It comprised aspects suited to the computer and aspects suited to the human. He thus described the need to "dissect out" from the diagnostic process those aspects that were routine and rote. Engle explained,

> Human beings . . . are able, in some unexplained way, to grasp subtle and complex relationships, recognize intricate patterns, recall integrated and interpreted facts, and originate new ideas. Computers have great potential for aiding thought if the mechanical facets of reasoning are identified and delegated to the computer. In order for computers to realize their full potential, the problem of interaction between human beings and computers must be approached from two sides. People must learn to analyze their thought processes so that they can dissect out the mechanical part and formulate the functions the computer is to perform.[45]

Here, it is clear how decisions about how to computerize diagnosis always implied certain ideas about humans and human nature—what kinds of work physicians were capable of, interested in, and suited for. As computers entered the arena of medical diagnosis, then, they not only came up against traditional ideas of professional identity; they also constructed new ideas about the physician's identity. Computers forced new discussions and thoughts about the physician's "appropriate" role in the diagnostic process and the clinical encounter.

## "A Sort of Psychoanalysis"

Questions about how doctors think, and whether computers ought to replicate such processes, pestered Zworykin's group almost from day one. What does clinical reasoning even look like? Can it be distilled, studied, or visualized? The hematology team believed they found a way of answering such questions in the clinicopathological conference (CPC), a formalized event where physicians reason aloud through a selected patient case. By analyzing published CPCs—and by staging their own—Zworykin and his colleagues hoped to purify and isolate the process by which the physician used medical information to reach a diagnosis.

The CPC evolved out of a broader late-nineteenth-century movement to introduce case studies into education. The so-called "case method" of medical education was an import from the legal academy. Under the direction of its visionary dean, Christopher Langdell, Harvard Law School pioneered the case method of legal instruction, whereby law professors, instead of relying on legal theory and abstract principles, would teach different areas of law by thinking through actual legal cases. Across the Charles River, reformers at Harvard Medical School's campus soon realized that an analogous method could be applied to medical education.[46] Medical instructors increasingly saw pedagogical value in presenting well-selected patient cases as a way of illuminating aspects of disease and diagnosis.

It was precisely this logic that motivated Richard C. Cabot, then a visiting physician at Massachusetts General Hospital, to begin scheduled performances of the CPC sometime around 1909.[47] At each conference, the featured physician would be presented with descriptions of a patient's symptoms along with laboratory and radiological information. Standing before an audience of physicians, and unwitting of the actual diagnosis, the physician would explicate their diagnostic reasoning and come to a diagnosis for the case before them.[48] The CPC was therefore a performative exercise, and it occasionally took on the character of a drama.

The purpose of the CPC was less about making a correct diagnosis than about simulating the diagnostic process itself. The editors of a 1960 volume of CPCs called the conference "an exercise in deductive reasoning," one in which "it is less important to pinpoint the correct diagnosis than to present a logical and instructive analysis of the pertinent conditions involved."[49] The complexity of solving many diagnostic problems justified this performance of the diagnostic process. Not only did physicians face vast amounts of patient information; they had to synthesize medical information coming from different sources and reconcile findings that seemed to point in different directions. In complex cases, it was rare for a patient's medical picture to map neatly onto any textbook description of disease. The CPC was a demonstration in how to navigate this complexity. Amid the bustle of medical work going on in the hospital, the CPC purported to isolate—and to stage—clinical cognition in its purest form. For some, the exercise promised a window into the inner workings of the physician's mind.

It was for these reasons that the hematology team took an interest in the CPC.[50] Yet the team ultimately concluded the CPC offered them little actionable insight. Engle later explained, "Obvious approaches to answer some of the questions concerning how a physician makes a diagnosis include analyses of published Clinical Pathological Conferences (CPC) such as those reported in the *New England Journal of Medicine* or the *American Journal of Medicine*, and interviews of physicians as they go through the diagnostic process during a real or simulated Clinical Pathological Conference. When our group first became interested in computer aids to decision-making in 1956 we used both of these approaches and came to a few conclusions."[51] Specifically, Engle and his colleagues realized that the conditions around CPCs were simply too sanitized and unrealistic to be of much use: "CPC's [*sic*] are carefully selected situations and are not representative of patients in general. They are more like games than like real life situations since the physicians know that the patients have died and that the decision reached will not have any effect on the treatment of the patients."[52] The exercise, to be fair, was not wholly fruitless. The CPCs did, Engle acknowledged, "give some indication as to how a physician approaches a particular problem"—namely, physicians "often pick from a multitude of findings certain ones of high significance and proceed to do a differential diagnosis related to those findings."[53] (This was the conclusion that Keeve Brodman had also reached in his own, more inwardly reflective, analysis of how doctors think.)

Ultimately, the hematology team found that, all too often, physicians were unable to explicate their decision-making processes. They could effectively navigate through some diagnostic maze, but they were not particularly good at describing *how* they got through—why, for instance, they made *this* assumption, and not *that* assumption. Different physicians, moreover, sometimes took different paths through the diagnostic process, even if they arrived at the same diagnosis. The team was left wondering: was one of these routes better, or more representative, than the other? As Engle elaborated, "The physician frequently could not give a rational reason for making certain inferences and certain decisions even though he may have been satisfied with his line of reasoning. There was considerable variation in approach from one physician to another and by the same physician in analyzing different cases. The physician often thought in the most general terms without much specific information. Occasionally, the basic information was erroneous."[54]

To many it was not self-evident that researchers should want to replicate human reasoning, even if they could. Computers, some believed, brought a different set of strengths and weaknesses to the table. Why replicate human reasoning when you can transcend it? At the 1963 Michigan conference, one attendee, Dr. Kossack, reasoned:

> I always seem to get the role of being the devil's advocate, not that I think it is a bad idea to try to get the computer to follow the human process. When I talk with business people I say that I am worried that when we do these things that we will find that in the computer we will have programmed the coffee break because we've copied what people do. In fact, is there any evidence that the diagnostic process, as an art practiced by the medical profession, is better than chance?[55]

Kossack's comment here was in response to Lipkin's claim at the conference that "the results of our [the hematology group's] studies demonstrate the feasibility of automating certain portions of differential diagnosis."[56] Lipkin answered Kossack's provocation, observing that while it may be true that his hematology program did not replicate the exact functions of the human mind, it was nevertheless worthwhile to "give some thought" to the possibility that mind and machine, at least in the context of this particular program, "bear some similarity."[57]

At the Rockefeller Institute's 1959 conference on Diagnostic Data Processing, two of Lipkin's colleagues—Russell Ebald and Robert Lane—similarly described the hematology "matching" program as a simulation of how doctors think. "To be more specific," they declared, "we attempted to simulate the thinking of the doctor." Ebald and Lane proceeded to outline their view of how clinicians reason: "Logically he would proceed as follows. Once the preliminary examination was complete and the results of appropriate tests had been recorded, the doctor would attempt to match these symptoms to some one disease or combination of diseases. He would do this either from his own experience or from the experience of his colleagues, or from texts of classical disease definition. This then is what we tried to do."[58] That is, the team defined and computerized certain disease definitions and developed an algorithm to match the individual patient findings to these larger pictures—just as the physician "matches" patient particularities to their own generalized definition of disease, created through their experience, study, colleagues, or some combination thereof.

In the discussion following Ebald and Lane's presentation, Engle pointed out other parallels between the program and his notion of clinical cognition. As Engle saw it, physicians, "when confronted with a large number of signs and symptoms, often picked from these one or a few key signs or symptoms, usually ones which were unquestionable. Then on the basis of this sign or symptom say, jaundice, he would automatically go into what we call a differential diagnosis, picking the diseases that would produce jaundice. Next the physician would consider these diseases in terms of all the signs and symptoms."[59] Engle felt that the program "paralleled" this human process of thinking by, first, matching patient findings to a broad disease class on the basis of key symptoms and only later homing in on the more specific disease diagnosis.

As the hematology project aged, however, the group came to side with Kossack's viewpoint. The hematology team presented this line of thinking in a 1975 paper:

> Like all other parts of the human body, the brain, the organ of thought, has become adapted to its environment through the evolutionary process. However, there are certain inherent limitations which restrict the development of organs and do not allow the optimum development of all aspects of function. For example, although animals have evolved legs and some have wings, none has evolved wheels, although we consider these essential for smooth and fast travel on the earth. Man has developed tools of all kinds to improve and extend his strength and endurance.[60]

As with automobiles, the group suggested, so too with automated diagnosis. The computer offered ways not just of replicating human abilities but of building upon and extending those capabilities.

Of course not all developers of early computerized diagnostic systems agreed that the explication and replication of diagnostic reasoning was so hopeless—or fruitless. As is clear in Brodman's case, the act of formalizing the diagnostic process forced physicians to think in new ways about the nature of the medical mind. Through his work computerizing diagnosis, Brodman clarified his own ideas about clinical reasoning—ideas that he then codified into the software of his diagnostic program. Others reported similar experiences. One crowning achievement of early efforts to computerize diagnosis, many later noted, was the explication and formalization of the medical decision-making process. The divide between enterprises in engineering (building a diagnostic system) and those in psychology (clarifying the nature of clinical reasoning) was a porous one, with ideas and individuals trafficking back and forth. Many of the same people who undertook research initiatives in the computerization of diagnosis also founded and populated some of the earliest medical societies dedicated to understanding the diagnostic process and to cultivating the emerging field of "decision science." Lee Lusted, for example, founded the Society for Medical Decision Making, and conferences like those on "The Diagnostic Process" were teeming with the likes of Lipkin, Engle, and Lusted.[61]

Historians have shown how the process of creating computer programs can give rise to new forms of reasoning and analysis that are then used outside of the context of computerization. In his history of Logic and Heuristics Applied to Synthetic Analysis, a computer program designed to help organic chemists with retrosynthetic analysis, historian Evan Hepler-Smith shows how the process of creating the program "shaped a way of thinking taken up by chemists, unaided by machines."[62] Such observations complement Lucy Suchman's arguments about the role of computers as "powerful disclosing agents," as tools that physicians and others used to reflect upon and better understand themselves (or at least what they believed to be true about themselves).[63]

Similar phenomena were at play in the computerization of diagnosis. The digital computer was an object that physicians began to think with, against, and alongside. The dynamics of "powerful disclosure" were particularly decisive in the creation of INTERNIST-I, a program at the University of Pittsburgh designed to make the majority of diagnoses in all of internal medicine. Developed under the auspices of the Stanford University Medical Experimental Computer for Artificial Intelligence in Medicine (SUMEX-AIM) (discussed in chapter 5 at greater length), INTERNIST-I grew out of a collaboration in the early 1970s between the computer scientist Harry Pople and the internist Jack D. Myers. Myers had just stepped down from his post as chairman of the Department of Medicine and taken up the role of "university professor," a supra-departmental appointment (modeled after similar professorships at Harvard) that gave faculty extraordinary levels of freedom to work and collaborate across disciplinary lines.[64] Deciding where to direct his energies during this new phase of his career, Myers was drawn to a set of concerns and challenges that almost seemed to be nagging at the medical field's collective consciousness. First, how to manage a knowledge base that had grown "vastly too large for any single person" to know, and second, how to ensure that the "busy physician" considered "the right answer particularly if the diagnosis was an unusual case."[65]

Through a mutual colleague, Myers (who "knew nothing about computer science") was connected with Pople (who "knew nothing about medicine").[66]

Together, they worked to develop a program that would incorporate the medical expertise and imitate the logical processes of this single physician, Myers. Of the internists in the United States at the time, Myers had a strong claim to be The One to be computerized. Myers enjoyed an eidetic memory (supposedly) and the reputation of being a "master diagnostician."[67] Their collaboration thus began with Myers analyzing—and performing—the diagnostic process before Pople. Pople's job was tripartite: to watch, to formalize, and then to program. Randolph Miller, an MD-PhD student who later joined the project, described the logic at play here: "find a genius and can their brain."[68] Myers described these sessions in greater detail: "I chose a goodly number of actual cases from clinical pathological conferences (CPCs) because they contained ample clinical data and because the correct diagnoses were known. At each small step of the way through the diagnostic process I was required to explain what the clinical information meant in context and my reasons for considering certain diagnoses. This provided to Pople insight into the diagnostic process."[69]

Because of INTERNIST-I's reliance on Myers, Pople characterized the system as an example of simulation, its heuristic rules and logical processes simply those that best resembled the reasoning he observed in action. In being "forced" to explain his diagnostic reasoning, Myers also felt himself changed. "After analyzing dozens of such cases," Myers wrote, "I felt as though I had undergone a sort of 'psychoanalysis.' "[70] The diagnostic process, once subconscious, was brought out into the open. The experience left a durable mark on Myers's "own diagnostic approaches and habits."[71]

Creating the hematology program likewise served as a kind of "psychoanalysis" for the hematology doctors. Even though Engle came to conclude that it was hopeless to have computers attempt to simulate the "uniquely human ability" of "intellectual synthesis," he and others in the hematology group acknowledged that their work with computers did much to clarify their own thinking about, and understanding of, the diagnostic process.[72] During the project's twilight years, Engle insisted (departing from the perspectives and goals of some of his earlier colleagues) that "the program was never intended to be a diagnosis machine."[73] Instead Engle defined the program's use in three other areas, one being its role "as a tool for studying the diagnostic process."[74] Engle expanded on this point at the 1963 University of Michigan conference. "Work on the problem of computer aids to diagnosis," he noted, "has forced us to try to define terms more precisely. It has also stimulated an interest in basic theoretical and philosophical questions which have some application to medical diagnosis; such questions as the theory of universals and the closely related problems of classification, definition, and nomenclature as well as induction and deduction."[75]

Having been forced to grapple with fundamental epistemological questions, Engle presented his conclusions in a three-part series of articles published in the *Archives of Internal Medicine* on the topic of "Medical Diagnosis: Present, Past, and Future."[76] The first of these articles, coauthored with B. J. Davis, dealt with the nature of diagnosis and the definitions of disease. Diagnosis, Engle and Davis argued, is essentially a two-sided coin: it refers both to the process of clinical decision-making and to the decision itself. Its functions, moreover, are multiple, involving not just "the naming and classification of disease" but also the communication of implicit theoretical frameworks about health and illness and "the construction of hypothesis by serving to stimulate investigation."[77] Engle and Davis proceeded to show how disease definitions can be just as amorphous as the concept of diagnosis. "At the present time," they observed, "there is no unified concept of disease and, therefore, no unified yet flexible and practical concept of diagnosis."[78] Instead, they argued, the nature of disease concepts varies considerably—ranging from diseases whose etiologies are well understood and whose clinical presentations are fairly uniform (such as certain congenital cardiac malformations), to diseases whose etiologies are not at all known and whose clinical presentations are highly idiosyncratic (such as "collagen diseases," "aplastic anemia," and other more syndromal disease categories).

The second article in the series turned largely to matters of philosophy. Engle argued that the process of diagnosis represented an instantiation of the philosophical concept of "the theory of universals," with physicians having to constantly negotiate and navigate between the particular (the individual patient) and the general (the disease concept). "Every time a physician thinks about a patient or makes a diagnosis, he must consider the patient as an individual and at the same time generalize as much as possible about his condition so that it can be classified and a diagnosis made."[79] Engle called the back-and-forth required of the physician a "psychic shuttle," borrowing a term from the English critic Herbert Read.[80]

In the final installment of the series, Engle, finally, addressed the computer's role in all of this. Engle saw a clear role for computers in medicine. It was a tool that boasted a unique suite of strengths: "We may conclude that electronic computers, because of their large data-storage capacity or memory, their accuracy and speed of data recall, and their ability to process rapidly large volumes of information, should be of great value to physicians for aiding in certain aspects of the thought processes required for medical diagnosis and even in aiding decision concerning therapy."[81] Yet he was careful to note that he saw their role as a limited one. Engle's reflections on the diagnostic process had convinced him that diagnosis included both deductive reasoning (down from general principles) and inductive reasoning (up from specific observations), and that the inductive modes of reasoning in particular contained an "intuitive" component that defied computerizability: "It is my opinion that intuitive induction cannot be performed by a machine and will remain solely within the physician's province."[82]

## Back to Bayes

The hematology group could not escape the magnetism of Bayes's theorem. By the late 1960s, the group had abandoned their "matching" approach, citing the method's "severe limitations."[83] In its place they returned to a method they had once eschewed: they developed a program called "HEME," which operated by a modified Bayesian algorithm. This shift in strategy in many ways reflected the group's shifting leadership. While the project's nucleus stayed in New York City throughout its existence, it bounced among different institutional homes.[84] After Zworykin relinquished leadership in 1961, the project moved from the Rockefeller Institute to the New York University College of Engineering, where it came under the direction of the statistician Max Woodbury (1961–1966) and later the sociologist Louis J. Gerstman (1966–1967). In 1967, the project moved from the NYU campus in Midtown Manhattan to Brodman's stomping grounds in the Upper East Side. There, at Cornell University Medical College, the project fell under the supervision of Engle who was joined at the helm by the mathematician Dr. Betty Flehinger a year later.

Flehinger was the driving force behind the model's substantive changes. Trained as a biostatistician, she worked as a research assistant in Columbia's Mathematics Department before joining the university's IBM Watson Laboratory in 1959.[85] She maintained this affiliation throughout her work on the hematology program. Flehinger's reputation preceded her. On learning of Flehinger's appointment, Woodbury wrote to Engle, "I am glad to see you have the cooperation of Betty Flehinger in your work. She is very good from what I know about her."[86] Flehinger delivered on these expectations and quickly began steering the group's research direction. The group spelled out her contributions in a 1972 grant application: "Because of our interest in the 'significance model' we did not start working with the Bayesian model until Dr. Betty Flehinger joined our group in 1967."[87]

Adopting a new strategy (and one that the group had once rejected) was not taken lightly. To make the new model more palatable, Flehinger drew out the parallels between her model and the group's prior approach. She noted that the same data that had been amassed for the significance model could be used to estimate the probabilities required for Bayes's theorem. "Dr. Flehinger," the team wrote, "pointed out that using most of the information accumulated for the significance model we would be able to apply a new version of Bayes' theorem, one which does not assume mutual exclusiveness of diseases."[88]

Early Bayesian models operated under the assumption that the patient in question only had one disease. The absurdity of this assumption drove many away from the theorem. But Flehinger proposed a work-around.[89] Whereas these earlier models took multiple diseases into consideration at once—assuming a universe of patients where each patient has but a single disease—the modified model only considered one disease at a time. The assumed universe of the modified algorithm also looked different, consisting of two groups of patients: those with the disease in question and those without the disease in question.[90] HEME, operating by this method, could iteratively compute the probability that the patient has each of the forty diseases presently considered by the system. The system could also marshal for the physician-user the findings that supported, and those that opposed, each of the diagnoses on the differential. Under this new model, the estimated probabilities of all diseases need not add up to one; that is, the model allowed for coexisting diseases in a patient.

Another selling point for the new model was what Engle and Flehinger called its "self-improving" nature.[91] As the computer saw more and more patients, it could incorporate these data and update its underlying conditional probabilities. With more and better data, the system should improve over time with experience—not unlike a practicing physician. The model wasn't just self-improving though. The team added their own improvements as well, expanding and updating the program's database to encompass 142 hematologic diseases and 667 findings.[92] The team also modified fundamental aspects of how the program worked. Indeed, as early as 1974, Engle and Flehinger had already started creating a new version of the program, HEME2. These changes were responsive to the team's investigations into the original HEME program's deficiencies: "After analyzing a number of diagnostic situations in which the computer went astray in the diagnostic process we decided that part of the problem related to the fact that HEME was a one-step system."[93] HEME2 functioned by two steps. In the first step, the program classified the patient into one or more of nineteen broad categories of hematologic disease; in the second, the program diagnosed the patient as having one of the diseases within the identified categories.[94] By classifying patients, first, into broad categories of disease and, only later, into the actual diagnosis, HEME2 carried forward the new ways of considering and classifying hematologic diseases that had been necessitated earlier on by the machine's material affordances.

Going back to Bayes, though a well-trodden path, presented its own challenges. Most pressingly, the approach remained vulnerable to many of the same critiques that members of the hematology team had leveled twenty years earlier. Woodbury, who had articulated the group's early critiques of Bayesian approaches, found the new, modified models developed by Flehinger nearly as restrictive as earlier ones articulated by Ledley and Lusted. Woodbury wrote in a note to Lipkin, describing his preliminary thoughts from his "investigation of the conditions for validity for the use of Flehinger's formulas."[95] Woodbury didn't pull any punches: "The conditions are quite severe and the more general formulas required to remove them are considerably harder to use and computer[ize]."[96]

He expounded upon his concerns in a letter to Engle. "I am a bit puzzled by the notes on the Bayesian Model used. It seems that you must have assumed that each finding was unique to a disease with what is, essentially, a uniform probability of 'false' positive for the finding for all other diseases. If this is even approximately true it represents an enormous simplification of the problem."[97] Woodbury had other concerns, too, but he merely directed Engle to his earlier paper on the "Inapplicabilities of Bayes' Theorem to Diagnosis": "Other than this," he wrote, "my criticisms are all pretty minor and are inferable from my article on 'Inapplicabilities.'"

Reviving another line of criticism against Bayes's theorem, others found HEME's new strategy questionable on the basis of its data requirements. In 1974, Engle and Flehinger lost a grant bid, in part because of these unresolved issues. Channeling many of the concerns about data judgment and bias discussed earlier, the grant reviewers felt that the group had not paid adequate attention to matters of data quality. "The applicant," they explained, "did not demonstrate that sufficient thought had been given to the critical issue of validating the input data."[98] Even if the quality of input data could be assured, the reviewers were skeptical that the group could harvest the appropriate quantity. The back-of-the-envelope mathematics didn't look promising. They broke it down: "A major reservation concerned the practicality of generating useful conditional probabilities for a system containing 120 diseases. With over 500 findings at present and perhaps 1,000 findings in the expanded system, the application would need to generate approximately 100,000 conditional probabilities. The number of cases required to estimate these conditional probabilities could number in the millions."[99] Alternatives to collecting such masses of "raw" data—namely, "textbook review or physician panel"—would still constitute a "tremendous effort" of their own. (One expects M. A. Atamer would have agreed.) The outcome of all this work, moreover, "would apply only to patients known to have hematologic disease"—a small fraction of patient diagnoses.[100]

Apart from these well-known challenges, a Bayesian approach to computerizing diagnosis had, by the late 1960s and early 1970s, lost the verve that it once enjoyed. As new faces in the field pioneered "expert systems" and self-avowedly "artificial intelligence" approaches to diagnosis (explored in Part III of this book), the Bayesian method came across as a bit outdated, ho-hum, even regressive. This view set the tone of a 1975 referee report for the *American Journal of Medicine*: "The manuscript is a rather typical example of the Bayesian statistical diagnosis programs that have been appearing for the past fifteen years. Although it purports to be different than prior attempts, it is not. It falls into the same old traps and limitations."[101] The reviewer thus concluded, "In summary, this manuscript would have been interesting 5–10 years ago, but now is just one of many like it."[102]

These troubles above the water reflected other troubles below. In their publications, the team boasted of HEME's "encourag[ing]" results during testing.[103] This outward optimism, however, belied ongoing uncertainties and challenges. The team had the frustrating sense that they had reached a point of diminishing returns: edits to the program solved some issues, only to introduce others. Modifications to the program and its database therefore frequently resulted in no net performance gains. "In HEME2 our attempts to correct the deficiencies were directed toward modifying the subjective information in the database of the program," they explained. "In doing so, we found that these changes resulted in improving some parts of the system, often at the expense of deterioration in other parts."[104]

The asymptote of performance that the HEME program reached wasn't even that impressive. The system did fine when fed simple cases. But when presented with more complex cases—the precise kind of cases for which physicians might need computerized decision support—the system seemed prone to choke. The group noted in a clear-eyed assessment of HEME: "If given relatively simple cases, the program does very well. If given very difficult cases it does poorly and it is sometimes difficult to be certain what the correct answers should be. Usually, however, the program gives a reasonable, though not necessarily correct answer. In moderately difficult cases, its performance is variable."[105] Thinking of these and related challenges, Engle concluded, "[I] don't believe we have evidence yet that 'accuracy often approaches that of a skilled hematologist.' We believe it is premature for this system to have any impact on clinical hematology."[106]

But Engle and Flehinger wondered: if not clinical hematology, perhaps there was another suitable home for the program. As they retreated from the hope that HEME would find its way into the rhythms of clinical care, they increasingly worked to define a new niche for the program in medical education. Toward this end, they introduced HEME as a teaching tool into the hematology elective for fourth-year medical students at Cornell University Medical College. The idea was that by working through a patient case alongside HEME, comparing one's own reasoning with that of the computer, early learners would more readily understand the intricacies of hematologic decision-making and the fundamentals of the diagnostic process.

But even medical students, a group accustomed to mindlessly grinding through curricular unpleasantries, resisted the program. Of the eight students invited to use the program, only four ended up using it and only one finished the syllabus.[107] The reasons behind this degree of attrition were variable and many, ranging from "obvious skepticism by many on the senior staff concerning the ability of a computer to aid teaching" and delayed response times due to "computer difficulties," to students being "very busy with their required work" and "unfamiliarity in the use of computers."[108] The matter ultimately boiled down to a matter of cost-benefit analysis for the students: "The students found it to be too unwieldy and time-consuming to sustain their interest and effort in using it."[109]

The team had high hopes for HEME: "It is hoped that the program ultimately will gain acceptance by physicians and will be used routinely as a step in the diagnostic process," the group wrote in 1976.[110] But by the 1980s, it was clear that this project, now ongoing for nearly three decades, would not gain clinical traction.[111] HEME had failed. It failed in its earlier quest to become a widespread aid in differential diagnosis, and it even failed in its later reformulations as a teaching aid. "For twenty-five years," the team reflected, "investigators have labored enthusiastically toward the development of computer aids to diagnosis. . . . At this point we have decided to end our labors in this field."[112] Having dedicated such a sizeable chunk of his career to the project, Engle was introspective about the possible reasons behind these persistent challenges. The hematology group's failures were surely overdetermined. Among the factors contributing to the project's demise, Engle identified poor user interfaces, unruly computing technologies, limitations of the program, and professional resistance to computerized diagnostic aids. Yet Engle concluded such factors, while contributory, were not really "critical."[113] Other factors were steering the ship.

Some wondered, for example, if computerized systems like HEME were really geared to the right problem—whether these systems excessively fetishized the act of "diagnosis" (assigning labels) at the expense of "decision-making," which they saw as the broader driving force of patient care. The physician William Bauman articulated this view in a 1969 letter to the editor of the *New England Journal of Medicine*: " 'Diagnosis' is the act of identifying a disease or giving a label to a set of medical findings. The major objective in patient care, however, is not 'Diagnosis' but rather 'Management.' A patient does not benefit from the label; he is helped by the physicians' recommendations, or actions. Nor is the diagnosis necessary to make a decision as to management. In fact, it is entirely possible to render good medical care without ever identifying the name of the illness."[114] Computerized systems, Bauman implied, should be less fixated on diagnosis. Instead they should take up the broader mission of helping physicians make better decisions of all kinds as they manage their patients. By this reasoning, such efforts may have failed because they weren't appropriately geared toward solving the more pressing problems in medicine. "Our major concern," Bauman concluded, "should be how to best treat the patient, not how to make a diagnosis."[115]

As Engle reflected on the fate of his work, he endorsed the possibility that programs like his were just not filling a real need. No matter how good the program got, perhaps it was not sufficiently well aligned with the needs of its users. Enumerating some of the reasons HEME "has received little use," Engle and Flehinger wrote, "It is rare that a purely diagnostic problem in which a name is to be given to a patient's ailment presents itself. Most of the physician's time is spent in the day-to-day management of patients of known diagnosis."[116] Even on the rare occasion when a narrow diagnostic task presents itself, it often involves practices and tools that defy computerization. They noted, "Many of the most important diagnostic tools, such as palpation of the spleen, bone marrow and blood smear examination, and general observations of the patient cannot be transferred to a computer. They require unique human pattern-recognition abilities."[117]

Ultimately, though, Engle's thirty-plus years of experience working on the program led him to the conclusion that the greatest obstacle to computerized diagnostic systems was nothing external to, or modifiable within, medicine. It was the nature of medicine itself—and of the diagnostic mind. Engle explained,

> In our estimation, the critical impediment to the development of decision programs useful in medicine lies in the impossibility of developing an adequate database and an effective set of decision rules. Any decision module contains only a small fraction of the data and of the intricate relationships that a physician learns in the course of education and practical experience. Personal experience over many years trying to develop a suitable diagnostic program for hematologic diseases confirms the great difficulty and even the impossibility of incorporating the complexity of human thought into a system that can be handled by a computer. A computer-based diagnostic system has three major components, each of which defies successful implementation: input, inference by means of an algorithm, and output.[118]

At every level, medicine and the mind were too slippery, too ill-defined, too complex.

In his three-part series on "Medical Diagnosis," Engle compared disease to light. By the Copenhagen interpretation, light can behave either like a wave or like a particle—depending on the questions one is asking. Similarly, disease definitions can take on different properties and characteristics—depending on one's frame of mind. Engle explained,

> At its heart, the question of qualitative disease versus quantitative disease is not unlike the quantum theory versus the wave theory of light. Either hypothesis can be invoked if need arises, and in this sense both are correct. At the most fundamental level in the chromosome or the DNA, we now think of changes as being discontinuous or qualitative. Nevertheless, because of the long chain of events between the chromosomes and the manifestations that we can interpret, the many interactions that occur at these stages produce effects which are quantitative.[119]

There are different ways of defining and conceptualizing disease entities. A purpose of chapters 3 and 4 has been to demonstrate the role of computers—and their material and mathematical basis—in shaping how we see and define disease entities. This part, when read together with Part I, yields insights into the process of disease definition—and the participation of computers and material culture in that process.

These cases illuminate the mechanisms by which material form shapes nosology. As two of the earliest efforts to computerize medical diagnosis, they reveal how the use of computers facilitated new ways of collating knowledge and defining disease. As soon as Zworykin and his colleagues started work on a diagnostic program in hematology, they began to generate new classifications and quantitative descriptions of disease. Similarly, in the process of creating the Medical Data Screen, Brodman translated subjective symptoms into the language of numbers and thresholds. The diagnosis of disease, in both cases, was the result of an algorithmically guided comparison between a numerical rendering of the patient's health status and population health data that was stored in the computer's memory.

PART THREE

# PHYSICIAN

CHAPTER FIVE

# MYCIN Explains Itself

Over four days in the summer of 1975, pioneers in the computerization of medical decision-making gathered in New Brunswick, New Jersey, to attend the First Annual Artificial Intelligence in Medicine (AIM) Workshop, hosted at Rutgers University. Present at the event were nearly thirty physicians, computer scientists, and mathematicians, affiliated with a range of early computerized decision support projects. Among them, Edward Shortliffe, Stanton Axline, and Randy Davis attended as the front men of MYCIN, a consultation system designed to aid physicians in the identification and treatment of bacterial infections; Harry Pople, Jack Meyers, and Randolph Miller brought their experience developing the expert system called INTERNIST-I, an ambitious system intended to recognize the majority of possible diagnoses in internal medicine; and Saul Amarel, Casimir Kulikowski, and Aran Safir discussed their work designing CASNET (causal-associational network), a program designed to assist in diagnosing optic nerve diseases.[1] These systems represented some of the first attempts to apply a self-avowedly "expert systems" technique to medical decision-making.

In addition to being some of the most promising—and hyped—efforts of their time, the systems represented at the workshop were unified by a more immediate and tangible connection: most had been developed under the auspices of the Stanford University Medical Experimental Computer for Artificial Intelligence in Medicine (SUMEX-AIM). Beginning in January 1974, SUMEX-AIM was established as a computing facility at Stanford to support research on medical applications of artificial intelligence (AI). The facility's scope, a 1974 prospectus observed, was national, with "a major part of its computing capacity . . . made available to authorized research groups throughout the country by means of a communications network."[2] This "communications network" was none other than ARPANET—the Department of Defense–sponsored forerunner to the Internet. Indeed, SUMEX-AIM was the first non–Department of Defense host on ARPANET's 63-node network.[3] In addition to describing SUMEX-AIM's national scope, the prospectus laid out its two main objectives: "(1) the specific encouragement of applications of artificial intelligence in medicine (AIM) and (2) the managerial, administrative, and technical demonstration of a national shared technological resource for health research."[4] The Rutgers workshop, then, was an occasion to celebrate SUMEX-AIM's early strides.

It was also an occasion to discuss common topics, challenges, and themes that cut across SUMEX-AIM-supported projects. The workshop broached topics that covered a spectrum that ranged from the technical to the philosophical. One topic in particular seemed to span both ends of this spectrum: the issue of explainability. How could advice generated by computerized algorithm be communicated, and made understandable, to human medical personnel? To many, this question begged a technical answer: communicability was a problem to be solved through technological innovations in natural language processing and human-computer interfaces. But philosophical considerations drove discussions around interpretability and communicability as well. To what extent were communicability and interpretability driving values in medicine and medical decision-making? Could they justifiably be sacrificed at the altar of other medical values—say, those of speed and accuracy?

Using the MYCIN system as its primary case study, Part III explores the interrelations among computing, authority, identity, and trust in postwar American medicine. It demonstrates that concerns about trust and transparency drove much of the development of, and responses to, the MYCIN system. Moreover, concerns about the extent to which a computer's advice could be understood, communicated, and trusted coexisted with concerns about authority and the physician's identity. The following chapters elucidate a dynamic that structured the creation and reception of computerized diagnostic systems through the second half of the twentieth century—a dynamic that endures today. This story begins in the arid foothills of the South San Francisco Bay Area, at a university that was just coming into its own.

## Knowledge Is Power

Today few universities are associated as strongly with the fields of medical informatics, biomedical computing, and computer science as Stanford University. Stanford's prominence in these areas, however, was not foreordained, as Joseph November has shown.[5] Indeed, in the 1940s and 1950s the university looked nothing like an optimal incubator for innovative work at the intersections of biology, medicine, and computing. Plagued by an inadequate flow of research funds, a medical school that rested on financially shaky grounds, and a research culture characterized by isolation and siloing, Stanford in the immediate postwar period lacked the basic ingredients required for a costly research enterprise that sought to bridge the computational and medical sciences.[6]

Over the next decade, all of this would change. This transformation was less the product of some natural or serendipitous evolution than a conscious effort to restructure and revitalize the university. Such an undertaking was spearheaded by the engineer and administrator Frederick Terman, who served as Stanford's academic dean beginning in 1946 and as its provost from 1955 to 1965.[7] From these perches, Terman laid the groundwork for the institution's transformation into a STEM (science, technology, engineering, and math) heavyweight. He attracted major grants from the Department of Defense; expanded the university's departments in the fields of science, engineering, and statistics; recruited top talent to Palo Alto; invested heavily in the idea of Stanford as a research-oriented institution; and forged new linkages between the university and the tech industry. By catalyzing this activity, Terman helped set into motion a series of developments that would culminate in the rebranding of "Santa Clara Valley" into "Silicon Valley."[8]

Important changes particular to the School of Medicine and the Department of Computer Science paralleled this larger institutional transformation. The School of Medicine, once financially strained and physically isolated, had, by 1959, found a firmer financial footing and moved from its former site in San Francisco to the main campus in Palo Alto.[9] A key motivation behind this relocation to the university's main campus was the hope that the School of Medicine's physical proximity to Stanford's larger research operation in the biological, physical, and engineering sciences would promote cross-fertilization between fields. As explained in a 1965 grant application, "Stanford made a calculated decision to move the medical school from San Francisco to the Palo Alto campus, and did so in 1959. This was a conscientious self-dedication to far-reaching communion of medical research and education with university life, based on the principle of mutual interdependence of medicine with the physical sciences and with human affairs."[10] The School of Medicine's move to Palo Alto reinforced Stanford's communal research culture and facilitated the sharing of tools, ideas, methods, and personnel among research groups.[11]

Atop the list of departments with which researchers at the School of Medicine would form new and significant collaborations was the Department of Computer Science, founded in 1965.[12] The department's rise to international prominence was short and swift. Its founding chair, George Forsythe, aggressively (and successfully) recruited some of the best and brightest minds in computer science and artificial intelligence to Palo Alto, from established leaders like John McCarthy at the Massachusetts Institute of Technology (MIT) to promising up-and-coming scholars like the Carnegie-trained Edward Feigenbaum.[13]

It was within this atmosphere that the university made its earliest forays into the area of biomedical computing. The most noteworthy of these early efforts was the creation of the Advanced Computer for Medical Research (ACME), a computer system "designed to provide powerful computing to research laboratories in the Medical School."[14] The vision behind the ACME was in many ways set by Forsythe, who saw computer science not as a mere subfield of mathematics but as its own discipline with manifold lessons and applications for manifold other fields of inquiry. By 1966, the ACME was operational, supporting a sundry of biomedical computing projects across the campus that ranged from the basic to the applied sciences—from "the analysis and interpretation of data on human white cell antigens" to the processing of data on the "effects of heart transplantation."[15]

Also among the computing projects supported by the ACME was one of the world's first expert systems, DENDRAL (Dendritic Algorithm). Expert systems are computer systems designed to emulate the decision-making processes of human experts. They comprise two main subsystems: a knowledge base—a store of facts and rules about a given problem domain—and an inference engine that performs the reasoning process with respect to these rules and facts. DENDRAL's problem domain was organic chemistry; the system aimed to assist organic chemists in identifying the structures of amino acids and new organic molecules from mass spectrometry data.[16]

DENDRAL was, like so many pioneering mid-twentieth-century enterprises in science and medicine, the brainchild of Joshua Lederberg, a Nobel laureate famous for his discovery of bacterial conjugation.[17] Lederberg's path to the field of biomedical computing was circuitous: a geneticist, he arrived at the fields of biomedical computing and artificial intelligence by way of an intermediary fascination with extraterrestrial life. As the head of the Instrumentation Research Laboratory (IRL) at Stanford, Lederberg became fascinated with several far-out questions.[18] Was there life on Mars? How might it be located, isolated, and analyzed? Might Martian life present risks of disease and contamination to life on Earth?

Lederberg initiated the DENDRAL project (or at least its early antecedents) in 1961 as part of this ongoing research into "exobiology."[19] At the IRL, Lederberg was developing an automated miniature laboratory for NASA that would test for signs of life on Mars. A computerized system, he hoped, would provide an important feature to this automated laboratory: using mass spectrometry data derived from a sample of Martian soil, such a system could help identify amino acids and organic molecules that suggested extraterrestrial life. Lederberg elaborated upon this vision in a draft proposal cowritten with John McCarthy. They wrote, trying to convince NASA of its interest in supporting "basic research" in artificial intelligence, "We believe that an automated biological laboratory in which a computer controls experimental apparatus according to programs that can be revised on earth [*sic*] is the key to the biological study of Mars. The effectiveness of this laboratory will depend in a large measure on how much 'intelligence' we can program into it."[20]

Though in many ways a product of Lederberg's vision, DENDRAL also benefited more circumstantially from its association with Stanford's intellectually rich environment. As Stanford grew through the 1960s into a massive research institution, countless prominent researchers across the life, physical, and medical sciences yielded to its pull. Lederberg tapped into this surge of intellectual activity. He recruited the eminent organic chemist Carl Djerassi as well as the young computer scientist Edward Feigenbaum to join the effort.[21] As the project gained intellectual energy, it reached a sort of escape velocity: the effort became a significant research program in its own right, no longer tethered to its origins in exobiology.

Others, like the philosopher of science Bruce Buchanan, came to DENDRAL from farther afield in the disciplinary landscape. Though trained as a humanist, Buchanan's background suited the DENDRAL project perfectly: in line with DENDRAL's early formulation as a project of scientific theory formation, Buchanan's academic expertise concerned the philosophy of scientific discovery. His doctoral dissertation advanced the proposition that discovery and theory formation in the sciences involved more of a systematic, formalizable process than had previously been recognized.[22] "I had some ideas,"

Buchanan explained, "that it shouldn't be as mysterious a process as the psychologists were making it out to be with a creative, 'Ah, ha, Eureka!' experience. It was totally mysterious. So I was trying to be somewhat systematic in looking at the process of discovery, but not from a psychological point of view, more from a logical point of view."[23] Many of the academic publications concerning DENDRAL described the system precisely in this vein: "More important," one such publication noted, speaking of the system's value to science, "is the contribution such computer assistance can make to scientific creativity . . . by providing new tools to aid scientists in hypothesis formation."[24]

A computer project with a narrow purpose—to assist organic chemists in identifying chemical structures—thus drew upon a wide spread of disciplines. It brought together an unlikely, and highly interdisciplinary, team comprising a geneticist, a computer scientist, an organic chemist, and a philosopher, among others. The interdisciplinarity and teamwork behind DENDRAL engendered an atmosphere of great excitement—albeit one that was male-dominated. Lederberg later singled out "the fraternity that came out of the DENDRAL effort" as "a high in [his] life experience, matching the gratifications of scientific excitement and . . . recognition."[25]

The excitement translated into a working system. DENDRAL functioned in two steps. First, the system used an algorithm in combination with mass spectrometry data to enumerate all topologically unique configurations of a given set of atoms that also followed the requirements of chemical valence. Second, to narrow this list of all possible configurations down to a list of all plausible configurations, the program then applied rules of thumb—a "knowledge base" of heuristics—to assess the chemical plausibility of each candidate structure.[26] Creating these rules was, in Lederberg's view, akin to "cramm[ing]" the program with chemical information. It was in the identification of such chemical information that Djerassi and his associates made distinctive contributions to the project, serving as "founts of chemical expertise."[27]

DENDRAL's reliance on domain-specific rules—that is, knowledge specific to the field of organic chemistry—heralded a new approach to artificial intelligence. Up to this point, most work in AI involved attempts to computerize and formalize some form of general human intelligence. This was the method pursued by Feigenbaum's doctoral advisor at Carnegie Institute of Technology, Herbert Simon.[28] Implicit in DENDRAL, however, was the view that human intelligence was little more than the domain-specific knowledge on which it rested. Lederberg recalled a revealing conversation with Feigenbaum on this very point—"a conversation when I was pressing Ed about the limitations of DENDRAL as general intelligence: he responded with the illumination that I may paraphrase: 'That's exactly the point! Knowledge, not tricks or metaphysical insight, is what makes the program effective—and that itself is an insight of general import.'"[29] If there was any slogan under which DENDRAL traveled, it was this: knowledge is power.

## Making MYCIN

In the fall of 1966, as Lederberg and his colleagues were working away on DENDRAL, a young student from Connecticut, Edward Shortliffe, moved to Cambridge, Massachusetts, to begin his freshman year at Harvard College. With the guidance of a mentor, Shortliffe discovered the recently founded Laboratory of Computer Science (LCS) at the Harvard-affiliated Massachusetts General Hospital, where he first encountered the fields of medical informatics and biomedical computing.[30] Directed by Octo Barnett, the LCS supported many lines of research at the intersection of computing and medicine: the lab did work on electronic health records, decision support, programming languages, medical education, and medical information systems.[31] At the LCS, Shortliffe became involved with research on a computer-based medical record system and brought, as one of Barnett's doctoral students remembered it, "a high degree of technical skill, and . . . boundless energy and enthusiasm" to one area of the larger research project.[32] This area, which would become the topic of Shortliffe's own honors senior thesis, concerned the implementation of "a structured input interface for composing research retrieval queries that could be run against the database of patients collected in the clinical system."[33]

As his Harvard career came to a close, Shortliffe began looking to the future. Interested in combining a clinical career in medicine with a research career in biomedical informatics, he decided to apply for MD-PhD programs, funded by the National Institutes of Health through its Medical Science Training Program, and commence training for a career as a physician-scientist. On learning of Shortliffe's wish to pursue a joint career at the nexus of medical informatics and clinical medicine, Barnett steered him to Stanford. There, Shortliffe could take advantage of not just its strong programs in computer science and medicine but also its more communal and laissez-faire research culture. "He decided he wanted to go to med school," Barnett later recalled, "and I told him to go to Stanford. At Stanford, he could get much more freedom to do what he wanted to do than [he could at] Harvard at the time."[34]

Shortliffe arrived in Palo Alto in 1970. Having dipped his toe into a career combining computers and medicine while at Harvard, once at Stanford he jumped in with both feet and completed his joint degree in only six years. He spent the first and last two years working toward the MD portion, and he allotted himself an astonishingly brisk two years in the middle to complete his PhD. His actual habits of work, however, did not perfectly obey such demarcations; even fresh into medical school, he was thinking about computer science, artificial intelligence, informatics, and the applications of these fields to medicine. Not long after arriving at Stanford, he set out to master contemporary research in artificial intelligence, enrolling in a course on the Introduction to Artificial Intelligence and joining the Heuristic Programming Project (HPP) laboratory, which had grown directly out of the DENDRAL project and supported research into expert systems.

In these environments, Shortliffe learned much through osmosis—through his proximity to exciting research into expert systems and to great minds like Lederberg and Feigenbaum. But Shortliffe was also, more than most dawning young medical students, the active author of his own educational and research program. Observing that there was no regular journal club at the HPP, Shortliffe established one himself. Initially called "SIGDoc," modeled after the well-known special interest groups (SIGs) of the Association for Computing Machinery, the group successfully brought together researchers at Stanford who were interested in the latest applications of computers to medicine.[35]

It was through SIGDoc that Shortliffe, in 1971, met Bruce Buchanan, who would become his closest collaborator and one of his primary dissertation advisors.[36] "I quickly identified Bruce as an ideal colleague and mentor. He was thoughtful, provocative, experienced, and highly interested in applying DENDRAL-like ideas to a problem with greater clinical emphasis," Shortliffe recollected. "Bruce was my closest advisor throughout this work and I still reflect fondly on the many hours that we spent in his office, working at the blackboard and devising new strategies for computational representation and control in that system."[37]

His other main advisor was the geneticist and clinical pharmacologist Stanley N. Cohen, whom Shortliffe had asked to work with upon his arrival at Stanford. While Cohen would later become famous primarily for his research into bacterial plasmids and his role in developing recombinant DNA methodologies, at the time he was a natural pick to be Shortliffe's primary advisor. In the early 1970s, Cohen was essentially pursuing two distinct research programs: he was doing the basic science research on bacterial plasmids that would make him famous, but he was also busy exploring the applications of computers to clinical pharmacology in his capacity as a pharmacologist.[38] As chief of the Department of Medicine's Division of Clinical Pharmacology, Cohen had been using the ACME to develop a computer-based reporting system that could monitor hospital drug use and alert doctors of possible drug interactions.[39]

With his advising structure in place, Shortliffe began to explore and define the parameters of a possible dissertation project. Given his interest in clinical medicine and his association with DENDRAL and the HPP, the possibility of bringing a DENDRAL-like system to the realm of medicine presented itself as the most natural path forward. Buchanan expounded, "We thought that clinical medicine was ripe for the technology, and Ted believed it and took the ball and ran with it."[40]

Although MYCIN drew on DENDRAL, the two teams approached their respective projects in divergent ways. DENDRAL, conceived by an eminent scientist, was more of a top-down project—moving with respect to the North Star of Lederberg's vision.[41] MYCIN, by contrast, was more of a bottom-up enterprise. To be sure, Shortliffe was brilliant, driven, and resourceful, and he wanted to explore computer applications in medicine. But within this broad domain, he was less prescriptive about the particulars: he was happy to go wherever his research or circumstance took him. As a result, the aims of the project that came to be known as MYCIN shifted over the course of its development.

Shortliffe, Buchanan, and Cohen initially planned to create a program that would evaluate decisions that had already been made at a hospital and flag those that were questionable. The program, in other words, was to help clinical practice review boards retrospectively determine when physicians had erred in their prescribing. As the team began to work on the program, however, they quickly decided that a forward-looking prospective program, one that offered advice about yet-unmade medical decisions, might be more productive, beneficial, and acceptable than the backward-looking retrospective program that they had originally envisioned. Why run around stomping out forest fires when there was an opportunity to prevent them from starting in the first place? Buchanan elaborated on this shift in an interview: "We decided that critiquing was not the right psychological model for a computer program with physicians' actions. But prospective systems to keep people out of trouble might be more acceptable."[42]

Having operationalized the project—having identified a problem domain and an approach to making decisions within that domain—now the team had to bring the program to life.[43] Among the most urgent orders of business was building MYCIN's knowledge base—its collection of rules about the domain of bacterial infections and antibiotic treatment. Such knowledge, however, fell outside the bounds of Shortliffe or Buchanan's area of expertise. "An important aspect of this work," a 1973 MYCIN report pointed out, "is its strong interdisciplinary nature—success in this project depends in part upon the integration of medical knowledge into a computation framework. This requires the participation of professionals with differing expertise, followed by the close coordination of the people from the various departments working with it."[44] If Shortliffe and his colleagues in the Department of Computer Science were going to get MYCIN to work, they were going to have to build connections with others at the School of Medicine, particularly those within the Division of Infectious Disease.

Luckily, Cohen already enjoyed personal and professional connections to Stanford's medical faculty. Exploiting this network, Cohen corralled Thomas Merigan, chief of the Division of Infectious Disease, and Stanton Axline, a physician in that division, into joining the project. (It was Axline who, in 1973, suggested that the system be named MYCIN, a gesture to the suffix attached to many antibiotics like streptomycin, tobramycin, gentamicin, and so forth.)[45] By March 1972, a semiformal, interdisciplinary group of researchers had coalesced around the MYCIN project. The group met on roughly a weekly basis to discuss all aspects of the MYCIN system, from the nature of decision-making in the context of antibiotic therapy, to more technical aspects of the system's programming and operation. Present at the initial meetings were Shortliffe, Buchanan, Cohen, Axline, Merigan, and the clinical pharmacologist Gil Hunn. Cordell Green—a computer science professor who taught the course at Stanford from which Shortliffe had learned LISP programming (CS 206: Symbolic Expressions)—also joined the meetings at a later time.[46]

An early plan for the antibiotic therapy program was for it to build directly upon existing computer-based operations at the School of Medicine. Perhaps, the group speculated, the program could simply extend the clinical pharmacology program that had already been developed by Cohen. Using organism and resistance pattern information obtained from the clinical microbiology laboratory, the MYCIN group wondered if Cohen's pharmacology program could be made to advise physicians on the appropriateness of antimicrobial therapy in addition to warning them about drug interactions. The team, however, soon came to appreciate that decision-making with respect to antibiotic therapy required far more than data from the clinical microbiology laboratory alone. As Shortliffe related in a 1972 memo and progress report, "It quickly became apparent . . . that the decision model used by an expert on antimicrobial therapy before he recommends treatment is highly complex and requires answers to questions only a few of which can be answered by the clinical microbiology lab culture and resistance pattern data."[47]

What, then, did antimicrobial therapy selection involve? This question fell to the group's infectious disease experts, chiefly Stanton Axline. In February 1972, Cohen sent a memo to Merigan and Axline on the subject of their "proposed computer project involving antibiotics therapy."[48] The memo summarized the early plans for MYCIN and outlined the role Merigan and Axline, as sources of human expertise, would play in the system's creation. The two infectious disease specialists would, the memo noted, play a central role in defining and identifying the kinds of knowledge that physicians use when identifying and treating infections: "It was agreed that Tom [Merigan] and Stan (Axline) would compile a list of major clinical factors to be considered in preparing the initial program for acquisition of the data base [*sic*] (i.e. the major branch point in the decision making process re: prescribing a specific antibiotic for a given situation)."[49] Within a few weeks, Axline responded to this charge. In a letter to the members of the original MYCIN group, Axline enclosed "a preliminary list of major clinical factors used in the decision-making process for antibiotic therapy of bacteremia."[50] He enumerated the principal clinical factors that physicians draw upon in making their decision—factors that came not only from the bacteriology laboratory (e.g., Gram stain result, recent cultures, antibiotic sensitivity) but also the pharmacy (e.g., drugs being taken at the time of culture collection), the patient's chart (e.g., age, recent operative procedures, the presence of catheters in place in any cavity), the patient's clinical status (e.g., temperature), and the patient's labs (e.g., hepatic and renal function).

Through the spring of 1972, the MYCIN team explored other existing systems off of which they might model MYCIN. Shortliffe and Buchanan met once or twice each week to study one such program—SCHOLAR, which had been developed by the electrical engineer Jamie Carbonell at MIT.[51] A tutoring program, SCHOLAR used semantic networks derived from AI research to help represent knowledge about South American geography in a way that was conducive to computer-aided instruction.[52] After working with SCHOLAR for a few months, however, Shortliffe and Buchanan threw in the towel: they concluded that "the SCHOLAR approach was inappropriate for the kind of problem area with which [they] were concerned."[53] The heart of the problem was the sharp difference between the world of medicine and the world of geography. They found the domain of infectious disease to be too ill-defined and ill-structured for representation by semantic network; infectious disease did not enjoy the same clear boundaries, borders, and demarcations that were characteristic of SCHOLAR's domain of South American geography.[54] By June the team had arrived at a different strategy. They garnered "an improved picture of the problems inherent in our task and decided that a modified theorem-proving approach based upon situation-action rules and multiple goals was the best way for us to proceed."[55]

MYCIN thus emerged as a "rule-based" expert system. This meant that MYCIN's knowledge base consisted of rules, hundreds of IF-THEN, premise-clause statements about the diagnosis and treatment of bacterial infections. Consider rule 047:

> IF: 1) The site of the culture is blood, and
> 2) The identity of the organism is not known with certainty, and
> 3) The stain of the organism is gramneg [gram negative], and
> 4) The morphology of the organism is rod, and
> 5) The patient has been seriously burned
>
> THEN: There is weakly suggestive evidence (.4) that the identity of the organism is pseudomonas.[56]

MYCIN used its collection of rules like this to reason through medical cases using a process called "backward chaining." In forward chaining, computerized systems start with the set of facts about a case, only later bringing the relevant rules to bear on these facts. Backward chaining goes in reverse: instead of starting with the facts at hand, the system begins with a goal—a piece of information to find out, a diagnosis to make, or some other end point—and then invokes the rules that can help the system reach that goal. For example, MYCIN may proceed with the hypothesis, or "goal," that the "identity of the organism is pseudomonas." The system would identify the rules that assist in making this conclusion. Each of these rules, such as rule 047 above, would have a series of premises (e.g., "the morphology of the organism is rod") that need confirmation and that other rules may address. The system thus proceeds backward, reaching back to these other rules, or reaching out to the physician, in order to establish the goal. MYCIN essentially worked through various hypotheses or goals in this fashion until it reached its conclusions about the case.

The initial batch of MYCIN rules came from the team's pharmacologists and infectious disease specialists, predominantly Axline and Cohen.[57] The team presented Axline and Cohen with actual patient infections as represented in patient charts. Before the team's computer scientists, Axline and Cohen performed their diagnostic and therapeutic reasoning with respect to these real cases, attempting to explicate their process of decision-making and distill their knowledge into discrete rules. "We reviewed several patient records," Shortliffe noted in 1972, "and began to examine what kinds of rules the experts in our group were using in an attempt to reach a therapeutic decision."[58] He elaborated on this process of rule extraction and creation during the 1975 Rutgers AIM workshop:

> All the rules we have in our system have been acquired at weekly meetings in which Dr. Axline and Dr. Cohen, two clinicians most closely associated with our project, took patient charts and with the end of those charts still unknown to them, began to review them. Those of us unfamiliar with the clinical aspects of what was being discussed would listen and try to pick out the underlying threads of reasoning. We would then code these into rules and use them to run patients' charts.[59]

Once formulated, the rules were shopped back to the medical experts, who judged the extent to which these preliminary rules were understandable and persuasive.

The development of MYCIN depended on the assumption that medical knowledge was communicable—that it could be extracted from medical experts, crystallized into discrete packets of information, and programmed into a computer system (Figure 5.1). Medical knowledge concerning antibiotic therapy was presumed to be explainable for the infectious disease specialists and comprehensible for the computer scientists. Certain social properties of the MYCIN project during these early stages facilitated the program's development. The MYCIN team was fairly intimate and small: every member knew every other member, and they all met regularly to touch base, trade ideas, and update the system.[60] Second, at the early stages of development, the MYCIN system itself, like the team that created it, was also pretty "small." By October 1972, MYCIN contained just seventy rules.[61] Thanks to the group's intimacy and the system's workability, a tight feedback loop formed between those who explicated the rules and those who encoded and tested them. The social characteristics would change as the project grew and matured.

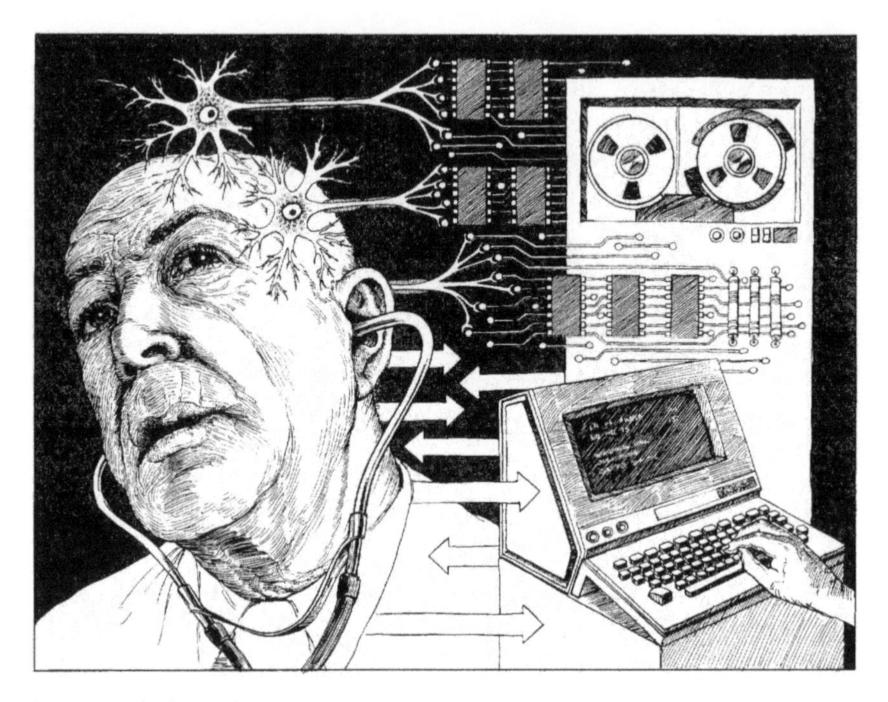

*Figure 5.1.* The logic of expert systems was one of knowledge extraction and transfer. Gregory Freiherr, "The Problems and Promises of Artificial Intelligence," *Research Resources Reporter* 3, no. 9 (1979): 1–6.

## Reasoning under Uncertainty

Medicine is an uncertain business. Doctors must make medical decisions with limited knowledge and imperfect data, and they must make these decisions with respect to individual patients who sometimes respond to equivalent treatments in surprising, divergent, and unpredictable ways. That a given therapy works in 95 percent of patients is no guarantee that it will work in the next patient. As the sociologist Renée Fox has noted, a central part of becoming a doctor is learning to live and cope with the limits of medical knowledge, the vagaries of individual patients, and one's own personal experiences of puzzlement, doubt, and ambiguity; training to become a doctor is often a matter of "training for uncertainty."[62] As they did medical trainees, the problems of uncertainty in medicine also plagued the MYCIN team. Few aspects of developing MYCIN consumed as much thought and energy as the question of how to formalize such uncertainty—how to convey, represent, and determine the strength of belief about a medical rule or proposition that is not definitively known.

Bayes's theorem offered one way forward. By the 1960s, many research teams had embraced Bayesian approaches to the task of computerizing diagnosis. The HEME project adopted such an approach, as did Shortliffe's own undergraduate mentor. In 1967, Octo Barnett, together with Anthony Gorry, developed an adapted Bayesian model of diagnosis for computer implementation.[63] Barnett and Gorry's diagnostic model developed upon the more prominent Bayesian system that had come out of the University of Utah a few years earlier (see chapter 3).[64] For all their promise, these Bayesian models employed certain simplifying assumptions that rarely held in the context of clinical medicine.

More problematic than the assumptions required for a functional Bayesian diagnostic system were its data requirements. For a Bayesian system to produce accurate results, it required large amounts of data—data that allow for the computation of the conditional probabilities on which the theorem rests. The data didn't just have to be big; they also had to be good: they had to reflect the true statistical properties of the disease in question. Homer Warner and his colleagues in Utah possessed such a dataset, with high-quality information on hundreds of patients with congenital heart defects. But Shortliffe—and countless other physicians—were not so fortunate: these clinicians were working in realms of medicine where clinical judgment, not hard data, was king. Shortliffe and his colleagues were thus presented with a conundrum: how, exactly, to formalize medical reasoning when that reasoning is itself inexact? As the problem of poor-quality data was ubiquitous in medicine, Shortliffe hoped that an alternative to the Bayesian approach might have wide appeal: "Although conditional probability provides useful results in areas of medical decision making such as those I have mentioned, vast portions of medical knowledge suffer from so little data and so much imperfect knowledge that a rigorous probabilistic analysis, the ideal standard by which to judge the rationality of a physician's decisions, is not possible."[65]

These weren't just different approaches to the computerization of diagnosis; they were also scaffolds upon which the groups constructed different professional identities. Members of Warner's group at the University of Utah viewed the efforts at Stanford as overly academic, theoretical, detached.[66] The Utah team thus fashioned themselves as Stanford's foil: pragmatic, data-driven, applied. Warner later reflected on this dynamic in an interview: "I'd always been sort of a critic of artificial intelligence, and the whole notion of it. I think it's far-fetched. . . . I think Ted's [Shortliffe] done some good things, even though they're more on the theoretical level, and we've been over on the practical end."[67]

In 1975, Shortliffe and Buchanan first described their solution to the problem of uncertainty in the landmark paper, "A Model of Inexact Reasoning in Medicine."[68] The uncertainty framework that they proposed and implemented rested on the concept of the certainty factor (CF). The certainty factor—a value that ranged from −1 to +1—reflected the change in belief in a hypothesis given certain evidence. Compared to Bayesian analysis and conditional probabilities, the CF concept, Shortliffe and Buchanan believed, was more intuitively accessible to physicians, who often had difficulties accurately estimating probabilities in the way a Bayesian system would require but who were quite comfortable expressing general "degrees of belief" about their medical conclusions. CFs, the team argued, captured and operationalized these degrees of belief. Put another way, the CF model more closely approximated how doctors actually thought.

Shortliffe and Buchanan were—despite how Warner may have framed it—pragmatic: they would not let the perfect be the enemy of the good. Their primary aim was producing a model that would work. When, in 1975, an MIT graduate student wrote to Shortliffe criticizing aspects of the CF model, Shortliffe defended his model not as an unassailable finished product but as a practical step in the right direction: "I guess you know that our own reaction to the CF model is based upon pragmatics and the need to have something that seems to work and to be at least mildly defensible within the domain for which it is designed."[69] Shortliffe and his colleagues, having found themselves navigating a terra incognita, improvised their way forward. Shortliffe continued, "We were left to follow our instincts with the goal of getting together a version of MYCIN that would work acceptably well. If another model is proposed that improves upon problems inherent in the CF approach, we would switch over in a minute. We have no vested interest in the CF's per se; we just don't see any real alternatives around."[70]

Their focus on the system's function did not mean the team was uninterested in its form. Even as the MYCIN team strove to create a system that worked, they also emphasized certain qualities of *how* MYCIN worked. MYCIN, they suggested, approximated—and gave a quantitative shape to—the "artistic" and "inexact" forms of reasoning used in medicine. A key contribution of MYCIN, the group argued, was to capture, formalize, and computerize this mode of reasoning that heretofore had seemed to defy quantitative analysis. They explained, "The purpose of this paper is to examine the nature of such non-probabilistic and unformalized reasoning processes and to propose a model by means of which such incomplete 'artistic' knowledge might be quantified."[71]

MYCIN therefore was developed to "reflect" (at least roughly) how experts reason with medical knowledge: "We look for ways to handle decision rules as discrete packets of knowledge and for a quantification scheme that permits accumulation of evidence in a manner that adequately reflects the reasoning process of an expert using the same or similar rules."[72] MYCIN aimed to convert the physician's artistic reasoning process into a quantified and programmable form.

## Technologies of Persuasion

Claims about the proximity of computerized reasoning to human reasoning often shaded into claims about trust, transparency, and communicability. Models of reasoning that approximated modes of human reasoning, many argued, could be better understood by, and communicated to, human users. The problem of how to create a computer system that physicians could understand and trust was one that consumed the MYCIN team. It was a question that led the team to hypothesize about the physician's nature and identity. And ultimately it was a question to which they proposed a technological answer. As part of the MYCIN system, Shortliffe and his group built communication technologies—technologies of persuasion—that served as a window for physicians into the opaque reasoning process of a novel machine.[73]

Designers of MYCIN and other computerized systems recognized the importance that machines be able to communicate, at least roughly, the steps by which they reached a given medical decision or diagnosis. The tight connection between the perceptibility and the credibility of an expert system's reasoning processes emerged as a theme of the 1975 Rutgers workshop. There, the Rutgers computer scientist Natesa S. Sridharan argued that a computer-generated diagnosis, even if accurate, is meaningless absent a mechanism by which to convey the logical processes underlying the diagnosis: "It is not enough for the system to produce right answers," Sridharan declared. "It has to be able to give reasons for those answers, in some sense explain its own processes. It has to be credible."[74] Many other participants agreed.[75]

To achieve this goal of transparent reasoning, designers of different decision support systems created technologies that adhered to a variety of strategies. What these technologies and strategies looked like depended in no small part on whether a given decision support system was built to supplement, imitate, or circumvent human diagnostic reasoning. Some systems sought to recreate the reasoning practices exhibited by physicians generally, and sometimes even the more particular forms of reasoning exercised by specific practitioners. INTERNIST-I, for example, aimed to incorporate the medical expertise and imitate the logical processes of a single physician, Jack D. Myers (see chapter 4). Other systems sought to anchor diagnostic logic in something more fundamental, and less mercurial, than human medical practices: causal, pathophysiological models of disease. A notable exemplar of this approach, Rutgers University's CASNET program, built its diagnostic logic around foundational knowledge about "the pathogenesis and mechanisms" of optic nerve diseases, represented "in terms of cause and effect relationships between pathophysiological states."[76]

The makers of MYCIN occasionally emphasized that their program was more ends-oriented than means-oriented. As Shortliffe said of the MYCIN program, "We are not necessarily trying to make the program perform the way a clinician does."[77] Rather, he continued, "We want the program to derive the right advice and whatever way we can come up with to do that is all right." Yet, even if the MYCIN team was not set on creating a system that replicated *exactly* human forms of medical reasoning, they remained intensely invested in the parallels between MYCIN's reasoning processes and those of physicians. The team believed that the similarities between MYCIN and human forms of reasoning would make their system more understandable and trustworthy to physicians. MYCIN's rule-based approach, with medical knowledge encoded into discrete information packets that took the form of production rules, promised "a straightforward mechanism for explaining decisions."[78]

As deeply as the principle of intelligibility was built into MYCIN's architecture, designers still believed that, in order to make the computer system convincing, it required a manner by which to accessibly explain its decisions. Even when first envisaging MYCIN through the early 1970s, Shortliffe appreciated that diagnostic accuracy alone would not be enough to secure acceptance among medical practitioners—that "other issues such as mode of interaction, transparency of the 'reasoning' behind a system's advice, and integration of a system into the physician's daily routine also seemed to be crucial determinants of acceptance."[79]

Of these "other issues" feeding into the system's clinical viability, Shortliffe and his collaborators quickly found themselves "particularly interested in explanation and . . . drawn to the techniques of artificial intelligence as potential methods for developing consultation programs that could justify their advice."[80] The clarity of discrete medical rules did not go far enough. Though Shortliffe discovered that MYCIN's production rules, "if translated into English, could provide explanations that were usually understandable," the mere "regurgitation of rules," he concluded, "is not always satisfactory."[81] The manner in which these rules were presented mattered as far as the system's intelligibility and credibility were concerned. This problem of explanation, the MYCIN team believed, had a technological solution in the "techniques of artificial intelligence."

The Stanford team was thus motivated to develop an explanation technology for the larger MYCIN system. This explanation technology came to be known as Subprogram 2.[82] The creators of MYCIN designed the system's explanation function such that physicians could tap these capabilities at two different points, either during the consultation session or after advice was given.[83] To examine MYCIN's reasoning chain during a consultation, physicians had a set of commands at their disposal, primarily intended to help them understand what the program was after in asking particular questions throughout the consultation.[84] By typing, for example, "WHY" into the MYCIN system, physicians could elicit an explanation of a particular question's "purpose"—that is, the question's relationship to the subgoal that MYCIN was trying to reach.

Understanding the purpose of a given question, however, did not guarantee full clarity: even if physicians grasped how a question served MYCIN in working toward a particular subgoal, they may not fully comprehend the program's reason for seeking that particular subgoal in the first place. To further inquire about the underlying subgoals, and their connection to the system's main goal, physicians could type "WHY" into the system a second (or third or fourth etc.) time (Figure 5.2). Physicians could also trigger explanations from MYCIN by using the HOW command. Unlike the WHY command, which elucidated MYCIN's active reasoning chain, the HOW command allowed users to explore other possible reasoning chains—to investigate, for instance, the different ways a given subgoal could hypothetically be achieved.

Even with explanatory support throughout the consultation phase, physicians might still be mystified by the system's eventual medical recommendation. Often MYCIN reached conclusions without having solicited any information from the physician, something that could happen, the MYCIN team explained, "either because the preconditions of a rule were satisfied by deductions from previous information (using other decision rules) or because the needed data had already been requested in the context of a different rule."[85] As a result, if physicians understood the meaning and purpose of each question in isolation, by no means did this assure that they would understand the system's final recommendation. The explanation capabilities initiated after the conclusion of the consultation session addressed this concern. MYCIN's post-

```
        .
        .  [preceded by the first 14 questions in the consultation]
        .
15) Is the patient's illness with ORGANISM-1 a hospital-acquired infection?
** WHY
[i.e. WHY is it important to determine whether or not the infection with
      ORGANISM-1 was acquired while the patient was hospitalized?]
[1.0] This will aid in determining the category of ORGANISM-1.
      It has already been established that
          [1.1] the gram stain of ORGANISM-1 is gramneg, and
          [1.2] the morphology of ORGANISM-1 is rod, and
          [1.3] the aerobicity of ORGANISM-1 is facultative
      Therefore, if
          [1.4] the infection with ORGANISM-1 was not acquired while the
                patient was hospitalized
      then
          there is strongly suggestive evidence (.8) that the category of
                ORGANISM-1 is enterobacteriaceae
      ALSO: there is weakly suggestive evidence (.1) that the identity of
                ORGANISM-1 is pseudomonas-aeruginosa]
      [RULE037]
** WHY
[i.e. WHY is it important to determine the category of ORGANISM-1?]
[2.0]... in order to determine the identity of ORGANISM-1.
      It has already been established that
          [2.1] this blood culture was taken from a sterile source
      Therefore, if
          [2.2] this current organism and at least one of the list of members
                associated with the category of the organism agree with
                respect to the following properties: air conformation
      then
          There is strongly suggestive evidence (.9) that each of them is the
                identity of ORGANISM-1
      [RULE003]
** HOW 1.3
[i.e. HOW was it established that the aerobicity of ORGANISM-1 is
      facultative?]
The following were used:
[3.1] RULE027 ndicated there is strongly suggestive evidence (.8) that the
      aerobicity of ORGANISM-1 is facultative
[3.2] RULE027 indicated there is weakly suggestive evidence (.2) that the
      aerobicity of ORGANISM-1 is anaerobic
Since this gave a cumulative CF of (.8) for facultative, and (.2) for
      anaerobic, it has been established that the aerobicity of ORGANISM-1
      is facultative
** HOW 1.1
[i.e. HOW was it established that the gram stain of ORGANISM-1 is gramneg?]
You said so [question 11].
```

*Figure 5.2.* A sample partial consultation with MYCIN. A. Carlisle Scott, William J. Clancey, Randall Davis, and Edward H. Shortliffe, "Explanation Capabilities of Production-Based Consultation Systems," Memo HPP-77-1 of the Stanford Heuristic Programming Project, and Report No. STAN-CS-77-593, February 1977, 14. Courtesy of Edward Feigenbaum papers (SC0340), Department of Special Collections and University Archives, Stanford University Libraries, Stanford, California.

consultation explanation capability took the form of a question-answering session, during which the physician could pose queries about a range of topics, including the current line of reasoning, MYCIN's production rules more generally, MYCIN's reasons for asking a previous question, or the accuracy of the physician's own knowledge (e.g., "Is chloramphenicol okay for *Salmonella* infections?").[86]

Designers and users of decision support systems commonly assumed that rule-based systems like MYCIN held a categorical advantage over purely statistical methods in the area of intelligibility. Simple rules were accessible to even the most arithmophobic of doctors. The Swedish linguist Hans Karlgren articulated this view, writing in reference to MYCIN, "The rule approach has its limitations but provides an impressive explanation capability."[87] Those who worked directly on rule-based approaches to computerized decision support in medicine similarly commented on the intrinsic intelligibility of this approach, especially when contrasted with earlier, statistical approaches. The CASNET team, for example, underscored the conceptual distinction between their rule-based diagnostic methods and alternative statistical methods, writing, "AI techniques attempt to capture decision making rules explicitly, while statistical methods may extract them implicitly from accumulated sample experience."[88] The former approach, involving "a more structured representation of the diagnostics and therapy selection problems," was far better suited to clear and effective explanation—these systems, the team reasoned, "are more likely to be accepted because they are expressed in a decision-making context familiar to the clinician."[89]

Despite its advantages, MYCIN's explanation capabilities were not without limitations, nor did these capabilities come without certain costs. Chief among such costs involved the fundamental trade-off between intelligibility and efficiency: improvements in the system's explanation competencies often came at the expense of its efficiency and speed. Shortliffe broached this dilemma in a paper delivered at the 1977 Annual Meeting of the Society for Computer Medicine: "The efficiency advantages of approaches relying more heavily on statistical theory must be weighed against the importance of the natural mechanism for explanation and knowledge modification that may be achieved through MYCIN's representation of knowledge in the form of production rules."[90] Achieving the appropriate balance between these competing values proved evasive, as intelligibility and efficiency, though clashing aims, both promoted the computer system's credibility in separate yet essential ways. The question of whether to pursue a system that was more accurate or more intelligible had no technological solution; this question occupied the realm of values and morals.

## Of Maintenance and Modularity

The Stanford team encountered several challenges as they worked to develop MYCIN's explanation capability. Some of these barriers were technical, such as the nascent state of natural language processing, the subfield of computer science concerned with the production and comprehension of natural human language. But the larger barriers were epistemological: they came from the nature of medical knowledge itself. MYCIN and its explanation technology rested on an understanding of medical knowledge as static and modular. Very quickly, however, the MYCIN group discovered that medical knowledge was more dynamic and interconnected than they had originally made out.

In Lewis Carroll's *Through the Looking-Glass*, the young Alice, a visitor to Looking-Glass Land, notices something odd while running. No matter how quickly she moved her feet, she realized that she wasn't moving with respect to the things around her. Perplexed, she bemoans to the Red Queen, "Well, in our country . . . you'd generally get to somewhere else—if you run very fast for a long time, as we've been doing."[91] The Red Queen interjects, explaining that the laws governing Looking-Glass Land were different from those governing Alice's country: "Now, *here*, you see, it takes all the running you can do, to keep in the same place."[92] Because everything in Looking-Glass Land was in a perpetual state of motion, one needed to continually move just to stay put.

Developers of computerized diagnostic systems like Shortliffe and his colleagues discovered that the world of medicine shared much in common with Looking-Glass Land. The MYCIN team was not working in a domain where knowledge, information, and data were frozen or fixed in time; knowledge about antibiotic prescribing, and about medicine in general, was growing and shifting in real time. Even after versions of MYCIN had been put forward, the system had to account for the fact that its knowledge base—that very thing that gave the system its power—was in a state of ongoing evolution and revision. The team was perpetually looking for ways to add new rules and tweak or improve the formulation of existing rules. To create the system and then step away would be to let the system fall into obsolescence—to let it fail.

Development of MYCIN was therefore less a singular act of invention than a continual process of maintenance. Historians of technology have long focused on innovation—on great individuals and their fleeting acts of creation and genius. But a recent turn within the historiography has shifted attention to the centrality of maintenance.[93] New technologies do not come into being through one-off strokes of genius but through the unglamorous work of tweaking, updating, cleaning, adapting, improving, editing, debugging—over and over again. Getting technologies built, and subsequently getting them to work, often falls at the feet not of "inventors" but of "maintainers."[94]

MYCIN bears these conclusions out. The system's knowledge base was under a constant state of construction. In 1973, the MYCIN team compared the growth and education of MYCIN to that of a medical trainee. Far from "complete," MYCIN was still in the process of acquiring medical knowledge and learning from its mistakes: "The program is currently at a stage roughly analogous to that of a medical student who, having completed his coursework, enters the clinic and encounters real and challenging cases. Like the student, the program will only gain a high level of broad competence by an extended period of being advised of its shortcomings and corrected in its errors."[95] A relatively young system, MYCIN still had much to learn. By exposing MYCIN to patient cases in controlled environments, the team believed the gaps in the system's knowledge base could be identified and addressed.

The need to maintain and update the system was not only a consequence of MYCIN's relative "youth" and "inexperience." It was also a side effect of the nature of the knowledge domain itself. Even if the team believed that MYCIN reached the level of an attending doctor, the work of maintenance would not be finished. Just as attendings must remain "up to date," incorporating new knowledge and evidence into their patterns of care, MYCIN too would have to incorporate new information about antibiotic therapy—new bugs, new drugs, new toxicities, new patterns of susceptibility. "Neither the CF model nor MYCIN," Shortliffe wrote in 1975, "is static."[96]

Beyond having to attend to MYCIN's knowledge base, the team also had to update and revise the system's code. The work of "debugging" accounted for a significant chunk of the group's time. Members of the team recalled "very bad debugging experiences"—experiences of "wading through code" in search of underlying causes of the system's problems.[97] The team reiterated these sentiments in a 1973 research proposal: "Vast amounts of work have been required for the derivation, encoding, and debugging of the knowledge bases."[98] Because code maintenance could easily burn through large amounts of time, the team created features that aimed to speed up the debugging process.[99]

Many believed that MYCIN's fundamental architecture was conducive to revision and change. With MYCIN being a collection of discrete IF-THEN rules, new rules could be easily added to the soup, and old, bad rules easily removed. Medical knowledge, in other words, was seen to be modular, consisting of individual building blocks that together amounted to the vast edifice of medical knowledge. The modularity of rules, some reasoned, meant that MYCIN's knowledge base could be easily understood, explained, and vetted—its errors and biases easily rooted out. The proposed introduction to a 1988 conference on the topic of "expert system knowledge transfer" adopted this view of rule-based expert systems like MYCIN: "The clinical expertise and interpretive rules in the knowledge base can be reviewed, modified and expanded independently by clinicians who are not required to have programming capabilities. Any biases, judgments, or logical errors remain exposed for scrutiny and discussion by the clinical, and not only by the programming community. This approach also allows the breadth and power of the system to be improved by adding to and modifying the knowledge base in a modular fashion."[100]

Early papers from the MYCIN group similarly listed "ease of modification" as a key advantage of the rule-based approach over different statistical approaches: "Since the rules are not explicitly related to one another and there need be no pre-structured decision tree for such a system, rule modifications and the addition of new rules need not require complex considerations regarding interactions with the remainder of the system's knowledge."[101]

This was the hope, at least. In reality things were more complex. Adding new rules to MYCIN's knowledge base sometimes produced unpredictable changes to the system's operation. This point was raised by the infectious disease fellow Robert Blum during a presentation at a MYCIN team meeting in September 1977. Blum's stance was summarized in the meeting minutes as "criticiz[ing] rule-based systems on the basis of lack of modularity." The notes include such details as "The chunks are not independent, statistically or otherwise. Pointed to problem associated with entry of new rules, i.e., that experts must be familiar with the entire corpus of rules to be able to enter 'independent' new ones."[102]

Challenges that the team encountered in building and refining MYCIN supported Blum's critique of modularity. The computer scientist William Clancey, for example, documented what he called the "rippling of CF's within the body of rules."[103] Such findings surprised Clancey, as they contradicted the conception of medical knowledge suggested by a rule's very look and feel. As he declared in a March 1976 memo, "For too long I have assumed that because a rule looks like a discrete object it is necessarily modular."[104] The rule-based expert system and a modular understanding of medical knowledge were mutually constitutive. The system arose out of ideas about the modularity of medical knowledge—ideas that the system in turn reinforced through its development and operation.

Shortliffe was sympathetic to these sentiments. On reading the draft introduction of the proposed 1988 conference on "expert system knowledge transfer," Shortliffe expressed surprise over the lack of critical discussion around modularity. He wrote to the conference organizers, "The nitty gritty syntactic details will only be worth pursuing if we have a common view of the big picture. I might mention, for example, that some of my students recently wrote a paper entitled 'the myth of modularity' which strikes at the very heart of the presumptions that knowledge can be created and stored in separable packets."[105] While Shortliffe did not disregard claims of nonmodularity, the view struck him as "too extreme."[106] Even if rules might occasionally interact in surprising ways, he felt that the modularity of rules could be defended—if only on a pragmatic basis. As Shortliffe wrote to his colleagues in 1976, "I still tend to believe that the claims of rule modularity can be defended although there are clearly examples of rules that are poor precisely because they do not conform to this requirement."[107]

The original MYCIN knowledge base concerned the infectious disease domain of bacteremia—bacterial infections of the blood. Soon, other members of the team—principally the infectious disease fellow Victor Yu—began developing a knowledge base that would allow MYCIN to operate in the area of acute meningitis (inflammation of the membrane around the brain and spinal cord). As MYCIN's knowledge base evolved, so too did the social dynamics of its creators. By the late 1970s, countless individuals had taken part in MYCIN's development, writing new rules, tweaking old rules, and debugging the code underlying all rules, new and old. Whereas one group of people was involved in developing MYCIN's bacteremia knowledge base, another group—headed by Yu—was involved in creating the meningitis knowledge base.

The methods and assumptions behind the bacteremia and meningitis rules were not always aligned. Yu, for example, wanted to use smaller gradations between different certainty factor values for the meningitis rule set. The decision sparked controversy among the MYCIN group. Some questioned whether such precise gradations carried any real clinical meaning. Could a physician truly defend that a given statement was known with a 0.45, as opposed to a 0.40, level of certainty? "What remains disturbing is the certainty factor model itself," protested Clancey. "Here we have no sure intuition about the performance meaning of .05 as opposed to .1, yet we are assigning them as if they were significantly different from one another."[108]

Particularly contentious was the way in which Yu used certainty factor values below the 0.2 cutoff. Below the 0.2 value, evidence was deemed to be "not known." Clancey worried that making CF assignments at these lower ranges might result in peculiar and nonsensical outcomes, with CF values in the "not known" range interacting to produce a "known" and actionable finding or observation. “I do not at all understand,” Clancey explained, “how a rule can be written which can at once stand on its own, and yet NOT be significant truth (i.e., believable observation, tangible conclusion).”[109]

For all of the debate around Yu’s approach, the meningitis rules seemed to outperform the original bacteremia knowledge base in at least one important respect: the meningitis rule set seemed to respond more favorably and predictably to subsequent additions and edits. The team summarized this finding in the minutes of a meeting on June 17, 1976:

> Meningitis appears to be more stable. Victor has run 60 patients through getting the correct answer for all of them. When a new patient was tried and the system did not get the right answer, Victor added new rules to make the patient run correctly—these additions were NOT detrimental to the system’s performance on the other patients that already worked. In contrast, the 21 evaluation and pre-evaluation patients uncovered a number of bugs in the bacteremia rules. When rules were added or changed to fix those patients on which the system did not perform well, other patients that had worked previously now got the wrong answer.[110]

Many of the challenges encountered during MYCIN’s development stemmed from the patchwork nature of its creation. Shortliffe described this phenomenon in a message to his colleagues: “I feel that comparisons of bacteremia and meningitis are suffering somewhat from the simple fact that no one has ever sat down to try to make the entire bacteremia rule base consistent and coherent—those rules have developed over several years through an evolutionary process involving several rule authors.”[111] The bacteremia and meningitis knowledge bases differed, in other words, because of the *social* circumstances surrounding their creation. The meningitis rule set was more amenable to revision because it was created by a small group of people in a relatively short period of time. Its makers had more of a global, synthetic understanding of the rule set and how it might respond to tweaks and edits. The bacteremia rule set, by contrast, came into being over a period of multiple years—the product of countless authors and revisions. Shortliffe continued, “Things could almost certainly be cleaned up if a single knowledgeable person devoted some time to revising the entire rule set. Meningitis, on the other hand, has been developed during a rather coherent short-term process during which the system itself has not undergone very many major changes.”[112]

Subprogram 2 was a technology developed to make MYCIN intelligible to its users. Yet threats to the system’s intelligibility loomed large. Some of these threats arose internally—from within the MYCIN project, its social organization, and the nature of its knowledge domain. One of these was epistemological: the realization that medical knowledge may not exist as modular packets. Another was social: the collaborative, ongoing, and socially distributed character of MYCIN's creation and coding. As the project matured, external limitations to MYCIN's explanation capabilities would emerge as well.

# "Hidden in the Code"

In a 1973 essay, the editor of the *New England Journal of Medicine*, Franz J. Ingelfinger, drew a provocative analogy. He compared physicians following clinical "algorithms" to children following the dice-roll and prescribed path in an imagined board game called "Triple-S." Guidelines, Ingelfinger suggested, stripped away from medicine all that gave the physician's work meaning and value: "If understanding is unimportant, judgment is prohibited, what need is there for some knowledge of biochemistry, physiology, pharmacology, diagnostic interpretation or therapeutic rationale? What need is there, moreover, for an MD diploma, or even a college degree? High-school students can play 'Triple-S'; they can also use clinical algorithms provided they have learned such skills as recognizing an abnormal eardrum."[1] For Ingelfinger, algorithms, like those underlying computerized decision support systems, and a physician's very identity were virtually incompatible; if one must stay, the other must go.

The development of MYCIN—and its offspring ONCOCIN, an oncology protocol management system—generated ideas about the role of the computer in shaping, reconfiguring, or reinscribing the physician's identity. This chapter follows the evolution of MYCIN through the 1970s and 1980s. It demonstrates how concerns about transparency and trust were entangled with ideas about the physician's identity and authority.[2] MYCIN's explanation capability was developed with ideas about the physician as a capable and autonomous actor who possessed a "self-sufficient, active, controlling personality." Yet in practice MYCIN often rendered physicians more as passive "users"—"ordinary folks" (to use the language of one team member) who received "the

Word" passed down from the MYCIN "priests" above. The team had difficulty squaring respect for the physician's authority on the one hand with arguments about their system's urgent clinical need on the other. Finally, the chapter shows how MYCIN's technological solution to the challenges of explainability fell short: they could not eliminate professional, moral, epistemological, and legal qualms about ceding medical decisions to a machine, nor did they adequately address the social and personal dimensions of medical decision-making.

## Authority and Identity

MYCIN's explanation capability was about more than transparency and trust. It was also about authority. If Subprogram 2 was a technology of persuasion, its arguments were twofold: first, that the system's decisions were correct and trustworthy, and second, that it presented no real threat to the physician's identity and authority. By opening up MYCIN's reasoning process to scrutiny, Shortliffe and his colleagues were affirming the physician's role as the ultimate decision-maker. To lay bare the computer's reasoning before the physician was as performative an act as it was a practical one. It communicated to physicians that, for all the complex medical decisions that the computer made, it was up to them to decide whether any given decision would stand.

In publications and user manuals, the MYCIN team frequently hinted at this connection between explanation and authority. Advice that could be understood, they often noted, was advice that could be reviewed and, ultimately, rejected. A 1976 version of the MYCIN User's Manual, for example, noted that the explanation feature not only "permit[ted] the program to justify its conclusions" but also "allow[ed] the user to reject the advice if he feels that some step in the reasoning process has been unsound."[3] Subprogram 2 was thus a way of "clarify[ing] and emphasiz[ing] the physician's role as the ultimate decision maker in patient management" and of "acknowledg[ing] that the users are ultimately making the decision and are using the computer program as an adjunct."[4] Once Shortliffe joined Stanford's faculty, some of his students carried forward this line of thinking. One of them, Greg Cooper, pursued, as a major thread of his PhD work, research into computerized explanation systems, the motivation behind which, he noted in a message to Shortliffe, "is the deeply held belief that physicians want active control of the diagnostic process."[5] A principal function of MYCIN's explanation capability was the inscription of hierarchy.

Because explanation signaled deference, MYCIN's creators saw the explanation capability as valuable even if it went unused. In 1974, Homer Warner, who was serving as the inaugural editor of the new journal *Computers and Biomedical Research,* wrote to Shortliffe about the necessary revisions to a manuscript that the MYCIN team had submitted to the journal. Of particular interest to Warner and his reviewers was MYCIN's explanation capability. "What is the basis," Warner probed, "for the statement that Doctors [*sic*] will not use advice given by a computer unless a thorough explanation of the basis for this advice is also provided? For instance, how often do they use the explanation program?"[6]

Shortliffe responded to Warner's inquiry candidly. He confessed that preliminary observations of the system in experimental settings seemed to classify MYCIN's explanation capability as marginal—at least as measured by the yardstick of direct utilization: "Based on observation of individuals who have experimented with the system to date, we do not expect that its ability to explain will be used with regularity by most users."[7] But the explanation capability, Shortliffe suggested, remained vitally important for ontological reasons: it dictated the kind of thing MYCIN was. Without an ability to explain itself, MYCIN risked becoming an inflexible, top-down dictator of medical advice. With such an ability, however, MYCIN became just another useful tool over which the physician retained control. As Shortliffe explained to Warner, "The capability is important, however, because it makes the program function as a tool to the physician rather than as a dogmatic advice giver."[8] Whether MYCIN could explain itself was more essential than whether MYCIN, in any given clinical encounter, *did* explain itself.

Despite all that was done to achieve deference, in reality MYCIN's relationship to the physician and their traditional authority was far more muddled. In a retrospective appraisal of the MYCIN project, programmer William Clancey argued that the system's mode of consultation was inescapably hierarchical, subordinating the physician's knowledge to that of MYCIN's architects. He wrote, "We viewed all interactions between people and program in terms of 'transfer': Experts had knowledge stored in their heads. The knowledge base was an objective inventory of expert knowledge. Users lacked knowledge. The role of consultation . . . was to transfer knowledge between experts, users, and students."[9] For Clancey, such a unidirectional model of transfer had an inherently tiered, even religious, character. "Knowledge engineers," he ventured, "are like priests; they receive 'The Word' from experts above, add nothing to the content, but codify it accurately into written rules, and pass it down to ordinary folks as commandments to live by. If you are not an expert, you learn by being told."[10] Such a view of knowledge transfer, Clancey maintained, reinforced an impoverished view of medical knowledge—it "lack[ed] any sense that the knowledge base could belong to a community of practitioners, the users and experts alike, and might be developed and maintained by them."[11] The identity of the physician imagined by MYCIN's creators was very different from the kind of physician the system created through its operation.

To a certain extent Clancey was selling himself and his Stanford colleagues short. The team did in fact see physicians as ancillary wells of medical knowledge and even designed features for physicians to edit and expand the existing body of rules. They also held informed, if not sophisticated, views about the nature of medical knowledge; they understood that MYCIN's rule-based formulation was imperfect and shallow—that not every aspect of medical expertise was explicit, transferrable, and rule-like. Arguments about the "tacit" and personal dimensions of knowledge, and even specific philosophers like Michael Polanyi and Thomas Kuhn, were not foreign to them.[12] The MYCIN team, then, did not espouse a wholly naïve and unchecked view about the nature of medical knowledge. Their attempts to explicate medical knowledge derived from a pragmatic impulse to build, under conditions of limited time and funding, a system that worked, as well as their view that medical knowledge, even if "tacit" in some regards, was at least partially formalizable.

Though an oversimplification, Clancey's retrospective critique still got a lot right. For all that the MYCIN team said publicly about deference, behind closed doors the creators sometimes did portray physicians as, to use Clancey's words, "ordinary folks." At times they presumed clinicians to be ignorant and unskilled. A significant internal consideration among the MYCIN team concerned the possibility of designing the system to minimize the physician's clinical judgment. The kinds of information that MYCIN requested from the physician arrayed along a spectrum of clinical discretion. Certain kinds of patient information required next to no clinical judgment to obtain. Data from the microbiological laboratory, for instance, could simply be transferred from the lab report into MYCIN. But other kinds of information about the patient derived from clinicians' own judgments.

Members of the MYCIN team questioned how much faith they could place in physicians' abilities to accurately obtain these more judgmental forms of patient information. MYCIN, after all, was predicated on the assumption that its user lacked expertise in the area of infectious disease diagnosis and treatment. If physicians needed assistance in the realm of infectious disease, could they really be trusted to discern, evaluate, and report clinical findings related to this area of medicine? Questions of this kind were, Shortliffe recounted in a 1976 message, the topic of "several sessions over the years when we have had to discuss the issue of how much judgmental information to request from the presumed non-experts using our system."[13] Much thought went into, as another MYCIN affiliate put it, "avoid[ing] the problem of user variability and fallibility."[14] The rationale for minimizing reliance on clinical judgment was best summarized in the minutes of a 1976 MYCIN meeting: "The closer the system is tied to objective information, and the fewer judgmental Q's it asks, the more reliable it will be. The MD's who most need help from MYCIN are the least likely to give sound answers to the judgmental Q's."[15] Such private renderings of the physician (unenlightened, reliant) flew in the face of the physician's identity as imagined by its explanation capability (capable, autonomous).

Considerations about the proper balance between judgmental and nonjudgmental forms of medical knowledge, often discussed in the abstract, gained a more concrete figure as MYCIN affiliates turned their attention to one particular finding used by MYCIN: a blood infection's portal of entry. The portal through which a given organism entered the human body—whether broken skin, the respiratory tract, mucous membranes, the genitourinary tract, or catheters—could help clinicians (and MYCIN) identify the infectious organism. Yet, some MYCIN affiliates worried that the portal concept demanded too much of the nonexpert physician: "The worst flaw is that its [the portal concept's] use requires clinical judgment and knowledge on the part of the user, which he may or may not have. . . . If the user selects an inappropriate portal, then Mycin and the patient will suffer the consequences of his error. The consultant (Mycin) then becomes dependent on the user."[16] The concern here was that MYCIN's reliance upon judgmental information left its performance up to chance: there, but for the physician's judgment, MYCIN goes.

For Shortliffe's part, he agreed that ideally MYCIN ought to rely upon as little judgmental information as possible: "In the ideal world we would like to ask the user only for LABDATA"—that is, nonjudgmental information that came from the microbiological laboratory.[17] But given that MYCIN would be operating under nonideal conditions, he was more willing than some of his colleagues to cut the physicians some slack. Shortliffe hastened to remind colleagues that the philosophy behind MYCIN—one of deference to physicians—aligned with the system's dependence, at least partially, on the user's judgment, skill, and competence: "I personally feel that we should give the nonexperts at least SOME credit for being able to make useful observations. It is, after all, consistent with our initial philosophy of MYCIN that we not try to replace entirely the physician's reasoning powers but rather to augment them."[18]

The discussion concerning judgmental knowledge highlights a version of the "dilemma of application" that Keeve Brodman and his colleagues faced some two decades earlier. The MYCIN team imagined the physician as controlling and atomistic, and they attempted to build a computer system that was consonant with this perceived physician identity. Yet the team had to navigate an inherent tension: at the very same time, MYCIN was premised on the notion that physicians needed help—that they were prescribing antibiotics irrationally. If physicians were truly independent, competent, and authoritative in the realm of antibiotic decision-making, there would be no need for MYCIN in the first place. MYCIN thus also turned physicians into "users," "ordinary folks" whose purpose was to receive and implement the antibiotic gospel from on high.

## MYCIN in the Antibiotic Era

The relationship between MYCIN and clinical authority must be understood against the backdrop of much larger tensions and transformations around antibiotics and their irrational use. While MYCIN was often thought of as a form of basic research in computer science and artificial intelligence (AI), a second aim of the enterprise was applied and clinical: to engender a rational approach to antibiotic prescribing. In its clinical objectives, MYCIN belongs to a larger and older reform effort, one whose origins date back at least two decades before MYCIN's creation. As Scott Podolsky has shown, antibiotic reform efforts first coalesced in the 1950s—as much the result of growing anxieties about antibiotic misuse as the emergence of the infectious disease specialist as a new category of medical expert.[19]

In these early years, antibiotic reformers directed their energies to a class of drugs that are now largely forgotten: fixed-dose combination antibiotics. Pharmaceutical companies promoted this class of drugs, combinations of multiple antibiotics into a single pill, on the basis that the whole was greater than the sum of its parts. But reformers remained skeptical. Infectious disease experts, led by Harvard's Maxwell Finland among others, pointed out that assertions about the drugs' worth rested on first-person testimonials rather than controlled clinical trials.[20] These critiques proved persuasive: reformers would see the fruits of their labor in 1962, with the enactment of the Kefauver–Harris amendments. The amendments granted the US Food and Drug Administration the power to remove from the market drugs, like fixed-dose combination antibiotics, that had not been proven (via "adequate and well-controlled investigations") to be efficacious.[21]

The passage of the Kefauver–Harris amendments freed antibiotic reformers to focus on a different aspect of medical practice that needed reforming: physicians' prescribing practices. By the 1970s, the attention lavished on the irrational prescribing practices of many physicians reached something of a crescendo, as reformers worked to underscore the problems associated with antibiotic overuse in medical, governmental, and popular fora.[22] In their appearances before these hearings, and in their broader campaign to change prescribing behaviors, antibiotic reformers frequently resorted to the rhetoric of "rationality."[23] Theirs was an effort to banish rampant "irrational" prescribing and to cultivate in its place a "rational" approach to antibiotic use. Although antibiotic resistance would later come to serve as the chief impetus driving such reform efforts, in the early 1970s reformers were motivated by a host of concerns beyond antibiotic resistance alone: reformers argued that irrational prescribing produced superinfections, adverse side effects, added costs, and even a broader "dumbing down" of the medical profession.

The topic of antibiotic misuse also received heightened attention in less public settings during this period. In medical journals, many researchers turned a critical—and empirical—eye to physicians' prescribing behaviors, producing studies that quantified the irrationality and regional variation in antibiotic use.[24] A 1974 *Journal of the American Medical Association* (*JAMA*) article concluded that "the gap between the actual antibiotic prescribing practices and the ideal practices recommended by infectious disease specialists appears to be widening."[25] Different regulatory bodies started to mobilize—and various guidelines, task forces, and committees started to materialize—in response to rising levels of concern about antibiotic misuse. The MYCIN team followed these studies closely and cited them as evidence of a need for a computerized consultation system such as theirs. The weight of empirical evidence, the MYCIN team observed, "reflects the need for improved therapy selection in patients requiring therapy." "This," they continued, "is precisely the decision task with which MYCIN is designed to assist."[26]

Such developments point to an important evolution in the nature of therapeutic reform efforts over the second half of the twentieth century, as Podolsky has demonstrated. In the 1950s and 1960s, therapeutic reformers primarily targeted irrational drugs, arguing that fixed-dose combination drugs were not just inefficacious but potentially dangerous. Having successfully worked to remove these drugs from the market, therapeutic reformers shifted their focus. Beginning in the late 1960s, reformers increasingly worried not about irrational drugs but about the irrational use of drugs that, in some contexts, were entirely warranted and efficacious.[27] The main target of reform, in other words, changed from the faulty drugs in the physician's armamentarium to the faulty behaviors of physicians themselves. As a decision support tool that aimed to intervene in physicians' prescribing practices, MYCIN aligned with this new reform emphasis.

The makers of MYCIN sometimes adopted the very vocabulary of therapeutic reformers, describing their system as a way of shoring up "rational," and reining in "irrational," prescribing behaviors. In March 1977, Richard DuBois of the US Department of Health, Education, and Welfare delivered news to Stanley Cohen that the MYCIN project was only recommended for a partial renewal of funding from the National Center for Health Services Research. The decision reflected concerns about the system's clinical utility. Specifically, reviewers believed that the selection of infectious disease as MYCIN's problem domain placed inherent limitations on MYCIN's potential usefulness in medical practice: "While regarding MYCIN as an excellent model of clinical decision-making for educational purposes, reviewers questioned its utility in medical practice. One factor contributing to reviewers' reservations is that the choice of antibiotics in practice is far more constrained than the choices built into MYCIN. Institutional norms and policies often dictate which antibiotics to use, and the necessity of protecting the patient against unidentified organisms often serves as justification for using a broad-spectrum antibiotic."[28]

This conclusion did not sit well with Cohen. Channeling the energies, insights, and even anger of the leading antibiotic reformers, Cohen shot back in a heated letter to the National Center's director, "I am astounded that the Center would officially take the position, as it seems to have done, that there is not really much need for developing a *rational* approach to antimicrobial therapy—since we can simply give broad-spectrum antibiotics."[29] When Cohen expanded upon these critiques in the same letter, he adopted the language of antibiotic reformers, contrasting MYCIN's "rational approach" with the reviewers' "irrational" position:

> This claim is complete rubbish; if selection of a broad-spectrum antibiotic to treat various infectious diseases is all that is necessary, there would be no need for diagnostic laboratories to culture organisms from diseased patients, and no need for infectious disease consultations by either human experts or computers.

> A major sub-specialty of Internal Medicine, Infectious Diseases, could simply disappear if the problem were as simple as some observers seem to believe. The view expressed is a prime example of the misinformation and ignorance that leads every year to the waste of billions of dollars of health care funds for *irrational* and unnecessary antibiotic use.[30]

According to Cohen, then, the center got things completely backward: the fact that "institutional norms and policies often dictate" antibiotic use was proof not of MYCIN's futility but of its clinical relevance and urgency. Physicians' irrational prescribing practices, driven by "misinformation and ignorance," were in need of correction.

Unsurprisingly, many physicians did not respond lightly to the suggestion that they were major contributors to the problem of antibiotic resistance. Indeed, many denied that there was a problem at all. "Yes, we *are* 'over-prescribing' antibiotics, and it is good that we are," opined one clinician in 1974. "My God, let's *not* go back to the 'good old days'!"[31] Of course, such sentiments represent the more extreme end of the spread of opinion, but they nevertheless highlight the resistance that reformers encountered as they set out to characterize, quantify, and ultimately tackle the challenge of antibiotic misuse. As tensions grew and pressure mounted, the medical community splintered along the familiar fault lines of "town" and "gown." Many doctors in private practice portrayed academic reformers as highfalutin ivory-tower types, divorced from the on-the-ground realities faced by time- and resource-strained doctors. "How many patients should you watch die from lack of prescribing before you give antibiotics?" challenged one physician. "Those idiots in Washington," he continued, "should try the practice of medicine for awhile, instead of doing it from the test tube."[32]

To a limited degree, the MYCIN project experienced similar pushback. In its mildest form, this pushback arose out of ignorance—a failure to appreciate the problem of antibiotic resistance, or this problem's connection to physicians' prescribing practices. Victor Yu encountered such resistance during a 1977 cross-country flight, when he found himself seated next to one of the very "site visitors" who had assessed the MYCIN project. On balance, the impressions from the site visit were favorable. The visitor reported being impressed by MYCIN's ability to justify itself. But one line of questions lingered in the visitor's mind. As conveyed in the minutes of a MYCIN team meeting, "His main questions were—'What is the WORTH of an Inf. Dis. Program?' (How often will it be used and for what sorts of consults) and 'What is the magnitude of the problem of the incorrect prescribing of antibiotics?' "[33] Clearly, as vigorously as therapeutic reformers campaigned to raise awareness of antibiotic misuse, a sizeable population of otherwise well-informed people remained oblivious to the magnitude of the problem.[34]

## "Hidden in the Code"

Yu's serendipitous meeting at thirty thousand feet, as well as Stanley Cohen's sharp exchange with the National Center for Health Services Research, together illustrate the extent to which ignorance presented a barrier to MYCIN's acceptance. A year later, Yu's colleague William Clancey encountered a different kind of barrier that threatened to be even more difficult to scale: calculated opposition. At an Artificial Intelligence in Medicine (AIM) banquet in 1978, Clancey had a conversation with one physician who seemed to suggest that "the problem of overprescribing antibiotics, which we argue is an important motivation for the MYCIN program, is not a real problem."[35] Mystified by the physician's stance, Clancey followed up with him after the banquet.

The physician, Harold Goldberger, took this subsequent exchange as an opportunity to clarify his position. As it turned out, Goldberger's view was not that antibiotic overprescribing was not a problem; rather, his view was that just as there are risks associated with overprescribing, there are also risks associated with underprescribing. Despite the cries of "irrationality" coming from antibiotic reformers, there was, Goldberger insisted, a logic—a *rationality*—to physicians' prescribing practices; these clinicians were in the difficult position of having to make medical decisions under conditions of uncertainty, delicately weighing manifold benefits and risks that cut in different directions. As Goldberger explained, "We can almost never be certain that the therapy we're prescribing is the appropriate one and we have to consider the consequences of erring in various directions. . . . So we have to consider the relative consequences of prescribing one or several extra antimicrobials that are ineffective against the actual pathogen that's growing and producing its destructive effect in the patient, against the possibility that nothing you're prescribing is going to be effective against the actual infective agent (assuming that an effective drug is available)."[36]

Goldberger developed these general observations into a more targeted critique of MYCIN. Central to Goldberger's critique was the observation that the developers of MYCIN and practicing physicians were invested in two different, and often conflicting, conceptions of health. Goldberger suggested that Shortliffe and his colleagues, much like leading antibiotic reformers, privileged a population-level conception of health, thus explaining the MYCIN team's concern with the problem of antibiotic resistance. Practicing physicians, by contrast, had no choice but to conceptualize health in terms of the individual—in terms of the person in front of them. Goldberger elaborated on this tension in his response to Clancey: "Another consideration that I don't think has been fully taken into account is the potential conflict between the interest of an individual patient and the epidemiological concerns that may be *hidden in the code* of a program such as MYCIN. If . . . one of the concerns of the developers of MYCIN is the proliferation of resistant organisms as a result of over-prescription of antibiotics, it would be reasonable for any physician or patient using the program to worry whether the recommendation of the program might be sub-optimal in a particular case because of that concern."[37] Goldberger's fear that MYCIN's alleged population-level bias might be "hidden in the code," invisible to the unsuspecting physician-user, is particularly instructive. Such sentiments illustrate how the values of trust, communicability, and transparency informed, often in very fundamental ways, the actions and concerns of both the MYCIN team and its critics.

Goldberger's point about individual- and population-level health in many ways reproduced the larger town-gown divisions discussed earlier. Many critics of antibiotic reform efforts came to similar conclusions: while those in the ivory tower, these critics argued, had the luxury of dealing with epidemiological abstractions of health, clinicians in the trenches had the obligation to deal with the well-being of the individuals before them. Viewing debates around antibiotic reform through the politics of town and gown goes a long way to making sense of how these reform efforts played out over the latter part of the twentieth century. But such a dyadic framework also elides important nuances. For one, a handful of leading academic clinicians lent support to so-called town physicians and criticized ideas about regulating prescribing behaviors. What's more, the views of reformers and their critics were far from homogeneous. Some reformers advocated for clear dictates and national guidelines. Others urged less heavy-handed approaches, favoring educational initiatives that simply augmented physicians' knowledge without curbing their autonomy.[38]

As with the larger national conversations taking place among reformers, the opinions of the MYCIN staff arrayed along a spectrum. Different members of the MYCIN project held differing views about the accuracy, universality, and helpfulness of clinical rules and guidelines—and about how rigidly such rules should be applied. These views, however, were not so much expressed outwardly as packaged implicitly in more technical conversations about MYCIN and its inner workings. In the spring of 1976, a debate emerged among MYCIN members around the possibility of rigidly defining what different certainty factors meant. What did it mean, clinically, to say that a certain medical proposition was known with a certainty factor of 0.9 as opposed to one of 0.7? Janice Aikins, one of the MYCIN programmers, outwardly wondered whether defining certainty factors in a standardized manner was, given the inexact state of medical science, impossible:

> Even if we could reach agreement among the infectious disease experts at Stanford as to the "right" CF's to put on our rules, the infectious disease experts on the east coast and other places would probably not agree with us. Now let's take this one step further. Say we are able to assign fairly straightforward meanings to our CF's. Now we have the problem of a doctor in some other part of the country who doesn't want to use MYCIN because our CF's don't agree with what he would use. In other words, by defining our CF's at all rigorously, we're inviting disagreement.[39]

From this discussion of clinical variability and its possible consequences for MYCIN's clinical viability, Aikins ventured that, even if it were possible to define certainty factors with great specificity, such rigid and prescriptive definitions "might not be such a good idea anyway." Why not, Aikins implied, give some wiggle room for physicians with varying inclinations and preferences? Aikins's suggestion was consonant with the views of some others in the field of biomedical computing, who argued that computerized decision support tools must "allow for a spectrum of knowledge and/or opinions instead of just one 'golden' standard."[40] Only by building in such flexibility would it be possible for a system developed at one locale to be adopted at another.

But to other members of the MYCIN team, Aikins's suggestion was preposterous, even heretical. "I need not remind all of us that we are dealing directly with human lives," Sam Ervin responded, showing little patience. "If another MD on the east coast disagrees with our CF's and has data (be it strong or weak) as to the basis for his disagreement, then we had better damn well know about it. I claim that one of the advantages of specific criteria for CF's is that it 'invites disagreement' (or to put it another way—critical analysis of the rules by non-MYCIN experts is possible)."[41] According to Ervin, the appropriate response to discordant clinical beliefs is not to throw one's hands up in the air and accommodate both beliefs. No, the responsible course of action is to drill down and figure out which belief is in the right. At stake was nothing less than human lives. This seemingly narrow and technical disagreement between

Aikins and Ervin about certainty factors was symptomatic of a much more fundamental disagreement concerning the authority of physicians and the epistemology of medicine. Whereas Ervin had confidence that there was a "correct answer" that could be revealed through medical science, Aikins was apparently less sure—or at least less sure that this correct answer could be discerned with much clarity or haste.

Behind these quarrels about certainty factors lay not just philosophical considerations but practical considerations as well. Aikins believed herself to be negotiating a perceived trade-off between precision and viability, accuracy and acceptability. By defining certainty factors rigidly, she argued, the makers of MYCIN would effectively be affixing to their system a ball and chain; they would be limiting how far their expert system could travel. Looser definitions, by contrast, made MYCIN more deferential to individual physicians, more attractive to a larger and more diverse clinical audience.

The notion that computerized systems like MYCIN could be flexible and adaptable to diverse local circumstances was held up as an advantage of new digital technologies over traditional analog ones. In a 1974 communication, Cohen enumerated what he saw as MYCIN's advantages over the existing information landscape: a computerized system could respond more nimbly to an ever-evolving base of medical knowledge; it was less prone to embarrass users (computers did not look down upon ignorance in the way human consultants might); it could accommodate uncertain and incomplete medical knowledge (textbooks, according to Cohen, contained only "well-codified, noncontroversial truths"); it was accessible on demand; it could pool the expertise of multiple infectious disease experts; and it did not tire, applying each rule with the upmost rigor and consistency, whether it was on the first or the one-hundredth consultation of the day. A computerized system also, Cohen argued, promised greater "local relevance." He noted, "Textbooks are designed to transmit general knowledge that is appropriate over a large geographical area, for 'typical' patients in various categories." MYCIN, by contrast, "applies its knowledge to specific clinical problems which must be dealt with in connection with particular patients."[42]

Notwithstanding debates about how to calibrate certainty factors, MYCIN was, on balance, highly deferential to the physician's authority and autonomy. There were many possible responses to the problem of antibiotic misuse, from compulsory governmental regulation to optional educational initiatives. Within this spectrum of possible reform policies, MYCIN represented a rather gentler intervention. This deference was not ancillary but fundamental to what MYCIN aimed to be. From the outset, concerns about clinical acceptance, autonomy, and authority were never far from the minds of MYCIN's developers. Such concerns even animated many technical debates and decisions about certainty factors and other aspects of MYCIN's inner workings, as the exchange between Aikins and Ervin demonstrates. It would be a mistake to conclude that MYCIN's explanation capabilities were built as a direct response to wider contemporaneous debates about antibiotic use and clinical autonomy; Shortliffe and his colleagues saw these capabilities as vital components of medical computer systems, irrespective of their problem domain. But the fact that MYCIN trafficked in the domain of infectious disease—an area of medicine that was a site of great tension, division, and resistance—was not unimportant either. This wider context gave the interwoven values of transparency, authority, and trust even greater weight.

## AI vs. MD

Shortliffe and his contemporaries regularly thought about whether the reasoning processes of computerized systems like MYCIN mimicked human forms of reasoning. Beyond such comparisons with respect to styles of reasoning, the Stanford team also compared MYCIN and physicians with respect to the endpoints of reasoning—their final diagnoses and therapeutic recommendations. In their efforts to build trust in MYCIN, Shortliffe and his colleagues pursued something of a two-pronged strategy. One prong was creating MYCIN's explanation capabilities—capabilities that aimed to open up the system's recommendations to scrutiny and cede authority to physicians. The second prong was proving, empirically, the accuracy of MYCIN's decisions. At first blush, systematic evaluation of MYCIN's decisions seemed like a straightforward enterprise, nothing more than answering a few simple questions. How did MYCIN's software stack up against the physician's wetware? Were the system's recommendations more, as, or less accurate than those generated by human physicians? But Shortliffe and his colleagues quickly discovered that behind such seemingly simple questions lay deeper complexities. In designing the evaluation study, the MYCIN team had to grapple with complicated questions of not just clinical trial design but also the philosophy of medicine.

The MYCIN team started brainstorming ways of formally evaluating the system within a couple years of starting the project.[43] As the MYCIN team thought through the logistics of evaluation, they identified a number of key sticking points. Most importantly, they were attempting to evaluate something for which there was no single, self-evidently "correct" answer. In medicine, the team realized, often multiple therapeutic approaches can be justified; the reason for choosing one approach over another can be as much a matter of values as empirics. Medical practice accommodates a host of different values and rationalities, and the "superior" therapeutic approach is often a consequence of how one opts to weigh these coexisting values, interests, and considerations. No clear-cut laboratory test can be ordered to tell one how to best assign these weights.

Shortliffe was acutely aware of these challenges, and he went out of his way to correct colleagues who failed to appreciate the complexities of clinical medicine. In reviewing a manuscript submitted to the *Annals of Internal Medicine*, Shortliffe critiqued the paper for its assumption that all medical knowledge could be sorted neatly into one of two buckets: "The discussion seems to assume that knowledge is either 'right' or 'wrong,' yet people in the field are aware that absolute gold standards of performance are difficult to define."[44] Buchanan similarly acknowledged how it could be "difficult to define precisely the term 'appropriate therapy.'"[45] Appropriate by what criteria, and by whose standards?

Even outside the realm of values, the MYCIN team discovered that medical decisions were difficult to evaluate in a binary, right-wrong fashion for a more practical reason: different experts believed different things. The MYCIN team worried about this possible lack of consensus from the outset. In a 1972 memo, Stanley Cohen noted, "In certain instances there might be so much difference of opinion that no reasonable hierarchy of recommended therapy can be defined."[46] By 1977, Cohen and his colleagues were no longer talking about expert variability in a speculative manner—in the realm of "mights" and "maybes." After five years of work, preliminary findings had confirmed Cohen's earlier suppositions. As Cohen and Yu reported in a 1977 letter, "We have observed considerable variability among different infectious disease specialists in their antimicrobial recommendations when presented with identical patients."[47] The challenges presented by expert variability were twofold. One, it smothered hopes of evaluating MYCIN's performance against a single, gold standard. And two, it meant that even if the team designed a study that evaluated MYCIN's performance against that of certified experts, the team would have to somehow account for disagreements among the experts themselves.

These were significant challenges, to be sure, but the MYCIN team viewed them as surmountable. "The real world problem area," Shortliffe explained in a 1975 letter, "is filled with disagreement and it was thus a challenge to try to develop an evaluation mechanism that would control for such lack of unanimity."[48] But try the MYCIN team did. The team published their first evaluation study—of the system's bacteremia knowledge base—in a 1979 issue of *Computer Programs in Biomedicine*.[49] In the study, the team sent MYCIN's recommendations for fifteen patients to ten experts, five infectious disease specialists from Stanford and five infectious disease specialists from other institutions. The experts then judged whether MYCIN's decision-making process and recommendations were identical or acceptable alternatives to their own recommendations. By this method of evaluation, a majority of experts found MYCIN's recommendations to meet the standards of acceptable practice in over 90 percent of cases.[50] This bacteremia study, however, left an important question yawning open before the MYCIN team. Where MYCIN and the physicians differed in their recommendations, who was in the wrong: the physicians, MYCIN, or both?

The team aimed to address this critical shortcoming in a subsequent evaluation, this time of MYCIN's meningitis, rather than its bacteremia, knowledge base. On August 9, 1977, Morton Swartz, an infectious disease expert at Massachusetts General Hospital, received an unsolicited letter from MYCIN's Victor Yu and Stanley Cohen: "We are asking for the participation of a group of distinguished academic infectious disease experts who have done clinical studies involving patients with meningitis. We would like you to look over 10 clinical summaries of patients with meningitis and complete a short questionnaire concerning antimicrobial recommendations."[51] Swartz was just one of at least eight such experts to receive the invitation. What Swartz and the other experts were not privy to was the real purpose of the study: they were not informed that one of these ten "clinical summaries" was of particular interest to the researchers. This summary had been produced by computer—by MYCIN. To serve as points of comparison, the other nine clinical summaries had been generated by medical personnel with varying levels of expertise and training.

Victor Yu first sketched the methodological outlines of this study, which would become the most rigorous evaluation of MYCIN, in a 1976 communication to his colleagues:

> Pick a selected number of interesting and/or challenging cases, 8 to 12 in number. . . . Have a 3rd year medical student, 4th year medical student, intern, resident, ID fellow, ID staff evaluate each case selecting his treatment recommendations, if any. Have 2 or 3 ID staff who are nationally recognized experts in

> Meningitis give their treatment recommendations. Then, they would "grade" the treatments given by our volunteers (students, housestaff, fellows, Stanford staff) plus MYCIN without knowing the identity of each volunteer (ie human vs MYCIN). Agree, Disagree, and Close call would be used.[52]

The entire purpose of this methodology—pooling MYCIN's recommendations together with the recommendations of various medical personnel and then subjecting that pool of recommendations to a *second* layer of evaluation—was "to achieve just the comparative power that the first two [evaluation studies] lacked."[53]

The evaluation as ultimately published hewed closely to Yu's proposal.[54] It had two phases. In the first phase, a physician, with no formal affiliation with the MYCIN project, selected ten patients with infectious meningitis according to predetermined criteria.[55] These patient cases were compiled into detailed summaries, which contained information concerning the patients' medical history, physical examination, laboratory data, and the immediately prior hospital course. These detailed summaries were then sent for evaluation to different medical personnel representing a range of expertise: a medical student, a medical resident, a senior postdoctoral fellow in infectious disease, five faculty members in Stanford's Division of Infectious Disease, and MYCIN. Using only the information contained in the patient summaries, each prescriber reported the optimal antimicrobial therapy regimen for each of the ten cases.

Having generated a pool of recommendations that could be compared and judged, the evaluation entered its second phase. The MYCIN team sent the ten patient summaries together with the resultant therapeutic recommendations to eight "super experts"—people, like Swartz, who were deemed experts in the management of meningitis and had published case reports dealing with the subject. The super experts were asked to review the patient cases and come up with their own prescriptions, before evaluating the therapeutic recommendations of the original prescribers. The super experts rated the original prescribers in a tripartite fashion: the prescription could be (1) "equivalent" to that of the super expert, (2) different from that of the super expert but nevertheless "acceptable," or (3) "not acceptable." Even if this new methodology of evaluating MYCIN against gradations of expertise did not fully eliminate the problem of the "gold standard," the team felt that it would demonstrate their system's accuracy to the greatest extent that medical knowledge would allow.

The results of the study, published in *JAMA* in 1979, looked pretty good for MYCIN.[56] The system's recommendation was deemed either "equivalent" or "acceptable" in 65 percent of the evaluations. While such a result surely left room for improvement, it compared favorably to the other prescribers evaluated in the study. Medical students issued acceptable prescriptions only 30 percent of the time—an outcome that residents bested by 15 percent. Even the five members of the Stanford faculty, some of whom were published experts in the field of infectious disease, sunk below MYCIN's level of performance, offering an appropriate recommendation in between 42.5 and 62.5 percent of cases.

For those already inclined toward computerized medicine, the study heralded a bright future. One Toronto-based laboratory technologist cited the MYCIN evaluation study (among others) as evidence that a digital revolution in medicine lurked just over the horizon. He concluded, "Computer applications in medicine will come of age in the 1980s. Despite resistance of many doctors to the use of these machines, the computer will lead to a new era in medical care. With the cooperation of physicians, computers may become to the medical system what the wheel was to mankind."[57] Yet, when the 1980s came, MYCIN remained confined to experimental settings, and Shortliffe and his Stanford colleagues had started to shift their attention to a different medical program. To show that a computerized diagnostic system could "beat" its human counterparts in controlled experimental settings was a far cry from demonstrating the system's use in the real world.

## "Algorithms, Anyone?"

After a decade's worth of effort, the firewall between the research side of medical AI and the clinical side of medical AI remained as strong as ever. Shortliffe and his colleagues were eager to break through. Shortliffe offered a sobering assessment of the situation in a 1982 memo to his colleagues at the Heuristic Programming Project: "Despite active research into the development of medical consultation systems over the last decade, no system from the AIM community has yet been introduced for ongoing use in a clinical setting."[58] In MYCIN's case, this distance from a real clinical setting was especially tragic. Many of the system's most prized features concerned its usability and acceptability within real world clinical environments. In branching out from the MYCIN project, Shortliffe and his colleagues thus prioritized the selection of a new domain that would allow them to fast-track a computerized consultation system into the actual clinic.

The team quickly settled on oncology protocol management. In the 1980s, as is the case today, many treatments in oncology were experimental. For many types of cancers, physicians and researchers did not have a clear sense of the comparative benefits and toxicities of different treatment regimens and modalities. As a result, oncologic treatment often involved enrolling patients into different experimental treatments, with the short-term hope of curing patients and the long-term hope of enriching medicine's understanding of comparative efficacy. Elaborate protocols—often spanning dozens or even hundreds of pages in length—were created to define the particulars of a given treatment plan, set certain eligibility requirements, and much else.[59] Strict adherence to the protocol was a must: because the protocols were not only treatment descriptions for individual patients but also key components of a larger experimental design, departure from the protocol could endanger the interpretability and analysis of treatment results.

The team also hoped that in selecting the domain of oncology they would be filling an unmet clinical need. Oncology protocols could be extraordinarily complex, delineating both the appropriate course of treatment and the appropriate management of countless events, problems, or complications that could arise during that treatment course.[60] The limitations of the human mind, combined with the hectic working environment of an oncologic clinic, nearly guaranteed deviation from protocol. The team explained in 1984: "Although an effort is made to have the documents [protocols] available in the oncology clinics when patients are being treated for their tumors, it is often the case that a busy clinic schedule, coupled with a complex protocol description, leads a physician to rely on memory when deciding on drug doses and laboratory tests. Furthermore, solutions for all possible treatment problems cannot be spelled out in protocols. Physicians use their own judgment in treating these patients, resulting in some variability in treatment from patient to patient."[61] A computerized system might thus help overstretched physicians adhere more closely to protocols of ever-increasing complexity.

But even beyond perceptions of clinical need, oncology protocol management gained favor among the team for a more self-interested reason: it was deemed supremely computerizable. "ONCOCIN's domain was selected," Shortliffe clarified in his 1982 memo, "precisely because its knowledge base is unusually well-formalized and highly structured. We wanted to develop a system that could be implemented for ongoing use in the short term, thereby allowing investigation into human issues that cannot be readily address when a system exists solely in a research environment."[62] The domain of antibiotic selection offered a nice playground for inventing a new kind of computerized system—the rule-based expert system. It would be the domain of oncology that would allow for the introduction of such a system in a real clinical setting. Their domain selected, the team began encoding a series of protocols for Hodgkin's and non-Hodgkin's lymphoma as part of a computerized system. ONCOCIN was born.

ONCOCIN came on the scene during a period of rapid regulatory and bureaucratic change in American medicine. Over the 1970s and 1980s, clinical practice guidelines and protocols—and the institutions for creating, evaluating, and regulating such guidelines—proliferated greatly.[63] The forces behind this surge were many. From above, administrators sought to leverage guidelines as a way of reigning in rising health care costs while also bringing order and uniformity to areas where variation seemed to reign. From below, clinicians and medical researchers themselves also fueled the proliferation of guidelines by participating in the booming post–World War II medical research enterprise. The magnitude (e.g., congressional appropriations to the National Institutes of Health ballooned in the decades following 1945) and nature (e.g., an emphasis on controlled clinical trials) of the postwar research enterprise made research protocols and clinical practice guidelines ubiquitous and indispensable.[64]

As guidelines spread through medical practice, they took on all sorts of meanings and were mobilized for various agendas. Given this complexity, it would be a mistake to view guidelines through a binary lens, with health administrators promoting them as tools for reducing costs or imposing standards and clinicians shirking them as overly blunt instruments that reduced the art of medicine into the language of a cookbook.[65] But it would also be a mistake to deny such tensions. Numerous physicians did interpret clinical practice algorithms and guidelines as intrusions into their professional jurisdiction, as impediments to humane and individualized care, or as gross simplifications of a highly complex and uncertain enterprise. Ingelfinger's 1973 editorial that opened this chapter, "Algorithms, Anyone?," characterized algorithms as threats to the very cornerstone of a physician's identity—clinical judgment.[66]

Ingelfinger's editorial was just one of many to criticize algorithmic approaches to medicine. In 1977, a team of researchers based out of the University of California, San Francisco (UCSF) published an article in *JAMA* detailing an algorithm to aid physicians in the evaluation and use of diagnostic laboratory data.[67] The article elicited an impassioned editorial from William H.

Crosby, a pioneering figure in the field of hematology. Crosby charged that algorithms approximate medical practice no more than the sanitized game of chess approximates the messiness of real war:

> Algorithms are to the practice of medicine as chess is to war, but with a difference: we can get hurt when results of the algorithm game are extrapolated into real life. When used as a teaching device, algorithms may provide students with ill-conceived or even dangerous simplifications. Furthermore, the algorithm is easily adapted to computer practice. Taken seriously by a looming bureaucracy, our algorithm might make its mark on American medicine by instructing us to order B12 analysis and forbidding serum iron analysis on the basis of one person's conception of how to play a game.[68]

Crosby's substantive critiques about the inability of algorithms to capture the complexity of medicine were motivated by deeper fears. In response to the UCSF team's discussion about what their algorithmic approach had to "offer" physicians, Crosby sounded the alarm. Clinical guidelines, he warned, were Trojan horses; they entered the clinic under the guise of being helpful, only to gradually chip away at the physician's autonomy: "It is a small step from 'offer' to 'provide.' It is another small step from 'provide' to 'require.' And all of this would finally be enforced with the clout of Medicare. Be alert. The first sproutings of this bureaucratic liana may be no farther away than your own clinical laboratory."[69] In Crosby's mind, "algorithmic medicine" and "bureaucratic medicine" occupied the same cognitive space.[70]

## ONCOCIN and the "Issue of Friendliness"

ONCOCIN's debts to MYCIN were clear. It was, after all, a rule-based system, containing IF-THEN rules that would be immediately recognizable to anyone with a passing familiarity with MYCIN. Above all, the two shared an emphasis on explanation.[71] The ONCOCIN system had two primary subsystems: the Reasoner, "a rule-based expert consultant that is the core of the system," and the Interviewer, "an interface program that controls a high-speed terminal and the interaction with the physicians using the system."[72] The group felt strongly that ONCOCIN's success hinged equally on the Reasoner and the Interviewer: a sharp computer system that could not compellingly engage with clinicians may as well be dull. As related in an early report on the project, "The actual mechanics of computer terminal interaction is as important to a clinical system's acceptance as the quality of the program's advice."[73]

As with MYCIN, ONCOCIN's user interface, and its explanation capability in particular, encoded certain ideas about the physician's identity and authority. "The physician generally has a rather self-sufficient, active, controlling personality," explained a 1980 report on ONCOCIN's user interface. "Thus, an unwanted intrusion on his lifestyle or environment is likely to be strongly resisted. Any machine that is designed to help him must be clearly and readily under his control."[74] Decisions about how to engineer a computer system and its user interface reflected and reinforced certain gendered notions about who a physician is, how *he* behaves, and where *he* stands in a medical hierarchy. The report continued, "While the issue of security and confidentiality is critical, so is the issue of friendliness to the physician. A system that is hard to get to use, that does not quickly and readily recognize the physician as does the secretary and nurses, is seen as hostile, harsh, and unpleasant." ONCOCIN's "interface program" contained cultural ideas about the identity of the physician—his gender, preferences, tendencies, and even personality ("self-sufficient, active, controlling").

The purpose of ONCOCIN's "Interviewer" was not simply to explain the system's reasoning. It was also to perform deference. One of the ONCOCIN project members, Cliff Wulfman, described how "there are two ways to view Oncocin's relationship to the physician using it. One way is to envision Oncocin as a Domain Expert Consultant. In this view, the Reasoner predominates; IT asks the questions, IT produces recommendations, and everything else is side effect. The other view (and the preferred one, I believe) makes Oncocin a Helpful Assistant, looking over the physician's shoulder as he fills out forms and decides what therapy to give on this visit. . . . In this view, the Interviewer is not an 'interviewer' at all; it is an archiving tool."[75] Here again, important to note is how the "Interviewer" components of ONCOCIN shaped the ontology of the system: ONCOCIN's ability to explain itself and to engage deferentially with the physician transformed its status from that of "Domain Expert Consultant" to that of "Helpful Assistant." Whether the system was conceived of as the former or the latter, its designers believed, would greatly influence its clinical acceptance.

To some degree, they were right. Their claim that computerized systems were purveyors of "advice" rather than "dogma" resonated with concerned physicians. In 1987, American Medical Association representative Daniel K. Harris wrote an editorial for *JAMA*, describing both the opportunities and the challenges introduced by new strides in the computerized decision support field.[76] *JAMA* readers saw Harris's piece expressive of "the fear that physicians may have that, if not vigilant, they will either abdicate, or somehow be forced to relinquish control of their diagnostic and therapeutic decision-making to computer software."[77] Yet Harris was reassured by Shortliffe's claim that computerized systems would remain under the dominion of the physician. Harris wrote, "Shortliffe expresses the same consideration: '. . . Decision-support programs are intended to serve as *tools* for the trained practitioners, who retain ultimate responsibility for determining diagnostic and therapeutic strategies.' "[78] Having marshaled this Shortliffe quote, Harris had little else to add beyond an "Amen": "As we take advantage of these exciting technologies, it would be well to heed these words."[79]

In certain respects, MYCIN was designed in a realm of projection, hypothesis, and theory: Shortliffe and his colleagues created the system thinking about how physicians *might* respond to a computerized system. ONCOCIN finally presented an opportunity to witness how physicians actually did respond. Yet even before implementation, the team was eager to understand what physicians wanted and expected from such a system. Prior to ONCOCIN's rollout, one member of the team, Paul Chang, conducted a series of "test interviews" with physicians "who have had direct experience with the oncology clinic and lymphoma protocols but will not directly interact with the ONCOCIN system in the clinical setting."[80] Many of the hopes for the computerized system revolved around reducing administrative burden. "Anything that the computer could do to reduce the amount of time spent on paperwork," Chang reported, "would be greatly appreciated by all interviewed."

Chang didn't just want a vague concept of administrative need among physicians at the oncology clinic. He dug deeper, asking physicians about their engineering concerns, design expectations, and criticisms of the plan. In response, some voiced a degree of skepticism that echoed of critiques leveled against computerized diagnostic systems decades earlier, during Keeve Brodman and Vladimir Zworykin's time. Many, for example, challenged the assumption that medical decision-making, in all of its messiness and complexity, could be fruitfully distilled into algorithms, flowcharts, or decision rules. Chang elaborated: "A few interviewees seriously doubted the ability for 'computer algorithms' to effectively deal with the 'art of medicine.' . . . Many questioned whether or not a program can ever get an 'adequate picture (gestalt) of a patient's state of health by the mere asking of a few questions.' "[81]

Despite such skepticism, Chang's interviewees happily delivered constructive feedback. They offered features and specifications that the system would need to have if it were to be functional and compelling in the clinical environment. Many of their recommendations concerned matters of workflow. As

Chang related, "All persons interviewed stressed that the computer 'must not give physicians something more to do or be excessively time-consuming.'"[82] Physicians also touched upon issues of understandability and trust. At least one physician emphasized to Chang that the system's explanations must be "intuitively reasonable" to the physician while also avoiding "Bayesian/probabilistic magic."[83]

For some, the importance of transparency extended beyond the mere medical knowledge within ONCOCIN to the *kind of people* who created the system in the first place. Were these people credible? Did they understand the on-the-ground realities of clinical practice? As Chang characterized one discussion, "One must also emphasize 'human input' into the system: the user must be convinced that 'sympathetic and experienced' physicians were involved in the design and implementation of the system."[84] Concerns about trust and transparency shaded into concerns about control and authority. Chang summarized the view among some of his subjects that "physicians must be able to always override the advice given by the computer—'the physician must always be in charge.'"[85] Attuned to these concerns, the makers of ONCOCIN hoped that their system—with its well-built knowledge base, elaborate interface, and explanation capabilities—would offer more than what some physicians worried it might represent: a "glorified algorithm."[86]

## ONCOCIN Goes Live

In May 1981, ONCOCIN went live at Stanford's Debbie Probst Oncology Day Care Center.[87] Three mornings per week, eight fellows in oncology used the system—implemented on a DECSYSTEM-20 computer—to help manage patients enrolled in lymphoma chemotherapy protocols. For all that the Stanford team had done technologically to make ONCOCIN explainable, they nevertheless encountered certain unanticipated (albeit interesting) challenges. One such challenge involved dealing with the temporal aspects of reasoning. Medical decision-making, the ONCOCIN team recognized, frequently depends upon the understanding, synthesis, and processing of time-related concepts. In what order did a patient's symptoms occur—and for how long did they last? How has the patient, over the full course of their disease, responded to the treatment? While physicians regularly made inferences based on temporal information, the ONCOCIN program had more difficulty doing so.[88]

Recognition that certain complex inferences ought to be protocolized did not mean that the task would be easy. "Our oncology collaborators," they reported, "are finding this aspect of their knowledge particularly difficult to distill, and we expect that our attempts to develop computer-based approaches to the problem will provide particularly stimulating challenges."[89] The view that medical knowledge could ultimately be isolated and translated into rule-based formalisms, a view first expressed during the MYCIN project, clearly carried into the ONCOCIN effort as well. Yet this difficulty distilling certain kinds of medical knowledge was seen more as a challenge to be overcome than an affront to the overall project of distillation.

A second major problem that the ONCOCIN team encountered derived from a phenomenon they had come to know well during their work on MYCIN: clinical variability. An implicit assumption made in the first iteration of ONCOCIN was that heterogeneous medical decisions (those that deviated from the protocol) were significant either for patient care or for research purposes. Indeed, clinical variability was the enemy of the protocol. As one team member wrote in 1980, "The purpose of a protocol is uniformity of care so that different treatment regimens can be compared more readily."[90]

However, the ONCOCIN team came to realize that, in practice, physician and protocol could differ in ways that were more stylistic than substantive. In these cases, physicians bristled at having to override a computerized system—and at having to provide a justification for doing so. The team elaborated on this realization in one of their annual reports:

> The second problem was unanticipated until the system was implemented, but it is having a major impact on our current work. . . . The changes they [physicians] make are frequently minor ones that are more stylistic than substantive (e.g., some physicians prefer always to give prednisone in multiples of 20 mgs when they are dealing with large doses; others prefer to be more precise in their dosing and will ask patients to take combinations of 5 and 20 mg tablets). In these cases, the physicians tend to be annoyed by requisitions for reasons that they have disagreement with ONCOCIN; they do not see the slight adjustments as being real disagreements.[91]

Recognition of "stylistic" differences among physicians highlighted certain tensions inherent in ONCOCIN's task. Eradication of clinical idiosyncrasy by computerized protocol might reduce clinically significant heterogeneity. But it also risked butting up against the physician's very identity—the personalized styles of practice with which many physicians came to identify.

Such realizations during the process of clinical implementation drove revisions to the system. Some of these revisions were geared toward identifying, and respecting, the so-called "stylistic" dimensions of decision-making. The

ONCOCIN team began "developing criteria for determining when a physician's preferred treatment is a clinically significant difference from what ONCOCIN has recommended."[92] Articulating a conceptual distinction between "substantive" and "stylistic" modes of medical practice was one thing; delineating the criteria that would actually differentiate between the two was another entirely.

The social circumstances around medical decision-making also tripped up ONCOCIN. Treatment decisions in medicine rest not just on medical evidence but also on the patient's values, goals, and circumstances. Yet it was impossible for the ONCOCIN team to formally encode all the possible social, moral, and personal drivers of therapeutic decision-making. This hole in ONCOCIN's knowledge base sometimes led the system to deliver recommendations that, while justifiable on the basis of oncologic protocol and medical evidence, were "wrong" considering the wider context of patients' life circumstances.

Shortliffe recounted one such case in 1987. On a typical Friday afternoon, a young woman with lymphoma was seen at the Stanford oncology clinic. ONCOCIN recommended business as usual: full, 100 percent continuation of the patient's current chemotherapy regimen. The physician, however, sharply disagreed, opting instead to give her no treatment. When the Stanford team encountered this discrepancy, they pressed the physician: what, they probed, could account for such a stark disagreement? As Shortliffe later described it, "The physician explained that the patient was to be a bridesmaid the next day and had asked to delay her treatment (which routinely caused a day or so of nausea) until after the weekend."[93] Shortliffe recognized that such a decision required knowledge that would be difficult, if not impossible, to incorporate into a computerized system like ONCOCIN: "Her request was eminently reasonable, but formulating a proper response required both medical expertise (to determine if a brief delay in treatment would be dangerous) and world knowledge (about bridesmaids, the nature of nausea, and why a patient would not want to be nauseated during a wedding)."[94]

As ONCOCIN went live, the Stanford team surveyed the oncology fellows for their early impressions of the system. Responses to the system were varied, with some fellows feeling "spoil[ed]" by ONCOCIN's advice and others complaining that the system was "so time-consuming" so as to "leave a sour taste in users' mouths."[95] Despite the system's technological capacity for explanation, some physicians could not shake the professional and moral discomfort with ceding medical decision-making to a machine. One fellow, for example, found it hard to imagine foregoing his own decision in favor of the computer's, no matter how crystal-clear its reasoning process: "I would use the system 'in parallel' with my own judgments. But, I wouldn't 'trust' the computer if there was some disagreement; I would never change my decision if the system differed from me."[96]

Reluctance to heed computer-generated decisions may have been fueled by legal uncertainties as well. Many raised questions regarding who would carry the burden of responsibility for a computerized decision that resulted in a poor patient outcome. The user of the system? Its developers? In the mid-twentieth century, this was uncharted legal territory. In an interview with *Computer Compacts*, Shortliffe highlighted the absence of formal legal precedents for many of these questions and noted, "It is unclear what the liability will be of those who built the system. But the physician will certainly be involved."[97] These legal issues remained unresolved even into the late 1980s. In 1987, the *Boston Globe* reported how a computerized diagnostic system is likely to "raise new ethical and legal questions, specialists say. Will the system, for instance, become so commonplace that a doctor who does not back up his diagnosis with a computer be considered negligent? On the other hand, might a doctor be held accountable for overrelying on the computer and underrelying on his own clinical skills and judgments?"[98] As one specialist in medical information systems quipped, "The lawyers could have us either way."[99] These questions would linger in the minds of physicians, no matter how slick MYCIN's or ONCOCIN's explanation technology and user interface.

Despite enduring uncertainties, ONCOCIN generated promising results. Shortliffe and his colleagues found that ONCOCIN promoted increased completeness in clinical data collection, with physicians collecting and reporting the data expected by oncology protocols at higher rates following the program's implementation.[100] Beyond promoting thoroughness of recordkeeping, the advice that ONCOCIN dispensed, the team discovered, also met reasonably high standards. In a study of 415 clinic visits involving ONCOCIN, the team found that the computer system's recommendations were identical to the treatment provided by physicians in 46 percent of cases. Where physicians and the system disagreed, an independent panel of expert oncologists found the differing recommendations to be equally acceptable.[101] Despite its promise, ONCOCIN never caught on widely.

The MYCIN project's legacy did not end with ONCOCIN. Even as its medical instantiations stumbled, its other descendants marched onward, reaching fields far outside that of medicine. The large demand for MYCIN's software inspired Edward Feigenbaum to found a company, Teknowledge, whose goal was "to migrate EMYCIN into the commercial domain, make it industrial strength, sell it, and apply it."[102] MYCIN's influence even extended beyond the successes of its immediate spin-offs. The project defined a new paradigm of research and practice—the rule-based expert system—that would dominate the field of AI through the 1980s. AI pioneer Allen Newell saw MYCIN as both the original impetus and the principal driver of this transformation toward expert systems approaches. It was, he believed, "the granddaddy of them all—the one that launched the field."[103]

But even this new field of AI, once ascendant, would ultimately fall out of favor. By the 1990s, researchers largely abandoned the expert systems approach to AI, returning to statistical approaches that did not require explicit enumeration of expert knowledge. The reasons behind this abandonment were many, but they largely centered on challenges that were already apparent during the field's early MYCIN years. Again and again, developers ran up against the challenge of having to render implicit forms of knowledge explicit, and of having to maintain unruly, ever-expanding knowledge bases. The struggles that plagued this next wave of expert systems engineers would have been familiar to members of the MYCIN team, who spent countless hours trying to "extract" and "crystallize" sometimes implicit and poorly defined areas of knowledge, and to update, modify, debug, and expand an untamed slurry of IF-THEN rules.

Despite the ultimate fate of MYCIN, and of the larger transformation it wrought, the history of the program brings out tensions, topics, and themes that transcend this particular computerized system, this particular approach to AI, and this particular time period. As computers entered the realm of medical diagnosis and decision-making for the first time, matters of trust and transparency emerged as sites of intense moral tension. How could human physicians hope to fully understand a computerized system that took many individuals, working across many years and many disciplines, to develop? How could physicians be expected to place matters of life and death in the hands of faceless algorithms? What kinds of biases might become calcified by an opaque, computerized algorithm? Such questions drove the development of, and responses to, MYCIN, as Part III has shown.

Almost from the outset, members of the MYCIN team were determined to create a system whose medical reasoning was clear and transparent, subject to the physician's appraisal and, ultimately, rejection. This determination stemmed not just from concerns about transparency but also from concerns about acceptance, identity, and authority. The purpose of explanation was to convey *both* medical and social information. In developing MYCIN and its explanation capabilities, the Stanford team inscribed certain assumptions about the nature of medical knowledge (explicit, modular)—and about the identity of physicians (atomistic, controlling).

The MYCIN group pursued technological solutions to this problem of trust and transparency—a problem that had moral, social, legal, and epistemological dimensions. Depending on the specific instantiation of the project, these technological fixes took on different names: with MYCIN it went by "Subprogram 2"; with ONCOCIN it was "the Interviewer." Yet these technological features invariably fell short. To deliver IF-THEN rules to physician-users, no matter how sophisticated the user interface, was not to instill a true understanding of MYCIN's reasoning process or its broader domain. Clancey spoke to this gap by referencing some of his past work: "In April 1975, I wrote an essay, 'Why is the Tetracycline rule so difficult to understand?' This simple rule presented itself as a puzzle: 'If the patient is less than 7 years old, then do not prescribe Tetracycline.' I knew what all the words meant, but I couldn't understand why the rule was correct. . . . What did it mean to understand a rule?"[104]

Clancey's reflections highlight some of the epistemological barriers to MYCIN's explanation capabilities. But other barriers existed as well. Medical diagnosis is not just about knowledge and information; diagnoses are made within a rich bureaucratic, moral, social, professional, and economic context, and they perform social and moral, as well as medical, work. As Charles Rosenberg has described, diagnosis "is a ritual that has always linked doctor and patient, the emotional and the cognitive, and, in doing so, has legitimated physicians' and the medical system's authority while facilitating particular clinical decisions and providing culturally agreed-upon meanings for individual experience."[105] Inevitably, then, relegating the task of diagnosis to machine was more than an informational challenge. MYCIN's technological capacity to "explain itself" did little to resolve the profound moral uncertainties of ceding important medical decisions to a machine, nor did it address broader legal and regulatory questions around blame, responsibility, and oversight. Transparent display of MYCIN's rules did not guarantee that certain assumptions and biases were not still "hidden in the code."[106]

# Conclusion

On April 11, 2018, the US Food and Drug Administration (FDA) granted marketing approval for the device IDx-DR, a software program developed by an Iowa-based biotech company that detects diabetic retinopathy. The press release announced, "The US Food and Drug Administration today permitted marketing of the first medical device to use artificial intelligence to detect greater than a mild level of the eye disease diabetic retinopathy in adults who have diabetes."[1] A noteworthy feature of IDx-DR is its diagnostic autonomy: the software's results do not need secondary approval or interpretation by a human physician. IDx-DR thus became the first FDA-approved fully autonomous diagnostic system in any area of medicine. The device uses an artificial intelligence (AI) algorithm to analyze patient retinal images captured by the Topcon NW 400 camera for signs of diabetic retinopathy. By allowing for diagnosis of this eye disease without a visit to the ophthalmologist—on the basis of images that can be captured at primary care offices—the developers hope that the device will save the vision of countless patients through earlier detection.

The FDA's decision followed the results of a multisite study of nine hundred patients known to have diabetes but with no known diagnosis of diabetic retinopathy. The device's performance was impressive. Compared to the gold standard of human grading of diabetic retinopathy, the device diagnosed with a sensitivity of 87.2 percent, a specificity of 90.7 percent, and an imageability rate of 96.1 percent, exceeding "all pre-specified superiority endpoints."[2] The findings, the clinical trialists concluded, demonstrated "AI's ability to bring specialty-level diagnostics to primary care settings."[3]

The US primary care setting hasn't been the only target for AI systems like IDx-DR. Similar technologies are being applied internationally to under-resourced settings. The Aravind Eye Hospital in Madurai, India, recently looked to automated AI systems to ease what it sees as a growing "bottleneck" problem, with massive numbers of diabetic patients and few trained ophthalmologists to evaluate them.[4] Partnering with a team of Google AI researchers, the hospital launched an algorithm that was developed to detect diabetic retinopathy. The system, Aravind's chief medical officer argued, would allow physicians "more time to work closely with patients on treatment and management of their disease while increasing the volume of screenings we can perform."[5]

This application of AI to ophthalmologic diagnosis, though notably far along, is by no means unique.[6] AI technologies are rapidly being developed to help dermatologists identify skin malignancies from skin images, radiologists diagnose pulmonary tuberculosis and other lung diseases from chest radiographs, and pathologists detect prostate cancer from biopsy specimens.[7] Others are applying these methods not just to diagnose but also to predict: to forecast which patients will end up in the intensive care unit, or which chemotherapy recipients will survive after treatment—and for how long.[8] Indeed, computers have already come to assist, sometimes with little fanfare, medical decisions of all kinds, such as the interpretation of electrocardiograms. "Big data," many opine, "will transform medicine," "improv[ing] the ability of health professionals to establish a prognosis," "improv[ing] diagnostic accuracy," perhaps even "displac[ing] much of the work of radiologists and anatomical pathologists."[9] With recent strides in AI and big data, some, like the prominent cardiologist Eric Topol, are forecasting (and hailing) the coming "creative destruction of medicine."[10]

Rather than rehashing this book's arguments and contributions, I have pulled together in this conclusion a number of themes that run through each of the book's sections and bear directly on contemporary efforts to integrate AI and machine learning into medical care. As engineers, physicians, tech companies, and policy makers look forward and try to bring AI tools into the clinic, it is also helpful to look back. The performance of computers today surpasses that of computers fifty years ago by orders of magnitude. Even the actors in this history dealt with evolving computing capabilities: Shortliffe's PDP-10 computer was very different from Brodman's IBM 704, which still relied on vacuum tubes. Yet amid all this change, many of the hopes, fears, challenges, and tensions that we face in this so-called era of "big data" are nothing new.

## Hopes

Medicine in the mid-twentieth century faced a series of perceived crises. There was a crisis of information. Medical knowledge, it seemed, was growing at an unmanageable rate and showed no sign of letting up; there was simply too much for the individual physician to know. There was a crisis of manpower. The number of physicians seemed stagnant, even as the US population and its health needs climbed steadily upward; there were simply too many patients for the individual physician to see. There was a crisis of distribution. Whereas metropolitan centers had easy access to health information and services, rural parts of the country seemed increasingly isolated and cut off; there was simply too much ground for the individual physician to cover.

For early developers of computerized diagnostic systems, the computer offered an alluring technological fix for the pressing social, economic, and distributional challenges of the time. By consolidating and bringing vast amounts of information to the physician's fingertips, computers promised to ease the cognitive load of physicians inundated by growing stores of medical knowledge. By taking over certain rote and routine aspects of clinical care, they promised to increase the physician's clinical capacity—allowing the physician to see more patients, or to focus more on the "human" aspects of medical care. By linking large medical centers with rural health clinics, they promised to facilitate the distribution of medical knowledge and care to underserved regions.

A half-century later little has changed. Medicine's crises—and the computer's imagined role as a solution—track closely to those during Keeve Brodman, Vladimir Zworykin, and Edward Shortliffe's times. In a 2017 issue of the *New England Journal of Medicine* (*NEJM*), two physicians argue that medicine has reached a tipping point, with the human mind newly outstripped by the vastness and complexity of medical knowledge: "The complexity of medicine," they write, "now exceeds the capacity of the human mind. Computers are the solution."[11] Others today see a future with computers taking over the routinized aspects of medical care and giving physicians more time to build relationships with their patients at the human level. In his 2019 book *Deep Medicine*, Topol argues that AI has the potential to reverse the progressive dehumanization of medicine and restore its "human side."[12] Beyond improving medical services where they already exist, AI, many argue today, also promises to bring medical care to places and patients without existing or adequate care. This historical analysis does not suggest that AI and other technological solutions to such challenges are misplaced or unimportant. But the persistence of these perceived problems—and the persistence of the computer as a perceived solution—suggests that other social and economic factors must be addressed as well.

## Fears

Though an exciting prospect for some, the notion of computers taking over the work of diagnosis stirred an inner disquietude among many physicians during the mid-twentieth century. These critics saw the computer as an agent of medicine's dehumanization. This was a technology, they warned, that would distance physicians from their patients, denigrate physicians' intuitive skills, hasten the bureaucratization of medicine, and treat patients as data rather than individuals. Animating many of these critiques were concerns about deskilling and replacement. When computers began making medical decisions, what parts of medicine would remain under the physician's remit?

Recent years have seen the amplification of similar fears. AI pioneer Geoffrey Hinton has claimed, "It's quite obvious that we should stop training radiologists"—a view that has received backing from leading computer scientists and clinicians.[13] Such claims have rippled widely through the medical profession. One recent study found that fears about displacement of radiologists by AI may be driving many medical trainees away from the field of radiology.[14] With digital enthusiasts prophesying the complete transformation, if not end, of entire fields of medicine—radiology, pathology, dermatology—many physicians and physicians-in-training have expressed concern over how AI will transform, remake, or even eliminate existing jobs and roles.

Others have expressed unease about the computer's potential role in the erosion of medicine's humanistic foundation. These commentators worry that the spread of AI through medicine will replicate many of the problems around the implementation of electronic medical records (EMRs). Now ubiquitous, EMRs have, many physicians believe, disrupted doctor-patient relationships, upended professional rituals, increased administrative burdens, and contributed to feelings of burnout. The physician-writer Abraham Verghese has documented what he sees as the EMR-driven dehumanization of the art of medicine, with physicians increasingly treating the "iPatient"—the patient of the EMR—at the expense of the real patient. Verghese writes,

> The patient is still at the center but more as an icon for another entity clothed in binary garments: the "iPatient." Often, emergency room personnel have already scanned, tested, and diagnosed, so that interns meet a fully formed iPatient long before seeing the real patient. The iPatient's blood counts and emanations are tracked and trended like a Dow Jones Index, and pop-up flags remind caregivers to feed or bleed. iPatients are handily discussed (or "card-flipped") in the bunker, while the real patients keep the beds warm and ensure that the folders bearing their names stay alive on the computer.[15]

Developers of AI systems, Verghese argues with colleagues, should pay heed: "The lessons learned with the EMR should serve as a guide as artificial intelligence and machine learning are developed to help process and creatively use the vast amounts of data being generated in the health care system."[16] Verghese's admonitions, while prescient, carry forward a line of thinking that has been in the making for more than half a century.

## Biases

The histories of the Medical Data Screen (MDS), HEME, and MYCIN all highlight how data get made. None of the actors in this book stumbled upon complete, cleaned, and fully formed data. Instead, they *created* these data, employing all kinds of assumptions and decisions in the process. The data on which the MDS was based, for example, reflected important decisions that Brodman had to make in developing the Cornell Medical Index (CMI): his choices about which questions to include, and his decisions about which population of patients on which to test the questionnaire. The data behind certain versions of the hematology program also rested on subjective human judgments. When, for example, the team looked to the medical literature for data on which to base their program, they discovered a remarkable absence of clarity and uniformity. Different clinicians and researchers reported medical data differently; they held to varying levels of quality, used different disease names, and fell at different places along the qualitative-quantitative spectrum. Making sense of such data—extracting, processing, and combining them—was no simple matter. It required the team to make subjective, ad hoc decisions about which studies to include and exclude, how to resolve contradictory reports, and whether and how to quantify qualitative data. The team turned to the medical literature to eliminate the need for human judgment—to do away with physician-generated estimates of significance in favor of objective significance data. Yet the need for subjective judgment remained. In the case of

MYCIN, data were made and constantly remade: the team was engaged in a process of relentless maintenance, always adding, subtracting, and tweaking the system's IF-THEN rules.

Attention to the contingencies and circumstances around the creation of data highlights the challenges of error and bias in computerized systems and medical algorithms. Although many mid-twentieth-century proponents of computerization viewed computerized systems as inherently objective, others were alive to possible problems of error and bias. These actors warned of the possibility of inaccurate reference data; they adopted the mantra, "garbage in, garbage out."

AI in health care today depends on the availability of massive, high-quality datasets. Yet insufficient attention is often paid to how these data get made. A historical perspective foregrounds the messy and monotonous, as well as contingent and consequential, work of data production. Medical data are extraordinarily complex. For them to be useful and meaningful, some kind of order must be imposed on them. In the process of imposing that order, however, decisions and judgments must be made, and biases and errors can be introduced. The use of big data in medicine has not erased the necessity for clinical and human judgment but rather defined new areas for its application. What assumptions, biases, and errors might a program encode and propagate? To what degree does a given program, and the data on which it was produced, apply to a given patient or patient population? These were questions that physicians grappled with in the mid-twentieth century, and they are questions that clinicians will continue to grapple with well into the twenty-first century.

These are not just hypothetical issues. Medical studies often suffer from relatively small numbers of racial and ethnic minorities. As a result, key sources of medical data often do not adequately represent all groups within society equally. AI systems based on such data may produce medical decisions suited for white patients, but not Black patients, for example.[17] Discrepancies between the data with which any AI system is created and the data on which it is applied leaves it vulnerable to the problem of "dataset shift."[18]

Similar scenarios of algorithms encoding racial bias and socioeconomic inequality have already been borne out by existing technologies, as Ruha Benjamin, Virginia Eubanks, and Safiya Noble have shown.[19] A machine-learning algorithm developed to predict the risk of criminal recidivism has displayed glaring racial biases.[20] Facial recognition software has performed worse on nonwhite faces because this software was developed with unrepresentative data.[21] Racialized algorithms for kidney function likely contribute to disparities in health care access and delivery.[22] A widely used commercial algorithm exhibited a racial bias that halved the number of Black patients identified for additional medical care.[23] A historical perspective alerts us to the real possibility of AI calcifying bias and exacerbating disparities in our health care system. To the extent that history helps us understand where data come from—how data "get made"—it also represents an important tool as we work to avert and remedy the problems of bias.

Issues of bias apply not just to data but also to the kinds of people permitted to work with these data. Anthropologist Diana Forsythe has described the gatekeeping around the people and perspectives accepted and valued in the field of medical informatics. As a participant-observer across five early medical informatics sites, Forsythe noted the "marginalization of women, their work, and their bodies, leaving men in symbolic possession of the Laboratory core."[24] The paucity of women and minorities in this book speaks to the "demographically and politically male" (and white) character of many of these spaces.[25] Despite efforts to increase equity and access, women and racial minorities remain underrepresented in biomedical informatics–related disciplines today.[26]

## Standards

It is a commonplace of evidence-based medicine to speak of "the gold standard"—of the randomized controlled trial as the gold standard of evidence, of *this* or *that* procedure as the gold standard of practice. The history of digitizing diagnosis demonstrates how elusive gold standards of diagnosis can be. After early developers created system prototypes, they frequently wanted to test them. How well did these systems perform compared to human physicians? Immediately, though, the developers realized that often in medicine gold standards of performance are difficult to identify and define. All too often there is no Supreme Court in medical decision-making. Instead, people like Brodman, Shortliffe, and Ralph Engle encountered a world of medicine where experts disagreed and varied in their judgments. In response to these realities, they pursued methodological innovations and clever research designs, for example, comparing the computer's performance against varying gradations of expertise and using "super experts" to evaluate the evaluators. Yet the fundamental fact remained that whether the computer was "correct" could not always be known with certainty.

Today, standards continue to present difficulties for those working to computerize medical decision-making. In machine learning systems, developers must use a training dataset that defines "ground truth" for the algorithm: the machine learning algorithm uses the training set to mathematically define borders between cases on the basis of already-known classifications in the training data. In medicine, confidently defining "ground truth," arriving at these already-known classifications, is no simple matter.[27] Because data about disease diagnosis can be messy and inaccurate, based in large part on subjective human judgments, the training data for ground truth can be off. Almost always, then, ground truth in medicine is fuzzy. Moving out from diagnosis in particular to decision-making more broadly, medical decisions are often not matters of black-and-white fact but rather matters of morals and values: the "right" treatment, for instance, depends not just on the results of randomized controlled trials but also on the goals and circumstances of the patient. If, how, and whether computers should be applied in such situations remain open and hotly contested questions.

The MYCIN team's methodological challenges around evaluation and validation also shed light on current problems. Certain characteristics of AI systems, both real and theoretical, have forced regulators to revisit best practices for designing, implementing, and reporting clinical trials. How should clinical trials report the handling of input and output data for AI systems so that researchers and consumers can critically appraise trial designs and outcomes? What is the best way to evaluate AI systems that can evolve and continuously train on new data even after they are first validated? Such questions have recently been taken up by multinational consensus committees, resulting in revised clinical trial reporting guidelines.[28] As AI technologies and applications rapidly change, these questions will need to be continually revisited by teams that engage not just their technical dimensions but their ethical, clinical, and social dimensions as well.

## Opacities

Through the mid-twentieth century, pioneers of computerized diagnosis debated different approaches to digitizing medical decision-making. Some looked inward, trying to define, explicate, and ultimately computerize how human physicians go about the process of making a diagnosis. Others looked outward—to new, nonhuman modes of reasoning. To this crowd, mimicry made little sense: not only are the strengths of the computer different from those of the human but humans may make medical decisions in suboptimal ways. Computerize diagnosis, they proposed, in a way that maximized the relative strengths of the machine and minimized the relative weaknesses of the human.

Central to the debate over the relative merits of these different strategies was the question of interpretability. Many argued that by replicating human reasoning processes, the computer would generate decisions that humans could understand, evaluate, affirm, or override. Other, more statistically oriented modes of reasoning, by contrast, risked looking opaque and foreign—uninterpretable. In the former scenario, some believed, physicians would be more willing to accept and adopt computerized systems, as these technologies would be more deferential to their authority and autonomy.

Much work went into unveiling the computer's reasoning before the physician, as the MYCIN case illustrates. Shortliffe and his colleagues developed sophisticated technologies that allowed MYCIN to "explain itself." Their hope was that by delivering to the physician the decision rules that MYCIN had used in its decision-making process, physicians would find the system more acceptable. Yet even with this technological capability, problems and concerns remained. Some questioned whether the display of IF-THEN rules really constituted meaningful explanation. Others continued to worry about possible biases "hidden in the code" of MYCIN and how these biases might undermine the physician's personal responsibility to the individual patient. These technological solutions, moreover, did not resolve open legal and regulatory questions concerning liability.

Interpretability has only become more of an ethical, legal, and professional flashpoint in recent years. Because machine learning algorithms create their own decision patterns and criteria on the basis of vast quantities of data, it is often impossible for humans to understand the processes by which AI systems arrive at their decisions. Motivated by novel digital challenges like those of the "black box," the European Union rolled out a General Data Protection Regulation in 2018 that established a "right to explanation."[29] In medicine, a domain where machine learning may be applied not to matters of advertising revenue and click-through rates but potentially to matters of life and death, the problem of interpretability is particularly salient. Many commentators believe that turning medical decisions over to uninterpretable machines runs counter to the physician's moral and professional duties. Others point out that additional core medical tenets, such as those of patient disclosure and safety, may also be challenged by AI systems that are making medical decisions in the dark.[30]

Not all, however, are so worried. Some have countered that concerns about interpretability are overblown—that the validity of computer-generated decisions should be held up as a higher social value.[31] Human intelligence, others point out, is often unintelligible and inexplainable, and society already tolerates all kinds of black boxes in medicine, such as the mechanisms of all kinds of drugs.[32]

While many researchers are pursuing promising technological solutions to the problem of interpretability—rolling out natural language processing technologies, developing AI systems to interpret the results of the original AI system, and defining the new research area of Explainable AI (XAI)—history suggests that the challenges introduced by opaque AI systems will not be solved through technological solutions alone. Interpretability is a value with ethical, legal, and professional valences. For example, if making an AI system interpretable comes at the expense of its predictive accuracy (as is sometimes the case), what should be done? The problems around interpretability can only be addressed through the collective moral, legal, and regulatory work of articulating, and implementing, societal standards of transparency and validation.

## Identities

The computer didn't just capture and implement preexisting notions of medical reality.[33] It also generated new notions about what medicine was and what it could be. It opened up a space where physicians and engineers began to rethink and redefine fundamental categories and roles. The computer's first forays into medical diagnosis prompted people like Brodman, Zworykin, Engle, and Shortliffe to reflect on the physician's identity—to carve out the aspects of medical work and medical thought that belonged to human physicians and those that belonged to machine. Always, ideas about the computer's "appropriate" role in the clinical environment reflected, reinforced, and displaced certain ideas about the nature and identity of humans. The patient's identity too was reconfigured and reimagined as data for computer processing.

Early computerized diagnostic programs were also mutually constitutive with respect to disease identities. The MDS, for example, both gave rise to and depended upon conceptions of disease that translated the "symptom complex" into the language of numbers, statistics, and thresholds. The hematology team similarly generated new ways of defining hematologic disease through their engagements with new digital media.

Questions about how computers may reconfigure disease, professional, and patient identities remain relevant today. As computers take on new clinical tasks, the kinds of work deemed "appropriately human" may shift. Already computing technologies have transformed how certain medical personnel are seen, and how they see themselves. In the 1990s, radiological reading rooms around the country adopted a technology called picture archiving and communication system (PACS). A medical imaging capability, PACS provides radiologists and other clinicians ready, digital access to radiological images and their associated interpretations and reports. Following the implementation of PACS, the radiological reading room—once a place bustling with activity, a place where physicians of all kinds would come to discuss a case—became removed and isolated from the rest of the hospital.[34] Because of PACS, the physical objects that drew clinicians of all stripes to this space—slides or film—were no more.

This transformation of social patterns within the hospital has influenced the radiologist's identity. Many radiologists have expressed concern about new limitations in their ability to "communicate clinical recommendations, relevant research, or alternate diagnostic options with the patient care team" following the adoption of PACS.[35] They have also felt increasingly disconnected. One senior radiologist opined, "We [radiologists] knew all the clinicians intimately before. And then with PACS, this intimacy disappeared. Before, I knew the face, name, wife's name, and kids' names of all the clinicians, but now I don't know who you are if you joined the medical staff after we got PACS. Now we're operating in a void because there's no history of the patient on the written image requests. Before, when a clinician showed up, I could ask them and find out what's really going on with the patient."[36]

Computing technologies can also shape the identities of patients and their diseases. How individuals experience disease today differs wildly from how individuals experienced disease in the past. More than ever before, our experience and understanding of disease is mediated through numbers. Though a patient may not subjectively feel sick, he might interact with the medical system as a prediabetic because his fasting blood sugar level falls between 100 and 125 mg/dL. Though a patient may not actually have breast cancer, she might make important health and life decisions knowing that, as a BRCA1 mutation carrier, she has a roughly 65 percent chance of developing breast cancer by the age of 70. Patients such as these experience health and disease not through any extant symptoms but through numbers—and through regimens of medical surveillance and management designed to minimize the health risks associated with these numbers.[37] Many patients today stand before what anthropologist S. Lochlann Jain evocatively calls "the firing squad of statistics."[38]

In addition to the experience of patienthood, the act of diagnosis is also an increasingly numerical enterprise. For most of history, patients' personal feelings and reports of their own health and body formed the basis of disease and diagnosis; in one way or another, a patient diagnosed with "dis-ease" really did subjectively lack ease. This is not always so for patients today. Whether a patient has a given disease is often a statistical question. Physicians and patients today inhabit a world in which medicine and statistics have converged—a world of "risky medicine."[39]

Computing technologies did not create this modern style of defining and experiencing disease. But this book prompts consideration of the ways in which they may have had a hand in shaping it. A number of pathways are readily apparent: these technologies permit the complex computations and administer the large databases that underlay a growing web of epidemiological knowledge; they, through automated health screenings and electronic health records, form much of the basis for our contemporary screening apparatus; and they have facilitated the intensification of diagnostic testing through phenomena like the automated processing of tests.

Such possibilities were on the front of the minds of people like Zworykin. In 1967, for example, an associate wrote to Zworykin about their shared interest in "how computer data processing [could be] used to obtain an 'early warning system' "—that is, a way of identifying and monitoring "at risk" patients.[40] Throughout his speeches and writings, Zworykin often spoke of computerized diagnosis and large-scale medical monitoring in the same breath. Zworykin foresaw a future in which computer centers storing medical records would collect "tremendous amounts of clinical data" and "provide the basis for medical statistical studies on an unparalleled scale."[41] Such information, he suggested, would allow physicians, researchers, and public health officials to make "many elusive correlations" among sundry clinical variables.[42] In many respects, the world Zworykin imagined is the world we live in today.

## Continuities

Computerization is often synonymous with change. It makes things faster and more efficient, alters fundamental workflows, and promotes a world of information and interconnection. This book has tracked important changes attendant to the computer's introduction into medical diagnosis—changes in how diseases are defined, how medical information is created and handled, and how professional roles and patient identities are imagined and constructed. It has also traced important continuities that link our current digital world dominated by computers to our former analog world dominated by pen and paper. Many of the earliest efforts to computerize medical diagnosis evolved directly from paper-based methods and tools. The hematology program had its roots in Firmin Nash's analog "Logoscope" as well as Martin Lipkin and James Hardy's punched card method of making hematologic diagnoses. The computer-based Medical Data Screen would have never come into being had the paper-based Cornell Medical Index not existed before it. To marshal another example, the International Classification of Diseases (ICD) coding system came into being long before either medical records or diagnoses were digitized, even though the ICD system is now a core part of the information infrastructure on which these digital tools rely.[43]

The pattern here is one of path dependency and constraint. Decisions made with respect to analog tools and technologies often carried over into their digital descendants. The fact that Lipkin and Hardy's analog device made diagnoses by way of "matching" informed and motivated the matching algorithm that Zworykin and his colleagues ultimately chose to implement as they worked to computerize hematologic diagnosis. Similarly, the nature of the CMI questionnaire affected the functioning of the computerized MDS method—from the questions it included to the syndromal clusters of symptoms it recognized.

Understanding these continuities has important implications for imagining and implementing digital medicine today. Discussions about the impact of computers in fields such as medicine are not confined to the academic historical literature. Physicians, policy makers, social critics, and others frequently extol the virtues, or bemoan the harms, of computerized medicine. Topol, for example, has hailed the arrival of digital technologies that promise to facilitate new modes of medical research and reconfigure the relationship between doctor and patient.[44] Thanks to computerization, some suggest, the medicine of today is (unlike the medicine of yesterday) a "data-driven science." While commentators may disagree about the appeal of medicine's digital transformation, few quibble about its magnitude: when medicine moved from the analog world of paper charts to the digital world of electronic medical records, everything changed.

This history instructs us not to discard these claims about medicine's digital transformation: there is no question that the introduction of computers has changed medicine in important, even fundamental, ways. Rather, the cases presented here invite us to engage with these well-worn claims with more thought, scrutiny, and skepticism. This history offers a sobering countermelody to a familiar tune of sharp discontinuity and "creative destruction." As narratives of discontinuity and disruption dominate headlines, this story helps us to see the continuities that link our present to the past, to engage with the promises of computerized medicine more critically, and to appreciate that many of the questions and challenges that medicine faces today are not entirely new.

From a practical standpoint, even in our increasingly digital clinical environments, older paper data practices have not only persisted to varying degrees but also shaped how existing digital infrastructures are imagined, built, and used.[45] EMRs have fallen short of their promise and potential, with physicians now spending increasing amounts of time on administrative tasks, wading through excessive "alerts," and battling climbing levels of burnout. These shortcomings reflect some of the issues of contingency, path dependency, and constraint that this book has highlighted. By and large, EMRs were not developed as part of the total hospital infrastructure but rather in a fragmented manner, geared more toward billing and administration than toward patient care. Attending to, and grappling with, the legacies of paper technologies and epistemologies in our current digital environment is an important step on the way to reimagining and better implementing EMRs today.

## Complexities

"The making of correct diagnostic interpretations of symptoms," Brodman confidently declared in 1959, "can be a process in all aspects logical and so completely defined that it can be carried out by a machine."[46] Yet behind the scenes Brodman struggled with colleagues to work out lingering kinks and imperfections in their computerized method—and to open up the black box of how human physicians actually think. Zworykin's group chose to create a diagnostic program in the field of hematology because of the field's supposed objective, quantitative, and straightforward nature. Yet they quickly found that the field was rich with complexity—and subjectivity. Shortliffe and his colleagues worked to codify much of the field of infectious disease into hundreds of IF-THEN rules. Yet they discovered that certain aspects of medical knowledge were difficult to formalize—and that even the nontacit aspects of knowledge were subject to considerable debate, disagreement, and contestation among medical experts.

The actors followed in this book repeatedly came up against, and underestimated, the complexity of medicine and medical decision-making. This complexity came from many places: the idiosyncrasy of the individual patient, the heterogeneity of medical data, health and health care's moral overlay, the opacity of the human mind, and the social construction of many of medicine's classifications. While today's era of "big data" involves very different technologies, capabilities, and actors than the "big data" moment of the mid-to-late twentieth century, these fundamental complexities remain.

In Brodman and Zworykin's time, conversations about the role of computers in medical diagnosis found their way into mainstream fora for the first time in history. Either could have picked up the *New York Times* on February 8, 1958, to read the headline "Diagnosis by Computer Envisaged for Patients."[47] In this way, their time is not unlike our own. Stories about the possible uses of computers in medical diagnosis swarm both medical journals and lay publications.[48] The questions that motivate these accounts tend to be questions of accuracy. To what extent does the computer "get it right"? What features of medical practice and medical knowledge limit their accuracy? What can be done—from engineering, behavioral, or health systems standpoints—to improve their effective use?

These are important questions. We must understand how to integrate computerized and machine-learning methods into the social world of medicine in ways that promote effective and humane medical care. But it is also important to recognize that computers and algorithms, in diagnosing disease, do not just identify predefined disease entities. They give shape to what disease is and how we think about it. They construct new professional roles and identities. They create profound moral tensions around values like precision, trust, and transparency. They eliminate some human biases, while at the same time replicating and extending others.

This history offers no clear path forward. It does, however, widen our perspective; it raises pressing questions, problems, and challenges that must be addressed as we work to harness AI for the benefit of the medical profession and its patients.

# NOTES

## *Abbreviations*

| | |
|---|---|
| CBI | Charles Babbage Institute Oral Histories, University of Minnesota |
| CDP | Carl Djerassi Papers, Stanford University Libraries |
| EFP | Edward A. Feigenbaum Papers, Stanford University Libraries |
| ESP | Edward H. Shortliffe Papers, National Library of Medicine |
| HKW | Homer Richards and Katherine Romney Warner Papers, University of Utah Libraries |
| HSP | Herbert A. Simon Papers, Carnegie Mellon University Archives |
| HWP | Harold Wolff Papers, Cornell University Medical Archives |
| JLP | Joshua Lederberg Papers, National Library of Medicine |
| KBP | Keeve Brodman Papers, Cornell University Medical Archives |
| MPC | Mayo Clinic Pamphlet Collection, Mayo Clinic Archival Collections |
| REP | Ralph L. Engle, Jr. Papers, Cornell University Medical Archives |
| RMP | The Regional Medical Programs Collection, National Library of Medicine |
| ROO | Regional Oral History Office, Bancroft Library, University of California, Berkeley |
| RUR | Rockefeller University Records, Catalogs and Directories, Rockefeller Archive Center |
| SCP | Stanley N. Cohen Papers, National Library of Medicine |
| SHP | Starke Rosecrans Hathaway Papers, University of Minnesota Archives |
| VZP | Vladimir K. Zworykin Papers, David Sarnoff Collection, Hagley Museum and Library |

## *Introduction*

1. Charles E. Rosenberg, "The Tyranny of Diagnosis: Specific Entities and Individual Experience," *Milbank Quarterly* 80, no. 2 (2002): 237–260.

2. Quoted in Rosenberg, "Tyranny of Diagnosis," 241.

3. Martin Campbell-Kelly and William Aspray, *Computer: A History of the Information Machine* (New York: Basic Books, 1996); Paul N. Edwards, *The Closed World: Computers and the Politics of Discourse in Cold War America* (Cambridge, MA: MIT Press, 1996); Agatha C. Hughes and Thomas P. Hughes, eds., *Systems, Experts, and Computers: The Systems Approach in Management and Engineering, World War II and After* (Cambridge, MA: MIT Press, 2000). Among more recent additions to the literature are Atsushi Akera, *Calculating a Natural World: Scientists, Engineers, and Computers during the Rise of US Cold War Research* (Cambridge,

MA: MIT Press, 2008); Stephanie Dick and Janet Abbate, eds., *Abstractions and Embodiments: New Histories of Computing and Society* (Baltimore: Johns Hopkins University Press, 2022); Michael S. Mahoney, "The Histories of Computing(s)," *Interdisciplinary Science Reviews* 30, no. 2 (2005): 119–135.

4. On artificial intelligence, see Stephanie Dick, "AfterMath: The Work of Proof in the Age of Human-Machine Collaboration," *Isis* 102, no. 3 (2011): 494–505; Stephanie Dick, "Artificial Intelligence," *Harvard Data Science Review* 1, no. 1 (2019); Stephanie Dick, "Of Models and Machines: Implementing Bounded Rationality," *Isis* 106, no. 3 (2015): 623–634; Matthew L. Jones, "How We Became Instrumentalists (Again): Data Positivism since World War II," *Historical Studies in the Natural Sciences* 48, no. 5 (2018): 673–684. On the challenges of writing the history of machine learning, see Aaron Plasek, "On the Cruelty of Really Writing a History of Machine Learning," *IEEE Annals of the History of Computing* 38, no. 4 (2016): 6–8. There are also more popular and less analytical accounts of artificial intelligence (many by individuals with personal ties to the field). See, e.g., Pamela McCorduck, *Machines Who Think: A Personal Inquiry into the History and Prospects of Artificial Intelligence* (New York: W. H. Freeman, 1979); Pamela McCorduck, *This Could Be Important: My Life and Times with the Artificial Intelligensia* (Pittsburgh: ETC Press, 2019); Nils J. Nilsson, *The Quest for Artificial Intelligence: A History of Ideas and Achievements* (Cambridge: Cambridge University Press, 2010). On bias and race, see, e.g., Ruha Benjamin, *Race After Technology: Abolitionist Tools for the New Jim Code* (Medford: Polity, 2019); Safiya Umoja Noble, *Algorithms of Oppression: How Search Engines Reinforce Racism* (New York: New York University Press, 2018). On gender, see, e.g., Janet Abbate, *Recoding Gender: Women's Changing Participation in Computing* (Cambridge, MA: MIT Press, 2012); Mar Hicks, *Programmed Inequality: How Britain Discarded Women Technologists and Lost Its Edge in Computing* (Cambridge, MA: MIT Press, 2017).

5. There is also a flourishing literature on the history of (big) data. See, e.g., Elena Aronova, Christine von Oertzen, and David Sepkoski, "Introduction: Historicizing Big Data," *Osiris* 32, no. 1 (2017): 1–17; Dan Bouk, *How Our Days Became Numbered: Risk and the Rise of the Statistical Individual* (Chicago: University of Chicago Press, 2015); Hallam Stevens, "A Feeling for the Algorithm," *Osiris* 32, no. 1 (2017): 151–174; Lorraine Daston, ed., *Science in the Archive: Pasts, Presents, Futures* (Chicago: University of Chicago Press, 2017); Rebecca Lemov, *Database of Dreams: The Lost Quest to Catalog Humanity* (New Haven, CT: Yale University Press, 2015); Theodore M. Porter, *Genetics in the Madhouse: The Unknown History of Human Heredity* (Princeton, NJ: Princeton University Press, 2018); Bruno J. Strasser, *Collecting Experiments: Making Big Data Biology* (Chicago: University of Chicago Press, 2019); Jacqueline Wernimont, *Numbered Lives: Life and Death in Quantum Media* (Cambridge, MA: MIT Press, 2019).

6. For helpful, albeit somewhat outdated, reviews of the literature, see Jennifer Stanton, "Making Sense of Technologies in Medicine," *Social History of Medicine* 12 (1999): 437–448; Harry M. Marks, "Medical Technologies: Social Contexts and Consequences," in *Companion Encyclopedia of the History of Medicine*, vol. 2, edited by W. F. Bynum and Roy Porter (New York: Routledge, 1993), 1592–1618. For some specific examples, see Joel D. Howell, *Technology in the Hospital: Transforming Patient Care in the Early Twentieth Century* (Baltimore: Johns Hopkins University Press, 1995); Thomas Schlich and Christopher Crenner, eds., *Technological Change in Modern Surgery: Historical Perspectives on Innovation* (Rochester: University of Rochester Press, 2017); Carsten Timmermann and Julie Anderson, eds., *Devices and Designs: Medical Technologies in Historical Perspective* (New York: Palgrave Macmillan, 2006); Keith Wailoo, *Drawing Blood: Technology and Disease Identity in Twentieth-Century America* (Baltimore: Johns Hopkins University Press, 1997).

7. There are important and notable exceptions. See Warwick Anderson, "The Reasoning of the Strongest: The Polemics of Skill and Science in Medical Diagnosis," *Social Studies of Science* 22, no. 4 (1992): 653–684; Marc Berg, *Rationalizing Medical Work: Decision Support*

*Techniques and Medical Practices* (Cambridge, MA: MIT Press, 1997); Brian Dolan and Allison Tillack, "Pixels, Patterns, and Problems of Vision: The Adaptation of Computer-Aided Diagnosis for Mammography in Radiological Practice in the US," *History of Science* 48 (2010): 227–249; Stanley Joel Reiser, *Medicine and the Reign of Technology* (Cambridge: Cambridge University Press, 1978); Stanley Joel Reiser, *Technological Medicine: The Changing World of Doctors and Patients* (Cambridge: Cambridge University Press, 2009).

8. Where November and Stevens focus primarily on the computer's role in biomedical research, this book focuses more on its impacts within clinical medicine. Joseph A. November, *Biomedical Computing: Digitizing Life in the United States* (Baltimore: Johns Hopkins University Press, 2012); Hallam Stevens, *Life Out of Sequence: A Data-Driven History of Bioinformatics* (Chicago: University of Chicago Press, 2013). Other works that explore the application of computation to biomedical research include Lily E. Kay, *Who Wrote the Book of Life? A History of the Genetic Code* (Stanford: Stanford University Press, 2000); C. Stewart Gillmor, *Fred Terman at Stanford: Building a Discipline, a University, and Silicon Valley* (Stanford: Stanford University Press, 2004).

9. See, e.g., Matthew Fuller, ed., *Software Studies: A Lexicon* (Cambridge, MA: MIT Press, 2008); Janet Vertesi and David Ribes, eds., *digitalSTS: A Field Guide for Science and Technology Studies* (Princeton, NJ: Princeton University Press, 2019).

10. Jeremy A. Greene, *The Doctor Who Wasn't There: Technology, History, and the Limits of Telehealth* (Chicago: University of Chicago Press, 2022); Kirsten Ostherr, *Medical Visions: Producing the Patient through Film, Television, and Imaging Technologies* (Oxford: Oxford University Press, 2013); Volker Hess and J. Andrew Mendelsohn, "Case and Series: Medical Knowledge and Paper Technology, 1600–1900," *History of Science* 48, no. 3–4 (2010): 287–314; Volker Hess and J. Andrew Mendelson, "Sauvages' Paperwork: How Disease Classification Arose from Scholarly Note-Taking," *Early Science and Medicine* 19, no. 5 (2014): 471–503; Hannah Zeavin, *The Distance Cure: A History of Teletherapy* (Cambridge, MA: MIT Press, 2021).

11. Mary Croarken, "Mary Edwards: Computing for a Living in 18th-Century England," *IEEE Annals of the History of Computing* 25, no. 4 (2003): 9–15. See also Martin Campbell-Kelly, William Aspray, Nathan Ensmenger, and Jeffrey R. Yost, *Computer: A History of the Information Machine*, 3rd ed. (New York: Routledge, 2014), 4.

12. Campbell-Kelly et al., *Computer*, 3rd ed., 21.

13. Howell, *Technology in the Hospital*, 40–42.

14. Indeed, intelligence obtained with the aid of Colossus informed the timing of the Normandy landings in 1944. Thomas Flowers, Alan Turing, William Tutte, and Max Newman are among the key individuals who worked on this early computer, as are many women "operators" whose critical work has often been overlooked. Abbate, *Recoding Gender*, 11–38; B. Jack Copeland, "Colossus: Its Origins and Originators," *IEEE Annals of the History of Computing* 26, no. 4 (2004): 38–45.

15. Campbell-Kelly and Aspray, *Computer*, 60–64.

16. Campbell-Kelly and Aspray, *Computer*, 63.

17. Campbell-Kelly and Aspray, *Computer*, 63. See also Kurt W. Beyer, *Grace Hopper and the Invention of the Information Age* (Cambridge, MA: MIT Press, 2009), 37.

18. For a detailed account of the events that culminated in the development of this computing device, see Harry Polachek, "Before the ENIAC," *IEEE Annals of the History of Computing* 19, no. 2 (1997): 25–30. Also see Campbell-Kelly and Aspray, *Computer*, 76–82.

19. The UNIVAC, for Universal Automatic Computer, was the direct descent of the ENIAC. On the emergence and maturation of the mainframe computing industry, see Campbell-Kelly et al., *Computer*, 3rd ed., 59–139.

20. Paul E. Ceruzzi, "When Computers Were Human," *IEEE Annals of the History of Computing* 13, no. 3 (1991): 237–244, p. 240.

21. Campbell-Kelly et al., *Computer*, 3rd ed., 203–225.

22. On the social history of computing, see Nathan Ensmenger, "Power to the People: Toward a Social History of Computing," *IEEE Annals of the History of Computing* 26, no. 1 (2004): 94–96.

## *Chapter 1 • Indexing the World*

1. Howard Bleich, himself a pioneer in biomedical computing, has written a short, encyclopedic overview of Brodman and the CMI. See Howard Bleich, "Keeve Brodman and the Cornell Medical Index," *MD Computing* 13, no. 2 (1996): 119–120, 122, 124. Brodman is also mentioned briefly in other histories of technology and biomedical computing. See Stanley Joel Reiser, *Medicine and the Reign of Technology* (Cambridge: Cambridge University Press, 1978), 215.

2. Keeve Brodman, "City College Alumni Association Medical Doctors Questionnaire," box 7, folder 4, KBP.

3. Antonio M. Gotto, Jr., and Jennifer Moon, *Weill Cornell Medicine: A History of Cornell's Medical School* (Ithaca, NY: Cornell University Press, 2016); Joseph C. Hinsey, "Cornell University Medical College," *Phi Kappa Phi Journal* 36, no. 1 (1946): 15–17.

4. Brodman to Headquarters, Second Corp Area, 90 Church Street, NY, October 4, 1940, box 7, folder 6, KBP.

5. The Adjutant General's Office, War Department to Brodman, July 3, 1942, box 7, folder 1, KBP; Henry Cave to Brodman, July 8, 1942, box 7, folder 6, KBP.

6. M. Chase to Commanding Officer, Station Hospital, July 8, 1943, box 7, folder 2, KBP.

7. Brodman to Arnold Albright, March 29, 1943, box 7, folder 2, KBP; Brodman to Patrick J. Madigan, May 11, 1943, box 7, folder 6, KBP. See also Brodman to Flanders Dunbar, June 1, 1943, box 7, folder 2, KBP.

8. Robert C. Powell, "Helen Flanders Dunbar (1902–1959) and a Holistic Approach to Psychosomatic Problems. I: The Rise and Fall of a Medical Philosophy," *Psychiatric Quarterly* 49, no. 2 (1977): 133–152; Robert C. Powell, "Helen Flanders Dunbar (1902–1959) and a Holistic Approach to Psychosomatic Problems. II: The Role of Dunbar's Nonmedical Background," *Psychiatric Quarterly* 50, no. 2 (1978): 144–157.

9. Brodman to Commanding Officer, Station Hospital, "Group Psychotherapeutic Clinics for Patients in the Cardiac Section, Station Hospital, Virginia," May 29, 1943, box 7, folder 2, KBP.

10. Brodman to Commanding Officer, Station Hospital, "Group Psychotherapeutic Clinics."

11. M. Chase to All Medical Officers, Station Hospital, Camp Lee, memorandum, n.d. (circa June 1943), box 7, folder 2, KBP.

12. M. Chase to Commanding Officer, Station Hospital, July 8, 1943, box 7, folder 2, KBP.

13. Keeve Brodman, "A Program for Psychosomatic Medicine in the Army," unpublished report, May 1943, p. 12, box 7, folder 6, KBP.

14. Surgeon General to Commanding General, Third Service Command, July 17, 1943, box 7 folder 2, KBP.

15. Brodman to Surgeon General (War Department), "Request for Assignment," January 28, 1944, box 7, folder 2, KBP.

16. Brodman to Surgeon General (War Department), "Request for Assignment."

17. Harold Wolff to Karl Menninger, January 22, 1944, box 7, folder 2, KBP.

18. Harold Wolff to Karl Menninger, January 22, 1944.

19. C. D. Bowen to Brodman, March 18, 1944, box 7, folder 2, KBP. See also Malin Craig, Proceeding of an Army Retiring Board in the Case of Major Keeve Brodman, Medical Corps, Army of the United States, Washington, DC, March 24, 1944, box 7, folder 2, KBP.

20. Keeve Brodman, *Men at Work: The Supervisor and His People* (Chicago: Cloud, 1947).

21. T. B. Campion to Brodman, n.d., box 3, folder 10, KBP.

22. Arthur Weider, Bela Mittelmann, David Wechsler, Harold G. Wolff, and Margaret Meixner, "The Cornell Selectee Index: A Method for Quick Testing of Selectees for the Armed Forces," *JAMA* 124 (1944): 224–228; Arthur Weider, Keeve Brodman, Bela Mittelmann, David Wechsler, and Harold G. Wolff, "Cornell Service Index: A Method for Quickly Assaying Personality and Psychosomatic Disturbances in Men in the Armed Forces," *War Medicine* 7 (1945): 209–213; Arthur Weider, Keeve Brodman, Bela Mittelmann, David Wechsler, and Harold G. Wolff, "The Cornell Index: A Method for Quickly Assaying Personality and Psychosomatic Disturbances, to Be Used as an Adjunct to Interview," *Psychosomatic Medicine* 8 (1946): 411–413; and Bela Mittelmann and Keeve Brodman, "The Cornell Indices and the Cornell Word Form: 1. Construction and Standardization," *Annals of the New York Academy of Sciences* 46 (1946): 573–578.

23. Arthur Weider, "Screening the Neuropsychiatrically Unfit Selectee from the Armed Forces" (PhD diss., New York University, 1945).

24. Weider et al., "The Cornell Selectee Index," 225.

25. On the history of federal regulation, repression, and penalization of homosexuality, see Margot Canaday, *The Straight State: Sexuality and Citizenship in Twentieth-Century America* (Princeton, NJ: Princeton University Press, 2009).

26. Harold J. Harris, "Cornell Selectee Index: An Aid in Psychiatric Diagnosis," *Journal Annals of the New York Academy of Sciences* 49, no. 7 (1946): 593–605, p. 599.

27. Roy A. Darke and George A. Geil, "Homosexual Activity: Relation of Degree and Role to the Goodenough Test and to the Cornell Selectee Index," *Journal of Nervous and Mental Disease* 108, no. 3 (1948): 217–240, p. 239. The literature on the problematic use of imprisoned, enslaved, dispossessed, and otherwise vulnerable populations in biomedical research is extensive. See, e.g., Allen M. Hornblum, *Acres of Skin: Human Experiments at Holmesburg Prison* (New York: Routledge, 1998); Harriet A. Washington, *Medical Apartheid: The Dark History of Medical Experimentation on Black Americans from Colonial Times to the Present* (New York: Doubleday, 2006). On the entangled histories of sexuality and carcerality, see Regina Kunzel, *Criminal Intimacy: Prison and the Uneven History of Modern American Sexuality* (Chicago: University of Chicago Press, 2008).

28. On the prehistory of algorithmic bias against gender and sexual minorities, see, e.g., Mar Hicks, "Hacking the Cis-tem: Transgender Citizens and the Early Digital State," *IEEE Annals of the History of Computing* 41, no. 1 (2019): 20–33.

29. Margo Anderson, *The American Census: A Social History* (New Haven, CT: Yale University Press, 1988).

30. Dan Bouk, *How Our Days Became Numbered: Risk and the Rise of the Statistical Individual* (Chicago: University of Chicago Press, 2015). On the interrelations between medicine and life insurance, see Audrey B. Davis, "Life Insurance and the Physical Examination: A Chapter in the Rise of American Medical Technology," *Bulletin of the History of Medicine* 55, no. 3 (1981): 392–406. The term "quantifying spirit" comes from Tore Frängsmyr, J. L. Heilbron, and Robin Rider, eds., *The Quantifying Spirit in the 18th Century* (Berkeley: University California Press, 1990).

31. Sarah Igo, *The Averaged American: Surveys, Citizens, and the Making of a Mass Public* (Cambridge, MA: Harvard University Press, 2007).

32. Harry M. Marks, *The Progress of Experiment: Science and Therapeutic Reform in the United States, 1900–1990* (Cambridge: Cambridge University Press, 1997). See also Robert Aronowitz, *Risky Medicine: Our Quest to Cure Fear and Uncertainty* (Chicago: University Chicago Press, 2015), 69–94.

33. See, e.g., Roderick D. Buchanan, "The Development of the Minnesota Multiphasic

Personality Inventory," *Journal of the History of the Behavioral Sciences* 30, no. 2 (1994): 148–161; Merve Emre, *The Personality Brokers: The Strange History of Myers-Briggs and the Birth of Personality Testing* (New York: Doubleday, 2018).

34. "Operation Medical Screen," draft proposal to Veterans Administration, March 3, 1961, p. 8, box 1, folder 7, KBP.

35. Keeve Brodman, Albert J. Erdmann, Jr., Irving Lorge, Harold G. Wolff, and Todd H. Broadbent, "The Cornell Medical Index: An Adjunct to Medical Interview," *JAMA* 140 (1949): 530–534, p. 530.

36. Keeve Brodman, "The Cornell Medical Index: A Health Questionnaire to Help the Doctor Help You," unpublished article for *Cosmopolitan Magazine*, n.d. (circa July 1949), p. 1, box 3, folder 10, KBP.

37. Brodman, "The Cornell Medical Index."

38. Brodman et al., "An Adjunct to Medical Interview," 530–534; Keeve Brodman, "The Cornell Medical Index-Health Questionnaire: II. As a Diagnostic Instrument," *JAMA* 145 (1951): 152–157; Keeve Brodman, Albert J. Erdmann, Jr., Irving Lorge, and Charles P. Gershenson, "The Cornell Medical Index-Health Questionnaire: III. The Evaluation of Emotional Disturbances," *Journal of Clinical Psychology* 8 (1952): 119–124; Keeve Brodman, Albert J. Erdmann, Jr., Irving Lorge, Charles P. Gershenson, Harold G. Wolff, and Todd H. Broadbent, "The Cornell Medical Index-Health Questionnaire: IV. The Recognition of Emotional Disturbances in a General Hospital," *Journal of Clinical Psychology* 8 (1952): 289–293; Albert J. Erdmann, Jr., Keeve Brodman, Irving Lorge, and Harold G. Wolff, "The Cornell Medical Index-Health Questionnaire: V. Outpatient Admitting Department of a General Hospital," *JAMA* 149 (1952): 550–551; Keeve Brodman, Albert J. Erdmann, Jr., Irving Lorge, and Harold G. Wolff, "The Cornell Medical Index-Health Questionnaire: VI. The Relation of Patients' Complaints to Age, Sex, Race, and Education," *Journal of Gerontology* 8 (1952): 339–342; Keeve Brodman, Albert J. Erdmann, Jr., Irving Lorge, Jerome Deutschberger, and Harold Wolff, "The Cornell Medical Index-Health Questionnaire: VII. The Prediction of Psychosomatic and Psychiatric Disabilities in Army Training," *American Journal of Psychiatry* 111 (1954): 37–40.

39. Brodman et al., "An Adjunct to Medical Interview," 530.

40. Lynn S. Bickley, Barbara Bates, and Peter G. Szilagyi, *Bates' Guide to Physical Examination and History Taking*, 11th ed. (Philadelphia: Lippincott, Williams, and Wilkins, 2013), 10.

41. For a rich engagement with the aesthetic dimensions of medicine, see John Harley Warner, "The Aesthetic Grounding of Modern Medicine," *Bulletin of the History of Medicine* 88, no. 1 (2014): 1–47.

42. The order and wording of these example questions come from the revised version of the CMI, as depicted in figure 1.1. The original 1949 version had a slightly different order and question content. See Keeve Brodman, Albert J. Erdmann, Jr., and Harold G. Wolff, *Manual: Cornell Medical Index-Health Questionnaire* (New York: Cornell University Medical College, 1956), 8–12, box 1, folder 3, KBP.

43. Brodman, "As a Diagnostic Instrument," 152.

44. See J. Andrew Mendelson, "The World on a Page: Making a General Observation in the Eighteenth Century," in *Histories of Scientific Observation*, edited by Lorraine Daston and Elizabeth Lunbeck (Chicago: University Chicago Press, 2011), 396–420; Volker Hess and J. Andrew Mendelsohn, "Case and Series: Medical Knowledge and Paper Technology, 1600–1900," *History of Science* 48 (2010): 287–314; and Volker Hess, "A Paper Machine of Clinical Research in the Early Twentieth Century," *Isis* 109 (2018): 473–493.

45. Hess and Mendelsohn, "Case and Series," 288–289.

46. Hess and Mendelsohn, "Case and Series," 291.

47. Hess and Mendelsohn, "Case and Series," 293.

48. See, e.g., Brodman et al., "An Adjunct to Medical Interview"; Brodman et al., "The Evaluation of Emotional Disturbances."

49. Brodman et al., "An Adjunct to Medical Interview," 530.

50. Brodman et al., "An Adjunct to Medical Interview," 531.

51. Brodman et al., "An Adjunct to Medical Interview," 531.

52. Brodman, "As a Diagnostic Instrument."

53. Brodman et al., "An Adjunct to Medical Interview," 532.

54. Brodman et al., "An Adjunct to Medical Interview," 532.

55. On the history of standardization in medicine, see Stefan Timmermans and Marc Berg, *The Gold Standard: The Challenge of Evidence-Based Medicine and Standardization in Health Care* (Philadelphia: Temple University Press, 2003).

56. Brodman, Erdmann, and Wolff, *Manual: Cornell Medical Index-Health Questionnaire*, 5.

57. Brodman, Erdmann, and Wolff, *Manual: Cornell Medical Index-Health Questionnaire*, 6.

58. On the history of taking a history, see Jonathan Gillis, "The History of the Patient History Since 1850," *Bulletin of the History of Medicine* 80, no. 3 (2006): 490–512.

59. Michael Mulkay, Trevor Pinch, and Malcolm Ashmore, "Colonizing the Mind: Dilemmas in the Application of Social Science," *Social Studies of Science* 17, no. 2 (1987): 231–256.

60. Brodman et al., "An Adjunct to Medical Interview," 534.

61. Brodman et al., "An Adjunct to Medical Interview," 534. Emphasis added.

62. Erdmann et al., "Outpatient Admitting Department of a General Hospital," 551.

63. "The Patient Tells His Story," *BMJ* 4796 (1952): 1246.

64. Brodman to Erich Meyerhoff, January 20, 1976, box 5, folder 1, KBP.

65. "The Patient Tells His Story," 1246.

66. "The Patient Tells His Story," 1246.

67. On the history of medical specialization in the United States, see Rosemary Stevens, *American Medicine and the Public Interest* (New Haven, CT: Yale University Press, 1971); George Weisz, *Divide and Conquer: A Comparative History of Medical Specialization* (Oxford: Oxford University Press, 2006).

68. R. Logan, "Correspondence: The Patient Tells His Story," *BMJ* (December 27, 1952): 1414.

69. Graham Grant and R. A. N. Hitchens, "Correspondence: The Patient Tells His Story," *BMJ* 4801 (January 10, 1953): 100–101, p. 100.

70. Eric Hodgins, "Listen: The Patient," *NEJM* 274 (1966): 657–661, p. 659.

71. Eric Hodgins, "Listen," 660. The patient was the novelist Eric Hodgins. He detailed his patient experience in his memoir *Episode: Report on the Accident Inside My Skull* (New York: Atheneum, 1964).

72. Multiphasic screening programs were also met with praise. Editorial, "Report on the Screening Clinic," *NEJM* 243 (1950): 275; Vlado A. Getting and Herbert L. Lombard, "The Evaluation of Pilot Clinics—The Mass Screening or Health-Protection Program," *NEJM* 247 (1952): 460–465. On the history of computing and multiphasic screening, see Jeremy A. Greene, *The Doctor Who Wasn't There: Telemedicine, History, and the Limits of Technology* (Chicago: University of Chicao Press, 2022).

73. E. M. Glaser and G. C. Whittow, "Experimental Errors in Clinical Trials," *Clinical Science* 13, no. 2 (1954): 199–210. For a sharp historical analysis of the "diagnostics of suspicion" around patients and their credibility, see Lakshmi Krishnan, "Person Under Investigation: Detecting Malingering and a Diagnostics of Suspicion in Fin-de-Siècle Britain," *Journal of Law, Medicine, and Ethics* 49, no. 3 (2021): 343–356.

74. "Questionaries in Clinical Trials," *BMJ* 4875 (June 12, 1954): 1366–1367.

75. Brodman to H. J. van Heyst, February 23, 1965, box 3, folder 13, KBP.

76. J. J. Fleminger to Brodman, January 20, 1965, box 3, folder 13, KBP.

77. Harold Braun to Brodman, September 26, 1966, box 4, folder 1, KBP; Henry Glah, Jr., to Brodman, October 9, 1966, box 4, folder 1, KBP.

78. Harriet Jean Anderson, "Questionnaire Helps Doctors Diagnose Ills; Cornell Medical's Health Form Proves Efficiency During Four-Year Test," *New York Herald Tribune*, March 9, 1951, p. 16.

79. Margaret Boomer to Brodman, April 14, 1953, box 6, folder 2, KBP. The quote comes from the introduction to an article—enclosed in the letter—that was to appear in a May 1, 1953, issue of *Vision*.

80. J. Anderson and J. L. Day, "New Self-Administered Medical Questionary," *BMJ* 4 (1968): 636–638, p. 636.

81. Brodman to Meyerhoff, February 11, 1976, box 5, folder 1, KBP.

82. See Cornell Medical Index translations, box 1, folders 5–6, KBP. See also Cornell Medical Index translation, box 2, folder 10, HWP.

83. Robert Turfbeer to Albert Erdmann, Jr., November 28, 1955, box 1, folder 5, KBP.

84. A. L. Cochrane, P. J. Chapman, and P. D. Oldham, "Observers' Errors in Taking Medical Histories," *Lancet* (May 5, 1951): 1007–1009. Cochrane became a forerunner and inspiration to the self-described "evidence-based medicine" movement of the late twentieth century, particularly following the publication of his 1972 book *Effectiveness and Efficiency: Random Reflections on Health Services* (London: Nuffield Provincial Hospitals Trust, 1972). David S. Jones and Scott H. Podolsky, "The History and Fate of the Gold Standard," *Lancet* 385, no. 9977 (2015): 1502–1503.

85. Cochrane et al., "Observers' Errors in Taking Medical Histories," 1008.

86. Philip Ball to Brodman, October 28, 1966, box 4, folder 1, KBP. Emphasis added.

87. Brodman, "The Cornell Medical Index: A Health Questionnaire to Help the Doctor Help You," pp. 1–2, box 3, folder 10, KBP.

88. Brodman to F. Chicou, March 29, 1971, box 5, folder 1, KBP.

89. Hirotugu Miyaki to Brodman, n.d. (circa March 1967), box 4, folder 2, KBP; Matilde de Dilva to Brodman, March 25, 1953, box 6, folder 2, KBP.

90. R. D. Verson to Brodman, June 12, 1962, box 6, folder 2, KBP.

91. Ludwig G. Laufer, "Cultural Problem Encountered in the Use of the Cornell Index among the Okinawan Natives," *American Journal of Psychiatry* 109, no. 11 (1953): 861–864, p. 862.

92. Norman A. Scotch and H. Jack Geiger, "An Index of Symptom and Disease in Zulu Culture," *Human Organization* 22, no. 4 (1963–1964): 304–311. H. Jack Geiger, then a newly minted physician with a strong activist bent, would go on to become a leader in the social medicine, community health, and civil rights movements. On Geiger, see Thomas J. Ward, Jr., *Out in the Rural: A Mississippi Health Center and Its War on Poverty* (New York: Oxford University Press, 2017).

93. Scotch and Geiger, "An Index of Symptom and Disease in Zulu Culture," 311.

94. Scotch and Geiger, "An Index of Symptom and Disease in Zulu Culture," 311.

95. Many other cross-cultural studies of the CMI were conducted during this period. See, e.g., Norman A. Chance, "Conceptual and Methodological Problems in Cross-Cultural Health Research," *American Journal of Public Health* 52, no. 3 (1962): 410–417; Esko Kalimo, Thomas W. Bice, and Marija Novosel, "Cross-Cultural Analysis of Selected Emotional Questions from the Cornell Medical Index," *British Journal of Preventive and Social Medicine* 24, no. 4 (1970): 229–240; Delbert M. Kole, "Cross-Cultural Study of Medical-Psychiatric Symptoms," *Journal of Health and Human Behavior* 7, no. 3 (1966): 164–174. The CMI's use outside of the United States reflects a broader postwar craze of using psychological and medical testing instruments (e.g., Rorschach inkblot test) to understand and catalog "remote" popu-

lations. See, e.g., Rebecca Lemov, *Database of Dreams: The Lost Quest to Catalog Humanity* (New Haven, CT: Yale University Press, 2015).

96. Brodman, "The Cornell Medical Index: A Health Questionnaire to Help the Doctor Help You," pp. 2–3, box 3, folder 10, KBP.

97. On "users" in science and technology studies and the history of science, see Nelly Oudshoorn and Trevor Pinch, eds., *How Users Matter: The Co-Construction of Users and Technologies* (Cambridge, MA: MIT Press, 2003).

98. Harold Wolff to Paul B. Magnuson, February 29, 1952, box 3, folder 5, KBP; Charles Glock to Irving Lorge, August 6, 1951, box 3, folder 5, KBP.

99. On the Bureau of Applied Social Research in the context of American survey research, see Jean M. Converse, *Survey Research in the United States: Roots and Emergence 1890–1960* (Berkeley: University of California Press, 1987).

100. Wolff to Magnuson, February 29, 1952.

101. Igo, *The Averaged American*, 16.

102. Wolff to Magnuson, February 29, 1952.

103. Unsigned letter to Irving Lorge, October 2, 1951, box 3, folder 5, KBP.

104. Unsigned letter to Irving Lorge, October 2, 1951.

105. Unsigned letter to Irving Lorge, October 2, 1951.

106. Notes on Oneonta Project, July 31, 1951, box 3, folder 5, KBP.

107. President's Commission on the Health Needs of the Nation, *Building America's Health: A Report to the President*, vol. 1 (Washington, DC: Government Printing Office, 1952), ix.

108. Harold Wolff to Joseph C. Hinsey, January 14, 1952, box 3, folder 5, KBP.

109. Magnuson to Wolff, February 18, 1952, box 3, folder 5, KBP.

## *Chapter 2 · The Statistical Patient*

1. For a discussion of this television appearance, see Lindsey M. Banco, "Presenting Dr. J. Robert Oppenheimer: Science, the Atomic Bomb, and Cold War Television," *Journal of Popular Film and Television* 45, no. 3 (2017): 128–138.

2. Einstein would die just a few months after Oppenheimer's January television appearance. Michael D. Gordin, *Einstein in Bohemia* (Princeton, NJ: Princeton University Press, 2020), 5.

3. Brodman to J. Robert Oppenheimer, January 12, 1955, box 3, folder 11, KBP.

4. Brodman to Oppenheimer, January 12, 1955.

5. Brodman to Oppenheimer, January 12, 1955.

6. Brodman to Oppenheimer, January 12, 1955.

7. Brodman to Oppenheimer, January 12, 1955.

8. Katherine Russell to Brodman, February 3, 1955, box 3, folder 11, KBP.

9. Brodman to Julian Bigelow, March 10, 1955, box 3, folder 11, KBP. Bigelow later published an essay on computing at the Institute for Advanced Study during this period. See Julian Bigelow, "Computer Development at the Institute for Advanced Study," in *A History of Computing in the Twentieth Century*, edited by N. Metropolis, J. Howlett, and Gian-Carlo Rota (London: Academic Press, 1980), 291–310.

10. Brodman to Bigelow, March 10, 1955.

11. Brodman to Bigelow, March 10, 1955.

12. Bigelow to Brodman, April 13, 1955, box 3, folder 11, KBP.

13. Bigelow to Brodman, April 13, 1955.

14. Brodman to Bigelow, April 26, 1955, box 3, folder 11, KBP.

15. Brodman to Howard Rusk, August 26, 1954, box 7, folder 6, KBP.

16. Brodman to Norbert Wiener, April 26, 1953, box 7, folder 6, KBP.

17. Brodman to Bigelow, April 15, 1955, box 3, folder 11, KBP.

18. On Wiener, Bigelow, and cybernetics, see Peter Galison, "The Ontology of the Enemy: Norbert Wiener and the Cybernetic Vision," *Critical Inquiry* 21 (1994): 228–266.

19. Norbert Wiener, *Cybernetics: Or, Control and Communication in the Animal and the Machine* (New York: J. Wiley, 1948).

20. Warren S. McCulloch and Walter Pitts, "A Logical Calculus of the Ideas Immanent in Nervous Activity," *Bulletin of Mathematical Biophysics* 5 (1943): 115–133.

21. On McCulloch and Pitts, see Tara H. Abraham, *Rebel Genius: Warren S. McCulloch's Transdisciplinary Life in Science* (Cambridge, MA: MIT Press, 2016). As Abraham has shown, the 1943 McCulloch-Pitts article preceded the cybernetics moment and should not be read *solely* as a proto-cybernetic idea or intervention. Nevertheless, McCulloch would become a leader in the cybernetics movement, and the ideas in the paper would serve as a foundation for a great deal of cybernetic thought.

22. For an account of the Macy Conferences on Cybernetics, see Steve J. Heims, *The Cybernetics Group* (Cambridge, MA: MIT Press, 1991).

23. This variability has led the historian Ronald Kline to refer to the "disunity" of cybernetics. Ronald R. Kline, *The Cybernetics Moment, Or Why We Call Our Age the Information Age* (Baltimore: Johns Hopkins University Press, 2015).

24. The significance of the Dartmouth conference to the emergence of artificial intelligence as a field has been hotly debated. McCarthy himself was disappointed that the conference did not coalesce into a unified research enterprise. Roland R. Kline, "Cybernetics, Automata Studies, and the Dartmouth Conference on Artificial Intelligence," *IEEE Annals of the History of Computing* 33, no. 4 (2010): 5–16.

25. John McCarthy, Marvin Minsky, Nathaniel Rochester, and Claude Shannon, "A Proposal for the Dartmouth Summer Research Project on Artificial Intelligence," *AI Magazine* 27 (2006): 12–14, p. 12. This is a reprint; the original is dated August 31, 1955.

26. Within this formulation of artificial intelligence, there remained significant variability. Researchers at Carnegie like Herbert Simon and Allen Newell pursued a heuristic ("rules of thumb") approach to artificial intelligence, whereas the MIT-based McCarthy and Marvin Minsky aimed for more algorithmic-driven conceptions. Hunter Crowther-Heyck, *Herbert A. Simon: The Bounds of Reason in Modern America* (Baltimore: Johns Hopkins University Press, 2005), 226–227.

27. Stephanie Dick, "Artificial Intelligence," *Harvard Data Science Review* 1, no. 1 (2019). Kline, *The Cybernetics Moment*, 179–185.

28. Andrew Pickering, *The Cybernetic Brain: Sketches of Another Future* (Chicago: University Chicago Press, 2010).

29. Quoted in Kline, *The Cybernetics Moment*, 12.

30. Brodman to Bigelow, July 23, 1955, box 3, folder 11, KBP.

31. Charles Robinson to Brodman, 1955, box 6, folder 3, KBP.

32. Robinson to Brodman, 1955.

33. For a brief, high-level overview of Van Woerkom's career, see his obituary in the *Bulletin of the American Astronomical Society (AAS)*. Raynor L. Duncombe and Morris S. Davis, "A. J. J. van Woerkom (1915–1991)," *Bulletin of the AAS* 23, no. 4 (1991): 1495.

34. Brodman to Van Woerkom, July 9, 1955, box 6, folder 3, KBP.

35. Brodman to Van Woerkom, February 3, 1960, box 6, folder 3, KBP.

36. Brodman to Van Woerkom, January 31, 1960, box 6, folder 3, KBP.

37. Brodman to Van Woerkom, February 3, 1960.

38. Brodman to Van Woerkom, February 4, 1960, box 6, folder 3, KBP.

39. Warren S. McCulloch and Walter Pitts, "How We Know Universals: The Perception

of Auditory and Visual Forms," *Bulletin of Mathematical Biophysics* 9 (1947): 127–147, pp. 127–128.

40. Wiener, *Cybernetics*, 133.

41. See, e.g., Oliver Selfridge, "Pandemonium: A Paradigm of Learning," in National Physical Laboratory, *Mechanisation of Thought Processes* (London: Her Majesty's Stationary Office, 1959), 511–529.

42. Kline, *The Cybernetics Moment*, 12.

43. Untitled notes, April, 20 1955, box 3, folder 11, KBP. No author is listed for these notes. Brodman's authorship can be inferred with a considerable level of confidence from the notes' content and style, which accord with that of his other writings, correspondence, and notes. See, e.g., Brodman to Van Woerkom, October 12, 1957, box 6, folder 3, KBP.

44. Brodman did, however, read materials that were rich in cybernetic thought. In 1960, he wrote to Van Woerkom, "I am sending you the books on *Mechanisation of Thought Processes*. You will find a great deal of material in it of interest to us" (Brodman to Van Woerkom, May 5, 1960, box 6, folder 3, KBP). These volumes were the published versions of a symposium held at the National Physical Laboratory in November 1958. The symposium brought together leading figures in the fields of cybernetics, artificial intelligence, pattern recognition, and other related areas. See, e.g., Andrew Pickering, "Psychiatry, Synthetic Brains, and Cybernetics in the Work of W. Ross Ashby," *International Journal of General Systems* 38, no. 2 (2009): 213–230.

45. Paul Edwards, *A Vast Machine: Computer Models, Climate Data, and the Politics of Global Warming* (Cambridge, MA: MIT Press, 2010), 83–110. Brodman noted to Van Woerkom in 1956, "As I told you yesterday, the listing you gave me on Friday indicates that the missing 10% of CMIs in the 1948 sample were not lost in a random manner as I had hoped" (Brodman to Van Woerkom, March 13, 1956, box 6, folder 3, KBP).

46. Brodman to Gerald Fleischli, October 2, 1970, box 5, folder 1, KBP.

47. Brodman to Van Woerkom, December 1, 1955, box 6, folder 3, KBP.

48. Brodman to Van Woerkom, December 21, 1955, box 6, folder 3, KBP.

49. Keeve Brodman, Adrianus J. van Woerkom, Albert J. Erdmann, Jr., and Leo S. Goldstein, "Interpretation of Symptoms with a Data-Processing Machine," *AMA Archives of Internal Medicine* 103 (1959): 116–122.

50. Keeve Brodman, "Diagnostic Decisions by Machine," *IRE Transactions on Medical Electronics* ME-7 (1960): 216–219, p. 217. On statistical aspects, see Adrianus J. van Woerkom and Keeve Brodman, "Statistics for a Diagnostic Model," *Biometrics* 17 (1961): 299–318.

51. Adrianus van Woerkom, "Program for a Diagnostic Model," *IRE Transactions on Medical Electronics* ME-7 (1960): 220.

52. Brodman, "Diagnostic Decisions by Machine," 216.

53. Brodman, "Diagnostic Decisions by Machine," 217.

54. Lucy Suchman, *Human-Machine Reconfigurations: Plans and Situated Actions* (Cambridge: Cambridge University Press, 2006), 226–240; Stephanie Dick, "AfterMath: The Work of Proof in the Age of Human-Machine Collaboration," *Isis* 102 (2011): 494–505.

55. Brodman to Van Woerkom, March 29, 1958, box 6, folder 3, KBP.

56. Brodman, "Diagnostic Decisions by Machine," 219.

57. This progression was not perfectly linear. For example, Brodman's musings about pattern recognition, discussed in the previous section, came after he and his colleagues published their first accounts of the "machine method" in 1959. These discussions about pattern recognition, however, would not amount to anything concrete, and Brodman and Van Woerkom soon returned to the machine method as originally published.

58. Keeve Brodman and Adrianus J. van Woerkom, "Computer-Aided Diagnostic Screening for 100 Common Diseases," *JAMA* 197 (1966): 179–183.

59. Brodman to Barbara Bates, October 18, 1967, box 4, folder 2, KBP.

60. Keeve Brodman, *Manual: Medical Data Screen Index (MEDIS)* (New York: Medical Data Corporation, 1964), p. 11, box 1, folder 11, KBP.

61. Brodman to Van Woerkom, July 30, 1964, box 6, folder 4, KBP.

62. Arnold Wander to Otto Wendel, November 4, 1967, box 4, folder 2, KPB.

63. On lay attitudes toward computers, see, e.g., Sarah Igo, *The Known Citizen: A History of Privacy in Modern America* (Cambridge, MA: Harvard University Press, 2018), 232–263.

64. "Operation Diagnostic Screen," "Rapid screening of VA patients for 100 diseases," draft application, n.d. (proposed project dates: May 1, 1961 to April 30, 1963), box 3, folder 12, KBP.

65. Max M. Kampelman to Brodman, February 13, 1962, box 3, folder 12, KBP.

66. Philip Sperling to Brodman, February 26, 1962, box 3, folder 12, KBP.

67. Ralph Bradley to Brodman, November 11, 1960, box 3, folder 12, KBP.

68. Brodman (likely) to Kampelman, January 12, 1960, box 3, folder 12, KBP. While the name Max Kampelman is written at the top of this letter, its author and recipient are not definitively clear. From its content and style—and its context within other letters sent between Brodman and Kampelman—I have inferred that it is a letter from Brodman to Kampelman.

69. Arnold Wander to Herbert Krasnow, December 5, 1967, box 4, folder 2, KBP. This letter was sent to Krasnow via his secretary. See also Wander to Krasnow, September 22, 1967, box 4, folder 2, KBP.

70. Brodman to Wander, September 27, 1967, box 4, folder 2, KBP.

71. "Computers Programmed to Sort Routine Symptoms," *Medical World News*, February 16, 1968, p. 61.

72. Wander to Krasnow, November 30, 1967, box 4, folder 2, KBP.

73. Wander to Krasnow, November 30, 1967.

74. G. W. Geelhoed and E. M. Druy, "Management of the Adrenal 'Incidentaloma,'" *Surgery* 92 (1982): 866–874. The term "incidentaloma" was coined in the 1980s, as computer tomography (CT) scans were becoming increasingly available. The term refers to incidental findings for which there exists no corresponding symptoms. It sheds light on the complexities around overdiagnosis and overtreatment.

75. Wander to Brodman, April 16, 1968, box 4, folder 3, KBP.

76. Brodman to Harold Dehner, April 28, 1972, box 5, folder 1, KBP.

77. Brodman to Charles Roland, May 23, 1966, box 4, folder 1, KBP. The reviewer comments are enclosed in this letter.

78. Robert Albrecht to Brodman, December 5, 1968, box 4, folder 3, KBP.

79. Wander to Krasnow, November 6, 1967, box 4, folder 2, KBP; Wander to Krasnow, January 22, 1969, box 4, folder 3, KBP.

80. In 1965, the *Medical World News* had an estimated circulation between 205,000 and 230,000. "Challenging the Leader," *Time* 85, no. 5 (1965): 71.

81. "Computers Programmed to Sort Routine Symptoms," 61.

82. Joseph A. Louis to Wander, March 22, 1968, box 4, folder 3, KBP.

83. Raymond D. Fowler, "Computer Interpretation of Personality Tests: The Automated Psychologist," *Comprehensive Psychology* 8, no. 6 (1967): 455–467. Computerized applications of the MMPI took hold at the Mayo Clinic. Wendell M. Swenson, David Osborne, and Robert C. Colligan, "A User's Guide to Mayo Clinical Computerized Scoring and Interpretive System for the Minnesota Multiphasic Personality Inventory (MMPI), Second Edition," p. 1, box 4, folder "User's Guide – Mayo Clinic MMPI," MPC. More generally, the MMPI, much like the MDS, sparked conversations about the possible mathematical basis of the medical mind. To what extent does statistical inference resemble clinical inference? A lively debate materialized

around this question within the realm of clinical psychology, especially following the publication of Paul Meehl's book *Clinical versus Statistical Prediction* (Minneapolis: University of Minnesota Press, 1954).

84. Marvin L. Miller to Brodman, April 26, 1968, box 4, folder 3, KBP.

85. Brodman to Van Woerkom, July 30, 1964.

86. Lyndon B. Johnson, "Special Message to the Congress on the Nation's Health," February 10, 1964.

87. Johnson, "Special Message to the Congress on the Nation's Health."

88. Nate Haseltine, "Experts Ask US War on 3 Diseases," *Washington Post*, December 10, 1964, A1.

89. On the history of the RMP, see Stephen P. Strickland, *The History of Regional Medical Programs: The Life and Death of a Small Initiative of the Great Society* (Lanham, MD: University Press of America, 2000). On the RMP in the context of Johnson's other health care reform efforts, see Paul Starr, *The Social Transformation of American Medicine: The Rise of a Sovereign Profession and the Making of a Vast Industry* (New York: Basic Books, 1982), 370.

90. The President's Commission on Heart Disease, Cancer, and Stroke, *Report to the President: A National Program to Conquer Heart Disease, Cancer, and Stroke*, vol. 1 (Washington, DC: US Government Printing Office, 1964), 29, 32, 34–35.

91. Daniel M. Fox, *Health Policies, Health Politics: The British and American Experience, 1911–1965* (Princeton, NJ: Princeton University Press, 1986).

92. President's Commission, *A National Program to Conquer Heart Disease, Cancer, and Stroke*, 28–29.

93. Because the RMP reorganized the delivery of medical care and not just its financing, many physicians at the time perceived the program to be more radical than Medicare. They responded accordingly. See Robert Dallek, *Flawed Giant: Lyndon Johnson and His Times, 1961–1973* (Oxford: Oxford University Press, 1998), 675.

94. On Billy Jack Bass and the Automated Physician's Assistant, see Arthur E. Rikli, Fred V. Lucas, and Fred Frazier, "The Automated Physician's Assistant," *Clinical Engineering News* 3, no. 4 (1975): 3–5; John G. Rogers, "Dr. Billy Jack Bass: He's 'Helping to Make Medical History,' " *Palm Beach Post*, July 11, 1971, p. 138. See also "Interview with Dr. Arthur E. Rikli," July 25, 1991, RMPC.

95. Brodman to Miller, April 30, 1968, box 4, folder 3, KBP.

96. Gerald Fleischli to Brodman, October 3, 1968, box 4, folder 3, KBP.

97. National Commission on Technology, Automation, and Economic Progress, *Technology and the American Economy*, vol. 1 (Washington, DC: US Government Printing Office, 1966), xiv.

98. Brodman to Roland, May 23, 1966. Reviewer comments are enclosed in this letter.

99. *Technology and the American Economy*, 78–83, 112.

100. Brodman to Charles Burger, September 24, 1969, box 4, folder 4, KBP.

101. *Physicians for a Growing America*, Report of the Surgeon General's Group on Medical Education, publication no. 709 (Bethesda: US Department of Health, Education, and Welfare, 1959.)

102. On trends toward specialization through the twentieth century, see Rosemary Stevens, *American Medicine and the Public Interest* (New Haven, CT: Yale University Press, 1971); George Weisz, *Divide and Conquer: A Comparative History of Medical Specialization* (Oxford: Oxford University Press, 2006).

103. "Notes on a method for preventative medicine by the early recognition of patients with symptoms of 100 diseases," typescript, June 1, 1962, box 3, folder 12, KBP.

104. Brodman to Marvin Sameth, October 6, 1967, box 4, folder 2, KBP.

105. "Machine Diagnostic Screening of 10,000 Patients," Application for Research Grant (RG-9116), National Institutes of Health, March 17, 1961, box 1, folder 7, KBP.

106. Brodman to Sameth, October 6, 1967.

107. "Adjunct for Comprehensive Medical Diagnosis," Application for Research Grant (No. GM 14382–01), Public Health Service, February 1, 1966, box 1, folder 7, KBP/1/7.

108. "Adjunct for Comprehensive Medical Diagnosis."

109. Wander to Krasnow, November 7, 1967, box 4, folder 2, KBP.

110. Wander to Krasnow, December 5, 1967.

111. Notes on conference with Dr. Koriter of Roche, August 16, 1968, box 4, folder 3, KBP.

112. Notes on conference with Dr. Koriter of Roche, August 16, 1968.

113. Brodman to H. J. van Heyst, February 23, 1965, box 3, folder 13, KBP.

114. Brodman to Van Heyst, February 23, 1965.

115. One of Brodman's interlocuters echoed these sentiments, suggesting that "electronic data processing and standardization of procedure" would allow physicians to address "the hidden segment of the 'iceberg' of human suffering." Van Heyst to Brodman, March 11, 1965, box 3, folder 13, KBP; Van Heyst to Brodman, February 19, 1965, box 3, folder 13, KBP. This phrase—the iceberg of human suffering—was one that Van Heyst borrowed from the famous Midtown Manhattan Study, a pioneering psychiatric and sociological study that aimed to unpack the relationship between urban health and the social community. Leo Srole, Thomas S. Langner, Stanley T. Michael, Marvin K. Opler, and Thomas A. C. Rennie, *Mental Health in the Metropolis: The Midtown Manhattan Study* (New York: McGraw-Hill, 1962).

116. List of significant items for the 100 diseases, box 3, folder 9, KBP.

117. Draft of proposal to Veterans Administration, February 28, 1961, box 3, folder 12, KBP. Emphasis added.

118. Brodman et al., "Interpretation of Symptoms," 120.

119. On the role of digitization in reducing data friction, see W. Patrick McCray, "How Astronomers Digitized the Sky," *Technology and Culture* 55 (2014): 908–944.

120. Robert Ledley, quoted in Brodman to Kampelman, January 12, 1960. This quote cannot be verified with certainty, as it comes (via Brodman) from an unpublished draft manuscript titled "The Federal Government and Medical Electronics," which was prepared by the Subcommittee on Reorganization and International Organizations of the US Senate Committee on Government Operations. Nevertheless, the sentiment (about the importance of a priori diagnostic criteria) is one that Ledley also expressed in other contexts. See discussion of Taffee Tanimoto, "IBM Type 704 Medical Diagnosis Program," *IRE Transactions on Medical Electronics* ME-7 (1960): 280–283, p. 283.

121. Brodman to Kampelman, January 12, 1960.

122. Katharine Boucot to Brodman, December 28, 1966, box 4, folder 2, KBP.

123. Brodman to Van Woerkom, February 4, 1960, box 6, folder 2, KBP.

124. Keeve Brodman, *Manual: Medical Data Screen*, 2nd ed. (New York: Medical Data Corporation, 1966), with handwritten revisions, December 15, 1971, box 2, folder 10, KBP.

125. Brodman to Van Woerkom, December 11, 1967, box 6, folder 4, KBP.

126. Physicians at the time associated symptoms with the subjective and signs with the objective. Walter Modell, "The Full Treatment—A Modern View of the Relief of Symptoms," *NEJM* 255 (1956): 1079–1084.

127. Jeremy A. Greene, *Prescribing by Numbers: Drugs and the Definition of Disease* (Baltimore: Johns Hopkins University Press, 2007), 230–231. Indeed, the move away from symptoms permitted the emergence of an entirely new disease category: asymptomatic prediabetes.

128. Keeve Brodman, Application for Research Grant (RG-4743), National Institutes of Health, Division of Research Grants, January 20, 1960, box 1, folder 7, KBP. The 1952 publication was the book's second edition; the first edition came out in 1947. Cyril Mitchell Mac-

Bryde, ed., *Signs and Symptoms: Applied Pathologic Physiology and Clinical Interpretation*, 2nd ed. (Philadelphia: Lippincott, 1952).

129. Brodman to Van Woerkom, February 16, 1960, box 6, folder 3, KBP.

130. Steven Shapin, "A Taste of Science: Making the Subjective Objective in the California Wine World," *Social Studies of Science* 46, no. 3 (2016): 436–460, p. 451.

131. Miller to Brodman, December 12, 1972, box 5, folder 1, KBP.

132. Miller to Brodman, December 12, 1972.

133. Brodman to Miller, December 15, 1972, box 5, folder 1, KBP.

134. Brodman, "City College Alumni Association Medical Doctors Questionnaire," box 7, folder 4, KBP.

135. Kline, *The Cybernetics Moment*, 179–185. On cybernetics in Chile, see Eden Medina, *Cybernetic Revolutionaries: Technology and Politics in Allende's Chile* (Cambridge, MA: MIT Press, 2011). On cybernetics in the Soviet Union, see Benjamin Peters, "Normalizing Soviet Cybernetics," *Information and Culture* 47, no. 2 (2012): 145–175.

## *Chapter 3 • The Disease Concept Incarnate*

1. "A Bizmac Program for Medical Data Processing," December 10, 1957, box 14, folder 10, REP.

2. Stacey V. Jones, "Computer Can Now Diagnose Ills," *New York Times*, November 6, 1965, p. 35.

3. Vladimir Zworykin, "New Frontiers in Medical Electronics: Electronic Aids for Medical Diagnosis," draft paper, September 27, 1963, box 78, folder 59, VZP.

4. Charles E. Rosenberg, "Framing Disease: Illness, Society, and History," in *Framing Disease: Studies in Cultural History*, edited by Charles E. Rosenberg and Janet Golden (New Brunswick: Rutgers University Press, 1992), xx. See also Charles E. Rosenberg, "The Tyranny of Diagnosis: Specific Entities and Individual Experience," *Milbank Quarterly* 80, no. 2 (2002): 237–260.

5. He officially retired from the RCA on August 1, 1954. On the retirement celebration event at Princeton University's McCosh Hall, see "Dr. Zworykin Is a 'Practical Dreamer' Sarnoff Declares at Testimonial Dinner," *Princeton Herald*, October 2, 1954, p. 8.

6. On Zworykin and the RCA in the history of television, see Albert Abramson, *Zworykin, Pioneer of Television* (Urbana: University of Illinois Press, 1995); Albert Abramson, *The History of Television, 1880–1941* (Jefferson: McFarland, 1987); Benjamin Gross, *The TVs of Tomorrow: How the RCA's Flat-Screen Dreams Led to the First LCDs* (Chicago: University of Chicago Press, 2018); Alexander B. Magoun, *Television: The Life Story of a Technology* (Westport: Greenwood Press, 2007).

7. "Address of Brig. Gen. David Sarnoff," Testimonial Dinner and Seminar in Honor of Vladimir K. Zworykin, box 87, folder 5, VZP.

8. On Zworykin's other work in medical electronics, particularly its telehealth dimensions, see Jeremy A. Greene, *The Doctor Who Wasn't There: Technology, History, and the Limits of Telehealth* (Chicago: University of Chicago Press, 2022).

9. Martin Lipkin and James D. Hardy, "Differential Diagnosis of Hematologic Diseases Aided by Mechanical Correlation of Data," *Science* 125, no. 3247 (1957): 551–552; Martin Lipkin and James D. Hardy, "Mechanical Correlation of Data in Differential Diagnosis of Hematological Diseases," *JAMA* 166, no. 2 (1958): 113–125.

10. Ralph L. Engle, Jr., "Attempts to Use Computers as Diagnostic Aids in Medical Decision Making: A Thirty-Year Experience," *Perspectives in Biology and Medicine* 35, no. 2 (1992): 207–219, pp. 208–209.

11. *The Rockefeller Institute Bulletin, 1960–1961*, volume 5, no. 2, pp. 36–37, box 1, folder FA207, RUR. On the history of the Rockefeller Institute and its research culture, see, e.g.,

Lily E. Kay, "W. M. Stanley's Crystallization of the Tobacco Mosaic Virus, 1930–1940," *Isis* 77 (1986): 450–472, pp. 452–432.

12. Vladimir Zworykin, "Medical Electronics," draft of presentation at the University of Bologna, October 1961, box 78, folder 27, VZP.

13. Engle, "Attempts to Use Computers," 209.

14. "A Bizmac Program for Medical Data Processing," December 10, 1957.

15. Engle, "Attempts to Use Computers," 208.

16. Engle, "Attempts to Use Computers," 209. Historians of medicine have also described how the findings of hematology cannot be isolated from their social and cultural contexts. See Keith Wailoo, *Dying in the City of the Blues: Sickle Cell Anemia and the Politics of Race and Health* (Chapel Hill: University of North Carolina Press, 1997).

17. Discussion of Martin Lipkin, "Correlation of Data with a Digital Computer in the Differential Diagnosis of Hematological Diseases," *IRE Transactions on Medical Electronics* ME-7, no. 4 (1960): 243–246, p. 246.

18. Discussion of Lipkin, "Correlation of Data with a Digital Computer," 246.

19. "A Bizmac Program for Medical Data Processing," December 10, 1957.

20. Stephanie Dick, "AfterMath: The Work of Proof in the Age of Human-Machine Collaboration," *Isis* 102, no. 3 (2011): 494–505; Stephanie Dick, "Of Models and Machines: Implementing Bounded Rationality," *Isis* 106, no. 3 (2015): 623–34; Stephanie Dick, "After Math: (Re)configuring Minds, Proof, and Computing in the Postwar United States" (PhD diss., Harvard University, 2015).

21. Stephanie Dick, "Of Models and Machines," 631.

22. "Detailed Report and Future Plans: January 1, 1962–December 31, 1962," box 14, folder 2, REP.

23. Application for Research Grant, US Department of Health, Education, and Welfare, "Trial of a New Bayesian Decision System for Diagnosis," October 1, 1972, box 5, folder 9 ("Teletype 1973"), REP.

24. Martin Lipkin and Max A. Woodbury, "Coding of Medical Case History Data for Computer Analysis," *Communications of the ACM* 5, no. 10 (1962): 532–534. See also Vladimir K. Zworykin to Howard Tompkins, draft letter, February 1, 1963, box 14, folder 2, REP; Vladimir K. Zworykin to Bertil Jacobson, January 28, 1965, box 84, folder 9, VZP.

25. Vladimir K. Zworykin and Carl Berkley, "Applications of Medical Data Processing," Paper No. VMe-3-57, box 77, folder 69, VZP.

26. Vladimir Zworykin, "The Future of Data Processing and World Health," June 8, 1961, draft of presentation at the meeting of the Panel on the Application of Physics to Biology and Medicine, Washington, DC, June 14, 1961, box 78, folder 34, VZP.

27. Vladimir K. Zworykin, "Welcome—Introduction to Conference," *IRE Transactions on Medical Electronics* ME-7 (1960): 239.

28. Discussion of Lipkin, "Correlation of Data with a Digital Computer," 246.

29. Discussion of Lipkin, "Correlation of Data with a Digital Computer, 246.

30. Taffee Tanimoto, "IBM Type 704 Medical Diagnosis Program," *IRE Transactions on Medical Electronics* ME-7 (1960): 280–283, p. 282.

31. Tanimoto, "IBM Type 704 Medical Diagnosis Program," 283.

32. Tanimoto, "IBM Type 704 Medical Diagnosis Program," 283.

33. For other early work by the hematology team, see R. Ebald and R. Lane, "Digital Computers and Medical Logic," *IRE Transactions of Medical Electronics* ME-7 (1960): 283–288; Martin Lipkin, "Correlation of Data with a Digital Computer in the Differential Diagnosis of Hematologic Diseases," *IRE Transactions of Medical Electronics* ME-7 (1960): 243–246; Martin Lipkin, Ralph L. Engle, Jr., B. J. Davis, Vladimir K. Zworykin, R. Ebald, M. Sendrow, and Carl Berkley, "Digital Computer as Aid to Differential Diagnosis: Use in Hematologic Diseases,"

*Archives of Internal Medicine* 108, no. 1 (1961): 56–72; Martin Lipkin, "Digital and Analogue Computer Methods Combined to Aid in the Differential Diagnosis of Hematological Diseases," *Circulation Research* 11 (1962): 607–613; Martin Lipkin and Max A. Woodbury, "Analytical Studies Related to the Differential Diagnosis of Hematologic Diseases," *Blut* 9, no. 7 (1963): 449–454; Ralph L. Engle, Jr., and B. J. Davis, "Medical Diagnosis: Present, Past, and Future; I. Present Concepts of the Meaning and Limitations of Medical Diagnosis," *Archives of Internal Medicine* 112, no. 4 (1963): 512–519; Vladimir K. Zworykin, "A Mechanized Matching Procedure for Computer Aided Differential Diagnosis," *Medical Electronics and Biological Engineering* 1, no. 1 (1963): 85–89; Martin Lipkin, Ralph L. Engle, Jr., Betty J. Flehinger, Louis J. Gerstman, and M. A. Atamer, "Computer-Aided Differential Diagnosis of Hematologic Diseases," *Annals of the New York Academy of Sciences* 161 (1969): 670–679.

34. Carl Berkley to Louis Gerstman, enclosed draft report, March 9, 1966, box 14, folder 2, REP.

35. "Progress Report: Electronic Data Processing in Hematology," Grant No. AM-06857-03, US Public Health Services, National Institutes of Health, January 1963, p. 2, box 14, folder 11, REP.

36. Eugene Kone to Kenyon Kilbon, n.d., box 14, folder 9, REP.

37. Lisa Gitelman, ed., *"Raw Data" Is an Oxymoron* (Cambridge, MA: MIT Press, 2013).

38. My discussion here is informed by Samuel Issacharoff and Pamela S. Karlan, "The Hydraulics of Campaign Finance Reform," *Texas Law Review* 77, no. 7 (1999): 1705–1738.

39. Carl Berkley to Vladimir Zworykin, October 22, 1962, box 81, folder 19, VZP.

40. Louis J. Gerstman, "Final Report: Electronic Data Processing in Hematology (AM-06857-05): January 1, 1966–February 28, 1967," p. 4, box 14, folder 13, REP.

41. Harry Marks, *The Progress of Experiment: Science and Therapeutic Reform in the United States, 1900–1990* (Cambridge: Cambridge University Press, 1997). Also on the limits and challenges of RCTs, see Laura E. Bothwell, Jeremy A. Greene, Scott H. Podolsky, and David S. Jones, "Assessing the Gold Standard—Lessons from the History of RCTs," *NEJM* 374 (2016): 2175–2181; Angus Deaton and Nancy Cartwright, "Understanding and Misunderstanding Randomized Controlled Trials," *Social Science & Medicine* 210 (2018): 2–21.

42. Marks, *The Progress of Experiment*, 197–228.

43. Marks, *The Progress of Experiment*, 213.

44. Algorithmic bias is a large and lively area of research in science and technology studies and the history of technology and computing. See, e.g., Ruha Benjamin, *Race After Technology: Abolitionist Tools for the New Jim Code* (Medford, MA: Polity, 2019); Safiya Umoja Noble, *Algorithms of Oppression: How Search Engines Reinforce Racism* (New York: New York University Press, 2018); Cathy O'Neil, *Weapons of Math Destruction: How Big Data Increases Inequality and Threatens Democracy* (New York: Crown, 2016).

45. More generally, many developers understood that their systems were limited by data quality. Homer Warner and his colleagues at the University of Utah (discussed later in this chapter) observed, "Our experience with this series of cases in computer diagnosis indicates that the computer's performance at this time is limited by two factors: (1) the accuracy of the input data from the patient as supplied by the examining physician and (2) the accuracy of the data matrix containing the coincidence of symptoms and diseases" (Alan F. Toronto, L. George Veasy, and Homer R. Warner, "Evaluation of a Computer Program for Diagnosis of Congenital Heart Disease," *Progress in Cardiovascular Disease* 5, no. 4 (1963): 362–377, p. 373). The team likewise noted that incidence figures derived from one patient might not apply to a different population. They cautioned, "The a priori incidence figures used are specific for this population and would not necessarily apply to patients with congenital heart disease referred to another laboratory or clinic" (p. 362).

46. "Medicine Faces the Computer Revolution: Electronic 'Brains' Are Heralding a New

Epoch of Improved Diagnosis, Timelier Treatment, and Far Less Medical Paper Work," *Medical World News*, July 14, 1967.

47. Keeve Brodman, "Diagnostic Decisions by Machine," *IRE Transactions on Medical Electronics* ME-7 (1960): 216–219, p. 219.

48. Brodman, "Diagnostic Decisions by Machine," 219.

49. Thomas D. Snyder, *120 Years of American Education: A Statistical Portrait* (Washington, DC: National Center for Education Statistics, US Department of Education, 1993).

50. Nancy Foner, "New York City: America's Classic Immigrant Gateway," in *Migrants to the Metropolis: The Rise of Immigrant Gateway Cities*, edited by Marie Price and Lisa Benton-Short (Syracuse, NY: Syracuse University Press, 2008), 51–68, p. 52.

51. Alvan R. Feinstein, *Clinical Judgment* (Baltimore: Williams and Wilkins, 1967).

52. For a nice review of Feinstein's ideas about epidemiology during this period, see, e.g., Alvan R. Feinstein, "Clinical Epidemiology I: The Population Experiments of Nature and of Man in Human Illness," *Annals of Internal Medicine* 69 (1968): 807–820.

53. Feinstein, *Clinical Judgment*, 380. An underlying point of the book was this: there is nothing mystical about clinical judgment—it is a process (made up of daily clinical "experiments") that can be studied, formalized, and improved.

54. Quoted in Harry T. Paxon, "The Computer: A Report on How It's Affecting the Hospital Physicians," *Hospital Physician*, September 1966, p. 37. For more on Feinstein's critiques of the application of hard data, Bayes's theorem, quantitative decision analysis, and other quantitative models to studying clinical reasoning, see Alvan R. Feinstein, "*Clinical Judgment* Revisited: The Distraction of Quantitative Models," *Annals of Internal Medicine* 120, no. 9 (1994): 799–805.

55. Edmund J. McTernan and Dean Crocker, "Push-Button Medicine Is No Pipe Dream!," *Hospital Physician*, January 1969, p. 86.

56. McTernan and Crocker, "Push-Button Medicine Is No Pipe Dream!"

57. Charles E. Lewis, "Variations in the Incidence of Surgery," *NEJM* 281 (1969): 880–884.

58. John Wennberg and Alan Gittelsohn, "Small Area Variations in Health Care Delivery," *Science* 182, no. 4117 (1973): 1102–1108.

59. R. John, C. Pearson, Björn Smedby, Ragnar Berfenstam, Robert F. L. Logan, Alex M. Burgess, Jr., and Osler L. Peterson, "Hospital Caseloads in Liverpool, New England, and Uppsala: An International Comparison," *Lancet* 292, no. 7567 (1968): 559–566.

60. Quoted in David S. Jones, *Broken Hearts: The Tangled History of Cardiac Care* (Baltimore: Johns Hopkins University Press, 2012). For a historical perspective on variation (geographic, racial, and otherwise) in medicine, see chapter 17, "Puzzles and Prospects," in Jones, *Broken Hearts*, 203–228. Alongside mounting speculation that medical care was inconsistent and ineffectual were anxieties that medical care might actually be injurious. Some of the first systematic studies of clinical error appeared in the 1960s. One of these studies, entitled "The Hazards of Hospitalization," found that in one hospital "deleterious episodes befell 20 per cent [*sic*] of all patients admitted to the service" and implored practitioners to remain "prepared to alter the procedures when imminent or actual harm threatens to obliterate their good" (Elihu M. Schimmel, "The Hazards of Hospitalization," *Annals of Internal Medicine* 60, no. 1 (1964): 100–110, pp. 108–09). Other formal studies of iatrogenesis that appeared during this time period include O. C. Philips, T. M. Frazier, T. D. Graff, and M. J. DeKornfeld, "The Baltimore Anesthesia Study Committee: Review of 1,024 Postoperative Deaths," *JAMA* 174, no. 16 (1960): 2015–2084; Max Schapira, Edith R. Kepes, and Elliott S. Hurwitt, "An Analysis of Deaths in the Operating Room and within 24 Hours of Surgery," *Anesthesia and Analgesia* 39, no. 2 (1960): 149–157; Robert H. Moser, *Diseases of Medical Progress*, 3rd ed. (Springfield: C. C. Thomas, 1969).

61. Stephen R. Yarnall and Richard A. Kronmal, "Computer Aids to Medical Diagnosis—

Problems and Progress," in *ACM '66: Proceedings of the 1966 21st National Conference* (New York: ACM, 1966), 269–274, p. 269. Emphasis original.

62. On (ir)rationality in the postwar period, see, e.g., Paul Erickson, *The World the Game Theorists Made* (Chicago: University of Chicago Press, 2015); Paul Erickson, Judy L. Klein, Lorraine Daston, Rebecca Lemov, Thomas Sturm, and Michael D. Gordin, *How Reason Almost Lost its Mind: The Strange Career of Cold War Rationality* (Chicago and London: University of Chicago Press, 2013); Jamie Cohen-Cole, *The Open Mind: Cold War Politics and the Sciences of Human Nature* (Chicago: University of Chicago Press, 2014); Hunter Crowther-Heyck, *Age of System: Understanding the Development of Modern Social Science* (Baltimore: Johns Hopkins University Press, 2015).

63. John von Neumann and Oskar Morgenstern, *Theory of Games and Economic Behavior* (Princeton, NJ: Princeton University Press, 1944); Leonard J. Savage, *The Foundations of Statistics* (New York: John Wiley & Sons, 1954).

64. On this challenge to Cold War rationality, see Erickson et al., *How Reason Almost Lost its Mind*, 159–181.

65. On Simon, his work, and his life, see Hunter Crowther-Heyck, *Herbert A. Simon: The Bounds of Reason in Modern America* (Baltimore: Johns Hopkins University Press, 2005).

66. On the origins of bounded rationality, see Dick, "Of Models and Machines."

67. Allen Newell, C. J. Shaw, and Herbert A. Simon, "Elements of a Theory of Human Problem Solving," *Psychological Review* 65, no. 3 (1958): 151–166, pp. 153–54.

68. Herbert Simon to John Horgan, February 21, 1991, box 26, folder 1789, HSC.

69. The early ideas of Simon and others would be carried forward into the 1970s by Daniel Kahneman and Amos Tversky, as well as others, who described and mathematized the various cognitive heuristics and biases that systematically distort human reasoning and judgment. See, e.g., Amos Tversky and Daniel Kahneman, "Availability: A Heuristic for Judging Frequency and Probability," *Cognitive Psychology* 5, no. 2 (1973): 207–232; Amos Tversky and Daniel Kahneman, "Judgment under Uncertainty: Heuristics and Biases," *Science* 185, no. 4157 (1974): 1124–1131.

70. Louis J. Gerstman, "Final Report: Electronic Data Processing in Hematology."

71. M. A. Atamer, *Blood Diseases* (New York: Grune and Stratton, 1963).

72. "The Rockefeller Institute Annual Report," July 1, 1961–September 1, 1962, Laboratory of V. K. Zworykin, box 81, folder 37, VZP.

73. Vladimir Zworykin, "The Need for Electronics in Medicine," n.d., box 82, folder 16, VZP.

74. Vladimir Zworykin and Carl Berkley, "Applications of Medical Data Processing," Paper No. VMe-3-57, box 77, folder 69, VZP.

75. Vladimir Zworykin, Ralph Engle, Max Woodbury, and Carl Berkley to Howard Tompkins, February 11, 1963, box 82, folder 32, VZP.

76. Zworykin, "The Future of Data Processing and World Health."

77. Quoted in Zworykin, "The Future of Data Processing and World Health." Originally from Byrd S. Leavell and Oscar A. Thorup, Jr., *Fundamentals of Clinical Hematology* (Philadelphia: W. B. Saunders, 1960), 321.

78. Zworykin et al. to Tompkins, draft of letter, February 1, 1963.

79. Peter C. English, "Emergence of Rheumatic Fever in the Nineteenth Century," *Milbank Quarterly* 67, no. 1 (1989): 33–49.

80. Joel D. Howell, *Technology in the Hospital: Transforming Patient Care in the Early Twentieth Century* (Baltimore: Johns Hopkins University Press, 1995), 48.

81. Stefan Timmermans and Marc Berg, *The Gold Standard: The Challenge of Evidence-Based Medicine* (Philadelphia: Temple University Press, 2003), pp. 30–54.

82. Ida M. Cannon, "Some Clinical Aspects of Social Medicine," *NEJM* 234, no. 1 (1946): 20–23, p. 21.

83. In this discussion on cognitive models, I am drawing upon John Harley Warner's regard of therapeutics as not just social or material practices but a "cognitive system" as well. See John Harley Warner, *The Therapeutic Perspective: Medical Practice, Knowledge, and Identity in America, 1820–1855* (Princeton, NJ: Princeton University Press, 1986). Warner has more recently extended these observations, discussing the "cognitive models" that both produced and emerged out of changing ways of organizing the medical record through the nineteenth century. John Harley Warner, "Vital Signs: The Transformation of the Medical Record in the Nineteenth Century," keynote address at Media Medica: Medicine and the Challenge of New Medicine, conference at Center for Medical Humanities and Social Medicine, Johns Hopkins University, Baltimore, MD, October 17, 2017.

84. This collaboration between Ledley and Lusted is masterfully, and more fully, recounted in Joseph A. November, *Biomedical Computing: Digitizing Life in the United States* (Baltimore: Johns Hopkins University Press, 2012), 56–66.

85. Robert S. Ledley and Lee B. Lusted, "Reasoning Foundations of Medical Diagnosis," *Science* 130, no. 3366 (1959): 9–21.

86. Ledley and Lusted, "Reasoning Foundations of Medical Diagnosis," 15.

87. Sharon McGrayne, *The Theory that Would Not Die* (New Haven, CT: Yale University Press, 2011). Bayesian probability theory was subsequently developed and popularized by Pierre-Simon Laplace. On Laplace, see Lorraine Daston, *Classical Probability in the Enlightenment* (Princeton, NJ: Princeton University Press, 1988).

88. McGrayne, *The Theory that Would Not Die*, 3. Andrew Hodges, "The Military Use of Alan Turing," *Mathematics and War*, edited by Bernhelm Booß-Bavnbek and Jens Høyrup (Basel: Birkhäuser, 2003), 312–325.

89. Stephan E. Fienberg, "When Did Bayesian Inference Become 'Bayesian'?," *Bayesian Analysis* 1, no. 1 (2006): 1–40.

90. Robert S. Ledley, "Medical Informatics: A Personal View of Sowing the Seeds," in *A History of Medical Informatics: Proceedings of the Association for Computing Machinery Conference on History of Medical Informatics*, edited by B. Blum and K. Duncan (New York: ACM Press, 1990), 84–110; Dean F. Sittig, Joan S. Ash, and Robert S. Ledley, "The Story Behind the Development of the First Whole-Body Computerized Tomography Scanner as Told by Robert S. Ledley," *Journal of the American Medical Informatics Association* 13, no. 5 (2006): 465–469. Prior to his stint at the Operations Research Office, Ledley had been at the National Bureau of Standards. There, he encountered the Standards Eastern Automatic Computer (SEAC), a first-generation digital electronic computer. It was this introduction to computers that reoriented his interests to questions of biomedical computing. "The SEAC," he wrote, "was my panacea"—the computer gave him hope that mathematical and physical formulas could be useful in solving, understanding, and representing complex biomedical phenomena (Ledley, "Medical Informatics," 90).

91. November, *Biomedical Computing*, 57–58. During his time at the NIH, Lusted accepted an invitation from the Airborne Instruments Laboratory to consult on the development of an optical electronic machine (the cytoanalyzer) designed to perform automated computer analysis of vaginal ("pap") smears. "Cytoanalyzer," *Public Health Reports* 72, no. 11 (1957): 1038. On the cytoanalyzer, see Peter Keating and Alberto Cambrosio, *Biomedical Platforms: Realigning the Normal and the Pathological in Late-Twentieth-Century Medicine* (Cambridge, MA: MIT Press, 2003), 63–66.

92. He first encountered Ledley's work through a presentation that Ledley gave at the 1956 annual meeting of the Operations Research Society of America. November, *Biomedical Computing*, 58; Rudolf Seising, "Robert S. Ledley, 1926–2012," *Artificial Intelligence in Medicine* 57, no. 1 (2013): 1–7.

93. Through the 1960s, and even into the 1970s, pioneers in biomedical computing

discussed the article frequently and circulated it widely. See, e.g., Joshua Lederberg to Luca Cavalli-Sforza, October 25, 1960, box 11, folder 81, JLP.

94. Ledley, quoted in "Planting the Seeds: Panel Transcript," in *A History of Medical Informatics: Proceedings of the Association for Computing Machinery Conference on History of Medical Informatics*, edited by B. Blum and K. Duncan (New York: ACM Press, 1990), 48–65, p. 61.

95. November, *Biomedical Computing*, 62–64.

96. Some examples include G. S. Lodwick, C. L. Haun, W. E. Smith, R. F. Keller, and E. D. Robertson, "Computer Diagnosis of Primary Bone Tumors: A Preliminary Report," *Radiology* 80 (1963); V. X. Gledhill, J. D. Mathews, and I. R. Mackay, "Computer-Aided Diagnosis: A Study of Bronchitis," *Methods of Information in Medicine* 11 (1972): 228–233; R. P. Knill-Jones, R. B. Stern, D. H. Grimes, J. D. Maxwell, R. P. H. Thompson, and R. Williams, "Use of a Sequential Bayesian Model in Diagnosis of Jaundice by Computer," *BMJ* 1 (1973): 530–533.

97. For more on this history, see Joseph A. November, "Early Biomedical Computing and the Roots of Evidence-Based Medicine," *IEEE Annals of the History of Computing* 33, no. 2 (2011): 9–23.

98. These efforts merged with the Intermountain Healthcare system, which in 2009 was cited by President Barak Obama as a model for health care reform. David Leonhardt, "Dr. James Will Make It Better," *New York Times Sunday Magazine*, November 8, 2009, p. MM31.

99. See Homer Warner interview: Dean F. Sittig, "Founder of the HELP System and the Utah Medical Informatics Program: 2005 Interview of Homer R. Warner, Sr.," in *Conversations with Medical Informatics Pioneers: An Oral History Collection*, edited by Rebecca M. Goodwin, Joan S. Ash, and Dean F. Sittig (Bethesda: National Library of Medicine, 2015), 6.

100. Homer R. Warner, Alan F. Toronto, L. George Veasey, and Robert Stephenson, "A Mathematical Approach to Medical Diagnosis: Application to Congenital Heart Disease," *JAMA* 177, no. 3 (1961): 177–183.

101. Warner et al., "A Mathematical Approach to Medical Diagnosis," 179.

102. Toronto, Veasy, and Warner, "Evaluation of a Computer Program for Diagnosis of Congenital Heart Disease"; Homer R. Warner, Alan F. Toronto, and L. George Veasy, "Experience with Bayes' Theorem for Computer Diagnosis of Congenital Heart Disease," *Annals of the New York Academy of Science* 115 (1964): 558–567.

103. Robert H. Plumb, "Computer Is Found Useful in Heart Diagnoses: Machine Taught to Analyze Symptoms Accurately, 3 Physicians Report," *New York Times*, May 28, 1963, p. 19.

104. Plumb, "Computer Is Found Useful in Heart Diagnoses."

105. On the history of HELP and biomedical computing at Utah and LDS Hospital, see, Gilad J. Kuperman, Reed M. Gardner, and T. Allan Pryor, *HELP: A Dynamic Hospital Information System* (New York: Springer-Verlag, 1991), 3–13.

106. Carl Berkley to Louis Gerstman, March 9, 1966.

107. For other discussions about the perceived disadvantages of Bayesian approaches, see, e.g., Eli Robins, "Categories versus Dimensions in Psychiatric Classification," *Psychiatric Annals* 6, no. 8 (1976): 39, 42–43, 46–47, 51, 55.

108. Max A. Woodbury, "Inapplicabilities of Bayes' Theorem to Diagnosis," in *Proceedings of the Fifth International Conference on Medical Electronics*, edited by C. C. Thomas (Springfield, IL, 1963): 860–868.

109. Woodbury, "Inapplicabilities of Bayes' Theorem to Diagnosis," 867.

## *Chapter 4 · The Medical Mind*

1. John A. Jacquez, "Preface" in *The Diagnostic Process: Proceedings of a Conference Held at the University of Michigan, May 9–11, 1963*, edited by John A. Jacquez (Ann Arbor: Malloy, 1964), iii–iv, p. iii.

2. William N. Hubbard, "Welcome and Prologue," in Jacquez, ed., *The Diagnostic Process*, 3–4.

3. Jacquez, "Preface," iii.

4. Zworykin, "The Need for Electronics in Medicine," p. 43, box 82, folder 16, VZP.

5. Discussion of Ralph L. Engle, Jr., "Medical Diagnosis," in Jacquez, ed., *The Diagnostic Process*, 20.

6. Gerald Goertzel, "Clinical Decision Support System," talk given at the New York Academy of Sciences' Conference on the Use of Data Mechanization and Computer in Clinical Medicine, January 16, 1968, box 3, folder "Clinical Decision Support System, 1967–1972," REP.

7. Ultimately the CDSS failed in large part because physicians had trouble building the database on which the system depended.

8. "Frederick J. Moore, IBM Diagnostician," *New York Times*, October 15, 1972, p. 72.

9. Frederick J. Moore, *Development of a Clinical Decision Support System* (Yorktown Heights, NY: IBM, 1968), p. 1, box 3, folder "Clinical Decision Support System, 1967–1972," REP.

10. Moore, *Development of a Clinical Decision Support System*, 3–4.

11. Moore, *Development of a Clinical Decision Support System*, 4. Emphasis added.

12. Moore, *Development of a Clinical Decision Support System*, 5.

13. Moore, *Development of a Clinical Decision Support System*, 5–6.

14. Moore, *Development of a Clinical Decision Support System*, 6.

15. Concerns about the threat of information overload were nothing new, as Anne Blair has shown. These anxieties were felt particularly, though, among twentieth-century physicians, who saw a host of biomedical breakthroughs. Anne Blair, *Too Much to Know: Managing Scholarly Information before the Modern Age* (New Haven, CT: Yale University Press, 2010).

16. Zworykin to Mary Lasker, "A Rapid Access Multi-Memory Unit for Medical Data Processing," October 21, 1960, box 78, folder 11, VZP.

17. Bryan Williams, "Personal View," *BMJ* 4 (October 1969): 165. See also George Pickering, "Medicine and Society—Past, Present, and Future," *BMJ* 1, no. 23 (January 1971): 191–196, p. 192. In 1963, Derek de Solla Price famously characterized the situation more empirically. Derek J. de Solla Price, *Little Science, Big Science* (New York: Columbia University Press, 1963).

18. David T. Durack, "The Weight of Medical Knowledge," *NEJM* 298, no. 14 (1978): 773–775, p. 773. The article was read widely by contemporaries, with many calling it "a classic." See Dr. Diane Madlon-Kay of the St. Paul-Ramsey Medical Center, quoted in "Science Watch; Heavy Reading," *New York Times*, October 3, 1989.

19. Durack, "The Weight of Medical Knowledge," 773.

20. "Computers and Clinical Medicine," *The Sciences* 8, no. 3 (1968): 32–38.

21. Richard Friedman, "Myths about Computers and Medicine," *Cornell University Medical College Alumni Quarterly* 47, no. 2 (1984): 9. See also Edmund McTernan and Dean Crocker, "Push-Button Medicine Is No Pipe Dream!," *Hospital Physician*, January 1969, p. 85.

22. Susan Sontag, *Illness as Metaphor* (New York: Farrar, Straus and Giroux, 1978); Susan Sontag, *AIDS and Its Metaphors* (New York: Farrar, Straus and Giroux, 1989). Whereas Sontag focused on the negative valence of medicine's metaphors (and argued for a stripping down of medicine to its mechanistic core), other historians have shown that many disease metaphors can also perform social, cultural, and political work in more nuanced ways. See, e.g., Benjamin J. Oldfield and David S. Jones, "Languages of the Heart: The Biomedical and the Metaphorical in American Fiction," *Perspectives in Biology and Medicine* 57, no. 3 (2014): 424–442; Keith Wailoo, *Dying in the City of the Blues: Sickle Cell Anemia and the Politics of Race and Health* (Chapel Hill: University of North Carolina Press, 1997), 3.

23. David S. Jones, *Broken Hearts: The Tangled History of Cardiac Care* (Baltimore: Johns Hopkins University Press, 2013), 28.

24. Marc Berg, "Turning a Practice into a Science: Reconceptualizing Postwar Medical Practice," *Social Studies of Science* 25, no. 3 (1995): 437–476.

25. Berg, "Turning a Practice into a Science," 455.

26. Marc Berg, *Rationalizing Medical Work: Decision-Support Techniques and Medical Practices* (Cambridge, MA: MIT Press, 1997), 45.

27. Jos De Mul describes "the informatization of the worldview" that resulted from engagement with new computing technologies. Jos De Mul, "The Informatization of the Worldview," *Information, Communication, and Society* 2, no. 1 (1999): 69–94. Building on De Mul, Sarah Nettleton has suggested that sociotechnical changes associated with the rise of computers facilitated the emergence of what she calls "e-scaped medicine"—a new medical cosmology akin to "laboratory medicine," "hospital medicine," "bedside medicine," and "library medicine." Sarah Nettleton, "The Emergence of E-Scaped Medicine?," *Sociology* 38 (2004): 661–679.

28. Homer Warner quoted in Robert H. Plumb, "Computer Is Found Useful in Heart Diagnoses: Machine Taught to Analyze Symptoms Accurately, 3 Physicians Report," *New York Times*, May 28, 1963, p. 19.

29. Quoted in "Biomedical Electronics: A Report on an Important New Bridge Connecting Mathematics, Engineering, and Medicine, with an Emphasis on Human Systems," n.d., box 3, folder "Computers in Medicine, 1959–1964," REP. See also "Medicine and IBM," *IBM World Trade News*, November 1959, p. 6.

30. Christopher Lawrence, "Incommunicable Knowledge: Science, Technology, and the Clinical Art in Britain 1850–1914," *Journal of Contemporary History* 20, no. 4 (1985): 503–520.

31. Lawrence, "Incommunicable Knowledge," 505.

32. Lawrence, "Incommunicable Knowledge," 505. Beyond Lawrence, for a synthetic historiographical discussion of skill and authority in the history of medicine, see Nicholas Whitfield and Thomas Schlich, "Skills through History," *Medical History* 59, no. 3 (2015): 349–360. For instructive case studies, see Warwick Anderson, "The Reasoning of the Strongest: The Polemics of Skill and Science in Medical Diagnosis," *Social Studies of Science* 22, no. 4 (1992): 653–684; David S. Jones, "Visions of a Cure: Visualization, Clinical Trials, and Controversies in Cardiac Therapeutics, 1968–1998," *Isis* 91, no. 3 (2000): 504–541.

33. Discussion of Martin Lipkin, "Data Processing in the Diagnostic Process," in Jacquez, ed., *The Diagnostic Process*, 275.

34. The resistance among traditional medical practitioners toward new medical technologies is a recurring theme in the history of medicine.

35. Stephen R. Yarnall and Richard A. Kronmal, "Computer Aids to Medical Diagnosis—Problems and Progress," in *ACM '66: Proceedings of the 1966 21st National Conference* (New York: ACM Press, 1966), 269–274, p. 271.

36. Ralph L. Engle, Jr., "Implications of Computer-Aided Medical Consulting," n.d., box 6, folder 5, REP.

37. Ralph L. Engle, Jr., "Medical Diagnosis: Present, Past, and Future. III. Diagnosis in the Future, Including a Critique on the Use of Electronic Computers as Diagnostic Aids to the Physician," *Archives of Internal Medicine* 112 (1963): 530–543, p. 540.

38. Hans Vaihinger, *The Philosophy of "As if": A System of the Theoretical, Practical, and Religious Fictions of Mankind*, translated by C. K. Ogden (New York: Harcourt Brace, 1925).

39. Engle, "Implications of Computer-Aided Medical Consulting," 4.

40. "Detailed Report and Future Plans, January 1, 1962–December 31, 1962," unpublished typescript, n.d., p. 5, box 14, folder 2, REP.

41. Vladimir Zworykin, Ralph Engle, Max Woodbury, and Carl Berkley to Howard Tompkins, February 11, 1963, box 82, folder 32, VZP.

42. Stephanie Dick, "Artificial Intelligence," *Harvard Data Science Review* 1, no. 1 (2019).

43. These same arguments have enjoyed a second life in recent years. See, e.g., Eric Topol, *Deep Medicine: How Artificial Intelligence Can Make Healthcare Human Again* (New York: Basic Books, 2019).

44. Cesar Caceres, "Computer Diagnosis, Off and Running," *Medical World News*, May 17, 1968.

45. Engle, "Implications of Computer-Aided Medical Consulting," 3.

46. In explaining the medical school's adoption of the case method, some accounts have emphasized the role of Walter Cannon, a fourth-year medical student at Harvard Medical School. Cannon's roommate at the time, a second-year student at Harvard Law School, was enthusiastic about the law school's use of specific legal cases in education. Inspired by his roommate's enthusiasm, Cannon advocated, in a 1900 article in the *Boston Medical and Surgical Journal*, for a similar style of teaching in medical education. This is an interesting story but it detracts from the broader cultural and ideological forces at play. See Nancy Lee Harris and Robert E. Sculley, "The Clinicopathological Conferences (CPCs)," in *Keen Minds to Explore the Dark Continents of Disease*, edited by David N. Louis and Robert H. Young (Boston: Massachusetts General Hospital and Harvard Medical School, 2011), 349–362.

47. Christopher Crenner, "Diagnosis and Authority in the Early Twentieth-Century Medical Practice of Richard C. Cabot," *Bulletin of the History of Medicine* 76, no. 1 (2002): 30–55, p. 37. On Richard Cabot more generally, see Christopher Crenner, *Private Practice in the Early Twentieth-Century Medical Office of Dr. Richard Cabot* (Baltimore: Johns Hopkins University Press, 2005).

48. In 1924, the *Boston Medical and Surgical Journal*—the precursor to the *New England Journal of Medicine*—started to publish the clinicopathological conferences as case records of the Massachusetts General Hospital. Richard C. Cabot and Hugh Cabot, eds., "Ante-mortem and Post-mortem Records as Used in the Weekly Clinico-pathological Exercises. Case 10271," *Boston Medical and Surgical Journal* 191, no. 4 (1924): 30–34.

49. Benjamin Castleman and H. Robert Dudley, eds., *Clinicopathological Conferences of the Massachusetts General Hospital, Selected Medical Cases* (Boston: Little, Brown, 1960), viii.

50. Others also viewed CPCs as "excellent windows through which to study the diagnostic process." David Eddy and Charles Clanton, "The Art of Diagnosis: Solving the Clinicopathological Exercise," *NEJM* 306, no. 21 (1982): 1263–1268, p. 1267.

51. Ralph Engle and Betty Flehinger, "The Diagnosis Process: I. Role of Physician," typescript, 1978, p. 14, box 11, folder 1, REP.

52. Engle and Flehinger, "The Diagnosis Process: I. Role of Physician," 14.

53. Engle and Flehinger, "The Diagnosis Process: I. Role of Physician," 14–15.

54. Engle and Flehinger, "The Diagnosis Process: I. Role of Physician," 15.

55. Discussion of Lipkin, "The Role of Data Processing in the Diagnostic Process," 276.

56. Discussion of Lipkin, "The Role of Data Processing in the Diagnostic Process," 255

57. Discussion of Lipkin, "The Role of Data Processing in the Diagnostic Process," 279.

58. R. Ebald and R. Lane, "Digital Computers and Medical Logic," *IRE Transactions on Medical Electronics* ME-7 (1960): 283–288, p. 283.

59. Ebald and Lane, "Digital Computers and Medical Logic," 286.

60. Ralph L. Engle, Jr., Betty J. Flehinger, Scott Allen, Richard Friedman, Martin Lipkin, B. J. David, and Leo L. Leveridge, "HEME: A Computer Aid to Diagnosis of Hematologic Disease," *Bulletin of the New York Academy of Sciences* 52, no. 5 (1976): 584–600, p. 585.

61. Arthur Elstein, "The Society for Medical Decision Making at 21," *Medical Decision Making* 21, no. 1 (2001): 75–77. Lusted also established the journal *Medical Decision Making*. J. Robert Beck, "*Medical Decision Making*: 20 Years of Advancing the Field," *Medical Decision Making* 21, no. 1 (2001): 73–75. Lee B. Lusted, *Introduction to Medical Decision Making* (Springfield: Charles C. Thomas, 1968).

62. Evan Hepler-Smith, "'A Way of Thinking Backwards': Computing and Method in Synthetic Organic Chemistry," *Historical Studies in the Natural Sciences* 48, no. 3 (2018): 300–337, p. 300.

63. Lucy Suchman, *Human-Machine Reconfigurations: Plans and Situated Actions* (Cambridge: Cambridge University Press, 2006), 226–240.

64. Jack D. Myers, "The Background of INTERNIST I and QMR," *HMI '87 Proceedings of ACM Conference on History of Medical Informatics* (New York: Association for Computing Machinery, 1987), 195–197, p. 195. Clark A. Elliott, "The Tercentenary of Harvard University in 1936: The Scientific Dimension," *Osiris* 14 (1999): 153–175. On Myers in the context of the University of Pittsburgh, see Edwin Kiester, Jr., "First Family of Medicine," *Pitt Med* 5, no. 4 (2003): 29–33.

65. Myers, "The Background of INTERNIST I and QMR," 195.

66. Myers, "The Background of INTERNIST I and QMR," 195.

67. On the idea of the "master diagnostician" and its evolution, see Gurpreet Dhaliwal and Allan S. Detsky, "The Evolution of the Master Diagnostician," *JAMA* 310, no. 6 (2013): 579–580. Dhaliwal himself enjoys the reputation of a master diagnostician. As the *New York Times* reported on his clinical reasoning: "To observe him at work is like watching Steven Spielberg tackle a script or Rory McIlroy a golf course" (Katie Hafner, "For Second Opinion, Consult a Computer?," *New York Times*, December 3, 2012).

68. Miller, quoted in "Dr. Jack Myers, 84, a Pioneer in Computer-Aided Diagnosis," *New York Times*, February 22, 1998, p. 39.

69. Myers, "The Background of INTERNIST I and QMR," 195.

70. Myers, "The Background of INTERNIST I and QMR," 195.

71. Myers, "The Background of INTERNIST I and QMR," 197.

72. Ralph L. Engle, Jr., "Attempts to Use Computers as Diagnostic Aids in Medical Decision Making: A Thirty-Year Experience," *Perspectives in Biology and Medicine* 35, no. 2 (1992): 207–219, p. 216.

73. "HEME2," draft, March 30, 1981, box 11, folder 8, REP.

74. "HEME2," draft, March 30, 1981. See also Jack D. Myers, "The Process of Clinical Diagnosis and Its Adaptation to the Computer," in *Logic of Discovery and Diagnosis in Medicine*, edited by Kenneth F. Schaffner (Berkeley: University of California Press, 1985), 155–180.

75. Engle, "Medical Diagnosis," 12.

76. Ralph L. Engle, Jr., and B. J. Davis, "Medical Diagnosis: Present, Past, and Future. I. Present Concepts of the Meaning and Limitations of Medical Diagnosis," *Archives of Internal Medicine* 112 (1963): 512–519; Ralph L. Engle, Jr., "Medical Diagnosis: Present, Past, Future. II. Philosophical Foundations and Historical Development of Our Concepts of Health, Disease, and Diagnosis," *Archives of Internal Medicine* 112 (1963): 520–529; Engle, "Medical Diagnosis: Present, Past, Future. III. Diagnosis in the Future, Including a Critique on the Use of Electronic Computers as Diagnostic Aids to the Physician."

77. Engle and Davis, "Medical Diagnosis: Present, Past, and Future. I," 516.

78. Engle and Davis, "Medical Diagnosis: Present, Past, and Future. I," 516.

79. Engle, "Medical Diagnosis: Present, Past, and Future. II," 521.

80. Herbert Read, *The Philosophy of Modern Art* (New York: Meridian Books, 1955).

81. Engle, "Medical Diagnosis: Present, Past, and Future. III," 541.

82. Engle, "Medical Diagnosis: Present, Past, and Future. III," 541.

83. "Critique on Computer Aids to Medical Diagnosis," n.d., box 4, folder 3, REP.

84. Engle, "Attempts to Use Computers as Diagnostic Aids," 209.

85. Jean F. Brennan, *The IBM Watson Laboratory at Columbia University: A History* (New York: IBM Corp., 1971).

86. Woodbury to Engle, March 12, 1970, box 4, folder 2, REP.

87. "Trial of a New Bayesian Decision System for Diagnosis," Grant Application (HL 15927-01), Department of Health, Education, and Welfare, October 1, 1972, box 5, folder 3, REP.

88. "Trial of a New Bayesian Decision System for Diagnosis," Grant Application.

89. The team's key studies on the HEME system include: Martin Lipkin, Ralph L. Engle, Jr., Betty J. Flehinger, Louis Gerstman, and M. A. Atamer, "Computer-Aided Differential Diagnosis of Hematologic Diseases," *Annals of the New York Academy of Science* 161 (1969): 670–679; Ralph L. Engle, Jr., and Betty J. Flehinger, "HEME: A Computer Program for Diagnosis-Oriented Analysis of Hematologic Disease," *Transactions of the American Clinical and Climatological Association* 56 (1974): 33–42; Betty J. Flehinger and Ralph L. Engle, Jr., "HEME: A Self-Improving Computer Program for Diagnosis-Oriented Analysis of Hematologic Diseases," *IBM Journal of Research and Development* 19 (1975): 557–564; Ralph L. Engle, Jr., Betty J. Flehinger, S. Allen, Richard Friedman, Martin Lipkin, B. J. Davis, and Leo L. Leveridge, "HEME: A Computer Aid to Diagnosis of Hematologic Disease," *Bulletin of the New York Academy of Medicine* 52 (1976): 584–600; Betty J. Flehinger and Ralph L. Engle, Jr., "HEME2: A Computer Based Responsive Reference Tool for Instruction and Consultation in Hematologic Diagnosis," in *The American Biomedical Network: Health Care Systems in America, Present and Future*, edited by S. B. Day, R. V. Cuddihy, and H. H. Fudenberg (South Orange, NJ: Scripta Medica and Technica, 1977), 283–285; Ralph L. Engle, Jr., and Betty J. Flehinger, "HEME2: A Long History of Computer-Aided Hematologic Diagnosis," in *Proceedings of the Sixth Annual Symposium on Computer Applications to Medical Care*, edited by Bruce I. Blum (Washington, DC: IEEE Computer Society Press, 1982), 763–767.

90. Engle et al., "HEME: A Computer Aid to Diagnosis of Hematologic Disease," 593.

91. Flehinger and Engle, "HEME: A Self-Improving Computer Program for Diagnosis-Oriented Analysis of Hematologic Diseases."

92. Engle, "Attempts to Use Computers as Diagnostic Aids," 214.

93. Engle, "Attempts to Use Computers as Diagnostic Aids," 214.

94. Engle and Flehinger, "HEME2," 765.

95. Woodbury to Lipkin, n.d., box 4, folder 2, REP.

96. Woodbury to Lipkin, n.d.

97. Woodbury to Engle, March 12, 1970.

98. Dorothy Reese to Engle, August 2, 1974, box 5, folder 4, REP.

99. Dorothy Reese to Engle, August 2, 1974. A reviewer for the *American Journal of Medicine*, criticized the HEME project in 1975 on similar grounds, writing, "One of the major limitations of this diagnostic approach has been the lack of availability of statistical data" (William Grace to Flehinger, January 29, 1975, box 4, folder 2, REP).

100. Dorothy Reese to Engle, August 2, 1974.

101. Grace to Flehinger, January 29, 1975.

102. Grace to Flehinger, January 29, 1975.

103. Tested on a series of thirty-one cases from the medical records of New York Hospital, HEME was found to have diagnosed fourteen cases as "excellent," seven as "good," one as "fair," three as "poor," and six as "not evaluable" by a panel of expert hematologists. ("Not evaluable" simply indicated that HEME did not include the ultimate diagnosis in its repository.) Engle et al., "HEME: A Computer Aid to Diagnosis of Hematologic Disease," 595.

104. Engle, "Attempts to Use Computers as Diagnostic Aids," 215.

105. "HEME2," draft, March 30, 1981, 14.

106. Ralph L. Engle, Jr., "Comments on Summary Reports," August 29, 1973, box 6, folder 7, REP.

107. Engle and Flehinger, "Report on Work Conducted Under the Biomedical Research Support Grant," June 22, 1977, box 6, folder 12, REP.

108. Engle and Flehinger, "Report on Work Conducted Under the Biomedical Research Support Grant."

109. Engle, "Attempts to Use Computers as Diagnostic Aids," 214.

110. Engle et al., "HEME: A Computer Aid to Diagnosis of Hematologic Disease," 598.

111. The group disbanded in 1972, but Flehinger and Engle continued their collaboration into the late 1980s.

112. Ralph L. Engle, Jr., handwritten draft of article on HEME2, n.d., box 11, folder 8, REP.

113. Engle, "Attempts to Use Computers as Diagnostic Aids," 216.

114. William Bauman to Franz Ingelfinger, July 11, 1969, box 8, folder 2, REP.

115. Bauman to Ingelfinger, July 11, 1969. Bauman was in fact enthusiastic about the possibility of applying computers to patient management. He simply saw the singular fixation on "diagnosis" as an iceberg; he was keen to redirect the ship. He wrote to Engle, "I believe that substantial proportion of patients' problems can be managed by the computer . . . better than they are now managed by the friendly druggist, the articulate TV announcer, the school or screening nurse, and even by some of our hard-working colleagues. I am not altogether sure that a disease diagnosis is needed. The cluster of findings, unlabeled, may be all that is required to give sound management advice" (Bauman to Engle, December 1, 1969, box 8, folder 2, REP).

116. Engle and Flehinger, "HEME2," 764–765.

117. Engle and Flehinger, "HEME2," 765.

118. Engle, "Attempts to Use Computers as Diagnostic Aids," 216.

119. Engle, "Medical Diagnosis: Present, Past, and Future. III," 535.

## *Chapter 5 • MYCIN Explains Itself*

1. Saul Amarel, Casimir A. Kulikowski, Natesa S. Sridharan, and Deirdre Sridharan, *Proceedings of the First Annual AIM Workshop, June 14–17, 1975*, box 94, folder 25, JLP.

2. "SUMEX-AIM Prospectus," June 22, 1974, p. 1, box 62, folder 29, JLP.

3. For discussion of SUMEX-AIM's configuration with ARPA, see, e.g., Tom Rindleisch to "SUMEX File," "Notes on First AIM Executive Committee Meeting (11/26/73)," December 3, 1973, box 62, folder 34, JLP. See also, Edward H. Shortliffe, "The Changing Nature of Telecommunications and the Information Infrastructure for Health Care," in *The Changing Nature of Telecommunications/Information Infrastructure* (Washington, DC: National Academy Press, 1995), 67–73, p. 67.

4. "SUMEX-AIM Prospectus," June 22, 1974, 1.

5. Joseph November, *Biomedical Computing: Digitizing Life in the United States* (Baltimore: Johns Hopkins University Press, 2012), 221–227. This section's discussion of Stanford, ACME, and DENDRAL draws on November's excellent work.

6. November, *Biomedical Computing*, 222.

7. On Frederick Terman and Stanford's postwar transformation, see, e.g., C. Stewart Gillmor, *Fred Terman at Stanford: Building a Discipline, a University, and Silicon Valley* (Stanford: Stanford University Press, 2004); Stuart W. Leslie, "Playing the Education Game to Win: The Military and Interdisciplinary Research at Stanford," *Historical Studies in the Physical and Biological Sciences* 18, no. 1 (1987): 55–88; Rebecca S. Lowen, "'Exploiting a Wonderful Opportunity': The Patronage of Scientific Research at Stanford University, 1937–1965," *Minerva* 30, no. 3 (1992): 391–421; Rebecca S. Lowen, *Creating the Cold War University: The Transformation of Stanford* (Berkeley: University of California Press, 1997); Cyrus C. M. Mody, *The Long Arm of Moore's Law: Microelectronics and American Science* (Cambridge, MA: MIT Press, 2017), 25–27.

8. The name "Silicon Valley" was popularized by a series of articles for the weekly trade

newspaper *Electronic News.* Don C. Hoefler, "Silicon Valley, USA," *Electronic News*, January 11, 1971.

9. November, *Biomedical Computing*, 224–225.

10. Joshua Lederberg, "Advanced Computer for Medical Research," Application for Research Grant, No. FR 00311-01, September 29, 1965, US Department of Health, Education, and Welfare, Public Health Service, p. 3, box 60, folder 25, JLP.

11. The historian Doogab Yi has characterized this communal culture—and its eventual unraveling through the second half of the twentieth century, as scientists and administrators "challenged, broke, and eventually redrew the boundary between academic research and industry." Doogab Yi, *The Recombinant University: Genetic Engineering and the Emergence of Stanford Biotechnology* (Chicago: University of Chicago Press, 2015), 214.

12. Before the Department of Computer Science developed into its own department, it existed as the Division of Computer Science within the Mathematics Department. George Forsythe founded the Division of Computer Science at Stanford in 1961. November, *Biomedical Computing*, 228.

13. Edward A. Feigenbaum, oral history by Pamela McCorduck, June 12, 1979, p. 13, CBI.

14. Gio Wiederhold, "A Summary of the ACME System," Notes for Presentation Given at the ONR Computer and Psychobiology Conference, the US Navy Postgraduate School, Monterey, CA, May 26, 1966, p. 1, box 60, folder 47, JLP.

15. "Advanced Computer for Medical Research (ACME)," Grant No. FR 00311-03, Special Research Resource Annual Report, August 1, 1968, to July 31, 1969, US Department of Health, Education, and Welfare, Public Health Service, pp. 91, 105, box 60, folders 30–31, JLP.

16. Bruce G. Buchanan, Georgia L. Sutherland, and Edward A. Feigenbaum, "Heuristic DENDRAL: A Program for Generating Explanatory Hypotheses in Organic Chemistry," in *Machine Intelligence*, edited by B. Meltzer and D. Miche (Edinburgh: Edinburgh University Press, 1969), 209–254.

17. On Lederberg's hand in shaping twentieth-century biomedicine, see Jan Sapp, *Genes, Germs, and Medicine: The Life of Joshua Lederberg* (London: World Scientific, 2021).

18. On Lederberg and contemporaneous research on extraterrestrial life, see Audra J. Wolfe, "Germs in Space: Joshua Lederberg, Exobiology, and the Public Imagination, 1958–1964," *Isis* 93, no. 2 (2002): 183–205. See also November, *Biomedical Computing*, 242–253.

19. Joshua Lederberg, "Signs of Life: Criterion System of Exobiology," *Nature* 207 (1965): 9–13.

20. John McCarthy and Joshua Lederberg, "A Proposal for the Study of Computer Control of External Devices and an Automated Biological Laboratory," draft proposal, October 15, 1964, p. 2, box 67, folder 69, JLP.

21. Joshua Lederberg, "How DENDRAL Was Conceived and Born," ACM Symposium on the History of Informatics, November 5, 1987, pp. 6, 9, box 86, folder 77, JLP. This paper was later published in Bruce I. Blum, ed., *A History of Medical Informatics: Proceeding of ACM Conference on History of Medical Informatics* (New York: ACM Press, 1990). On Stanford and Djerassi in the history of modern chemistry, see Carsten Reinhardt, *Shifting and Rearranging: Physical Methods and the Transformation of Modern Chemistry* (Sagamore Beach, MA: Science History Publications, 2006).

22. Bruce G. Buchanan, "Logics of Scientific Discovery" (PhD diss., Michigan State University, 1966).

23. Bruce G. Buchanan, oral history with Arthur L. Norberg, June 11–12, 1991, Philadelphia, PA, p. 4, CBI.

24. Bruce G. Buchanan and Edward A. Feigenbaum, "Dendral and Meta-Dendral: Their Applications Dimension," *Artificial Intelligence* 11 (1978): 5–24, p. 7.

25. Lederberg, "How DENDRAL Was Conceived and Born," 13.

26. Robert K. Lindsay, Bruce G. Buchanan, Edward A. Feigenbaum, and Joshua Lederberg, *Applications of Artificial Intelligence for Organic Chemistry: The DENDRAL Project* (New York: McGraw-Hill, 1980), 2.

27. Lederberg, "How DENDRAL Was Conceived and Born," 11.

28. Hunter Crowther-Heyck, *Herbert A. Simon: The Bounds of Reason in Modern America* (Baltimore: Johns Hopkins University Press, 2005).

29. Lederberg, "How DENDRAL Was Conceived and Born," 12.

30. Lucila Ohno-Machado, Donald Ellison, and Edward H. Shortliffe, "Presentation of the 2008 Morris F. Collen Award to Robert A. Greenes," *JAMIA* 16, no. 3 (2009): 413–418, p. 414.

31. G. Octo Barnett, "Report to the National Institutes of Health Division of Research Grants Computer Research Study Section on Computer Applications in Medical Communication and Information Retrieval Systems as Related to the Improvement of Patient Care and the Medical Record—September 26, 1966," *JAMIA* 13, no. 2 (2006): 127–135. This is a printing of a formerly unpublished historical report on the LCS from 1966. See also G. Octo Barnett, "History of the Development of Medical Information Systems at the Laboratory of Computer Science at Massachusetts General Hospital" in *HMI '87: Proceedings of ACM Conference on History of Medical Informatics*, edited by Bruce I. Blum (New York: ACM Press, 1987), 43–49.

32. Robert A. Greenes, Bruce G. Buchanan, and Donald Ellison, "Presentation of the 2006 Morris F. Collen Award to Edward H. (Ted) Shortliffe," *JAMIA* 14, no. 3 (2007): 376–385, p. 376; Robert A. Greenes, "A Computer-Based System for Medical Record-Keeping by Physicians" (PhD diss., Harvard University, 1969).

33. Greenes, Buchanan, and Ellison, "Presentation of the 2006 Morris F. Collen Award," 376. Edward H. Shortliffe, "A Computer-Based Medical Record System: Approaches to the Interface Problem" (AB thesis, Harvard University, 1970).

34. Octo Barnett, "From 'Farm Boy' to Director of the Laboratory of Computer Science: 2004 Interview of Octo Barnett," interviewed by Joan S. Ash and Dean F. Sittig, in *Conversations with Medical Informatics Pioneers: An Oral History Collection*, edited by Rebecca M. Goodwin, Joan S. Ash, and Dean F. Sittig (Bethesda, MD: US National Library of Medicine, 2015), 10.

35. "SIG" for Special Interest Group. Greenes, Buchanan, and Ellison, "Presentation of the 2006 Morris F. Collen Award," 377.

36. Buchanan, oral history with Norberg, June 11–12, 1991, 27.

37. Shortliffe to Shi-Kuo Chang, December 5, 1990, box 2, folder "Buchanan, Bruce, 1975–94," ESP.

38. Stanley N. Cohen, "Science, Biotechnology, and Recombinant DNA: A Personal History," an oral history conducted by Sally Smith Hughes, 1995, p. 23, ROO.

39. Stanley N. Cohen, Marsha F. Armstrong, Linda Crouse, and Gilbert S. Hunn, "A Computer-Based System for Prospective Detection and Prevention of Drug Interactions," *Drug Information Journal* 72 (1972): 81–86, p. 81. During this period, Cohen also published an influential handbook on drug interactions: Stanley N. Cohen, *Drug Interactions: A Handbook for Clinical Use* (Baltimore: Williams and Wilkins, 1974).

40. Buchanan, oral history with Norberg, June 11–12, 1991, 27.

41. Buchanan, oral history with Norberg, June 11–12, 1991, 27.

42. Buchanan, oral history with Norberg, June 11–12, 1991, 27.

43. Some of the key early writings from the MYCIN team include Edward H. Shortliffe, "MYCIN: A Rule-Based Computer Program for Advising Physicians Regarding Antimicrobial Therapy Selection" (PhD diss., Stanford University, 1972); Edward H. Shortliffe, Stanton G. Axline, Bruce G. Buchanan, and Stanley N. Cohen, "Design Considerations for a Program to Provide Consultations in Clinical Therapeutics," in *Proceedings of the 13th San Diego Biomedical Symposium* (1974), 311–319; Edward H. Shortliffe and Bruce G. Buchanan, "A Model

of Inexact Reasoning in Medicine," *Mathematical Bioscience* 23, no. 3–4 (1975): 351–379; Edward H. Shortliffe, Randall Davis, Stanton G. Axline, Bruce G. Buchanan, C. Cordell Green, and Stanley N. Cohen, "Computer-Based Consultations in Clinical Therapeutics: Explanation and Rule Acquisition Capabilities of the MYCIN System," *Computers and Biomedical Research* 8, no. 4 (1975): 303–320; Edward H. Shortliffe, Stanton G. Axline, Bruce G. Buchanan, Thomas C. Merigan, and Stanley N. Cohen, "An Artificial Intelligence Program to Advise Physicians Regarding Antimicrobial Therapy," *Computers and Biomedical Research* 6 no. 6 (1973): 544–560. The group also published much of this work in book-length collections. Edward H. Shortliffe, *Computer-Based Medical Consultations: MYCIN* (New York: Elsevier, 1976); Bruce G. Buchanan and Edward H. Shortliffe, eds., *Rule-Based Expert Systems: The MYCIN Experiments of the Stanford Heuristic Programming Project* (Reading, CA: Addison-Wesley, 1984).

44. "Computer Acquisition of Medical Judgmental Knowledge," research proposal, December 1973, box 10, folder "MYCIN History, 1972–78," ESP.

45. Buchanan and Shortliffe, *Rule-Based Expert Systems*, 10.

46. Edward Shortliffe to Stanley N. Cohen (S. Axline, B. Brown, B. Buchanan, C. Green, G. Hunn, T. Merigan, B. Raphael, J. Rulifson, R. Schimke, P. Suppes, H. Sussman, and R. Waldinger copied), "Progress Report on the Antimicrobial Therapy Project," memorandum, October 13, 1972, box 10, folder "MYCIN History, 1972–78," ESP. See also Greenes, Buchanan, and Ellison, "Presentation of the 2006 Morris F. Collen Award," 378.

47. Shortliffe to Cohen, "Progress Report on the Antimicrobial Therapy Project."

48. Stanley N. Cohen to Thomas Merigan and Stanton Axline, "Proposed Computer Project Involving Antibiotics Therapy," memorandum, February 25, 1972, box 10, folder "MYCIN History, 1972–78," ESP.

49. Cohen to Merigan and Axline, "Proposed Computer Project Involving Antibiotics Therapy."

50. Stanton Axline to Cohen, Merigan, Buchanan, Hunn, and Shortliffe, "Proposed Computer Project Involving Antibiotics Therapy," memorandum, March 13, 1972, box 10, folder "MYCIN History, 1972–78," ESP.

51. Shortliffe to Cohen, "Progress Report on the Antimicrobial Therapy Project."

52. Jamie R. Carbonell, "AI in CAI: An Artificial-Intelligence Approach to Computer-Assisted Instruction," *IEEE Transactions on Man-Machine Systems* 11, no. 4 (1970): 190–202.

53. Shortliffe to Cohen, "Progress Report on the Antimicrobial Therapy Project."

54. Buchanan and Shortliffe, *Rule-Based Expert Systems*, 9.

55. Shortliffe to Cohen, "Progress Report on the Antimicrobial Therapy Project."

56. Shortliffe, *Computer-Based Medical Consultations: MYCIN*, 52.

57. Buchanan and Shortliffe, *Rule-Based Expert Systems*, 9.

58. Shortliffe to Cohen, "Progress Report on the Antimicrobial Therapy Project."

59. Amarel et al., *Proceedings of the First Annual AIM Workshop*, 23.

60. On the mutually constitutive nature of a research group's social form and its knowledge production, see Alma Steingart, "A Group Theory of Group Theory: Collaborative Mathematics and the 'Uninvention' of a 1000-Page Proof," *Social Studies of Science* 42, no. 2 (2012): 185–213.

61. Shortliffe to Cohen, "Progress Report on the Antimicrobial Therapy Project."

62. Rene C. Fox, "Training for Uncertainty," in *The Student Physician*, edited by Robert K. Merton, G. Reader, and P. L. Kendall (Cambridge, MA: Harvard University Press, 1957). See also Rene C. Fox, "The Evolution of Medical Uncertainty," *Milbank Quarterly* 58, no. 1 (1980): 1–49.

63. G. Anthony Gorry and G. Octo Barnett, "Experience with a Model of Sequential Diagnosis," *Computers and Biomedical Research* 1 (1968): 490–507.

64. Homer R. Warner, A. F. Toronto, and L. G. Veasy, "Experience with Bayes' Theorem for Computer Diagnosis of Congenital Heart Disease," *Annals of the New York Academy of Science* 115 (1964): 558–567.

65. Shortliffe, *Computer-Based Medical Consultations: MYCIN*, 160.

66. This dynamic is one that played out more widely across the fields of mathematics, statistics, and computer science, particular in the postwar period. See, e.g., Matthew L. Jones, "How We Became Instrumentalists (Again): Data Positivism since World War II," *Historical Studies in the Natural Sciences* 48, no. 5 (2018): 673–684.

67. Homer R. Warner, "Founder of the HELP System and the Utah Medical Informatics Program," interviewed by Dean F. Sittig, in *Conversations with Medical Informatics Pioneers: An Oral History Collection*, edited by Rebecca M. Goodwin, Joan S. Ash, and Dean F. Sittig (Bethesda, MD: US National Library of Medicine, 2015), 20.

68. Edward H. Shortliffe and Bruce G. Buchanan, "A Model of Inexact Reasoning in Medicine," *Mathematical Biosciences* 23 (1975): 351–379.

69. Shortliffe to William Mark, July 21, 1975, box 10, folder "MYCIN, 1973–77," ESP.

70. Shortliffe to Mark, July 21, 1975.

71. Shortliffe and Buchanan, "A Model of Inexact Reasoning," 353.

72. Shortliffe and Buchanan, "A Model of Inexact Reasoning," 356.

73. On the use of "literary technologies" to persuade and establish matters of fact, see Steven Shapin, "Pump and Circumstance: Robert Boyle's Literary Technology," *Social Studies of Science* 14 (1984): 481–520; Steven Shapin and Simon Shaffer, *Leviathan and the Air-Pump: Hobbes, Boyle, and the Experimental Life* (Princeton, NJ: Princeton University Press, 1985).

74. Amarel et al., *Proceedings of the First Annual AIM Workshop*, 30.

75. The ophthalmologist Aran Safir, for example, commented, "Given a data base and a set of numbers it is very important to be able to explain to a physician who is using them how these numbers were arrived at and their relative importance and how the system goes about reaching a decision or a hypothesis" (Amarel et al., *Proceedings of the First Annual AIM Workshop*, 37).

76. Sholom M. Weiss, Casimir A. Kulikowski, Saul Amarel, and Aran Safir, "A Model-Based Method for Computer-Aided Medical Decision-Making," *Artificial Intelligence* 11, no. 1–2 (1978): 145–172, p. 147

77. Amarel et al., *Proceedings of the First Annual AIM Workshop*, 23–24.

78. Shortliffe and Buchanan, "A Model of Inexact Reasoning in Medicine," 357.

79. Edward H. Shortliffe, "Clinical Consultation Systems: Designing for the Physician as Computer User," in *Proceeding of the Annual Symposium on Computer Applications in Medical Care* (Silver Spring, MD: IEEE Computer Society Press, 1981): 235–236, p. 235.

80. Shortliffe, "Clinical Consultation Systems," 235.

81. Shortliffe, "Clinical Consultation Systems," 235.

82. The consultation system was Subprogram 1. Shortliffe, *Computer-Based Medical Consultations*, 195–204.

83. A. Carlisle Scott, William J. Clancey, Randall Davis, and Edward H. Shortliffe, "Methods for Generating Explanations," in *Rule-Based Expert Systems: The MYCIN Experiments of the Stanford Heuristic Programming Project*, edited by Bruce G. Buchanan and Edward H. Shortliffe (Reading, CA: Addison-Wesley, 1984), 338–362, p. 340.

84. Shortliffe et al., "Explanation and Rule Acquisition Capabilities of the MYCIN System," 310–314.

85. Shortliffe et al., "Explanation and Rule Acquisition Capabilities of the MYCIN System," 314.

86. Shortliffe et al., "Explanation and Rule Acquisition Capabilities of the MYCIN System," 314.

87. Hans Karlgren, "*Computational Linguistics in Medicine*: Werner Schneider and Anna-Lena Sågvall Hein (eds.), Amsterdam: North-Holland. 1977", book review, *Journal of Pragmatics* 4, no. 2 (1980): 183. See also G. Anthony Gorry, "Computer-Assisted Clinical Decision Making," *Methods of Information in Medicine* 12 (1973): 45–51.

88. Weiss et al., "A Model-Based Method for Computer-Aided Medical Decision-Making," 146.

89. Weiss et al., "A Model-Based Method for Computer-Aided Medical Decision-Making," 146.

90. Edward Shortliffe, "MYCIN: A Knowledge-Based Computer Program Applied to Infectious Diseases," in *Proceeding of the Annual Symposium on Computer Applications in Medical Care* (1977): 66–69, p. 67. See also Shortliffe, *Computer-Based Medical Consultations*, 203.

91. Lewis Carroll, *Through the Looking-Glass* (Mineola, NY: Drover, 1990), 20.

92. Carroll, *Through the Looking-Glass*, 20.

93. See, e.g., Andrew L. Russell and Lee Vinsel, "After Innovation, Turn to Maintenance," *Technology and Culture* 59, no. 1 (2018): 1–25; David Edgerton, *The Shock of the Old: Technology and Global History Since 1900* (Oxford: Oxford University Press, 2007). Maintenance has also long been an enduring and vibrant theme of certain feminist histories. See, e.g., Susan Strasser, *Never Done: A History of American Housework* (New York: Pantheon Books, 1982).

94. Andrew L. Russell and Lee Vinsel, "Make Maintainers: Engineering Education and the Ethics of Care," in *Does America Need More Innovators?*, edited by Matthew Wisnioski, Eric Hintz, and Marie Stettler Kleine (Cambridge, MA: MIT Press, 2019).

95. "Computer Acquisition of Medical Judgmental Knowledge," research proposal, December 1973.

96. Shortliffe to Mark, July 21, 1975, box 10, folder "MYCIN, 1973–77," ESP.

97. Clancey to Greg Cooper (Shortliffe and Buchanan copied), email printout, October 6, 1980, box 2, folder "Clancey, William (1), 1978, 81," ESP.

98. "Computer Acquisition of Medical Judgmental Knowledge," research proposal, December 1973.

99. Carli Scott, "BATCH," email printout, November 13, 1978, box 11, folder "MYCIN–General, 1973–82," ESP.

100. Ove B. Wigertz to Shortliffe, email printout, October 3, 1988, box 3, folder "Columbia Presbyterian Med Ctr Retreat, (Arden Homestead, 6/89), 1989," ESP.

101. Shortliffe and Buchanan, "A Model of Inexact Reasoning in Medicine," 357.

102. Robert Blum, "Blum's presentation," email printout of minutes from September 21, 1977, meeting, October 6, 1977, box 10, folder "MYCIN–Current, 1975–82," ESP.

103. Clancey, "MYCIN's Sensitivity to CF Changes," unpublished report, September 1975, box 10, folder "Certainty Factors, 1976–84," ESP.

104. Clancey, unpublished memo, March 1, 1976, box 10, folder "Certainty Factors, 1976–84," ESP.

105. Shortliffe to Paul Clayton, email printout, April 21, 1989, box 3, folder "Columbia Presbyterian Med Ctr Retreat, (Arden Homestead, 6/89), 1989," ESP. See David Heckerman and Eric Horvitz, "The Myth of Modularity in Rule-Based Systems for Reasoning with Uncertainty," *Machine Intelligence and Pattern Recognition* 2 (1986): 23–34; Eric Horvitz and David Heckerman, "Modular Belief Updates and Confusion about Measures of Certainty in Artificial Intelligence Research," in *Proceedings of the First Conference on Uncertainty in Artificial Intelligence*, edited by Laveen Kanal and John Lemmer (Arlington, VA: AUAI Press, 1985), 283–286.

106. Shortliffe to Clayton, email printout, April 21, 1989.

107. Shortliffe to Carli Scott (Yu, Buchanan, David, Van Melle, Clancey, Fagan, Axline,

Wraith, and Aikins copied), email printout, July 8, 1976, box 10, folder "MYCIN–Current, 1975–82," ESP.

108. William Clancey, "<CLANCEY>CF.TWOCUTOFF;1," email printout, box 10, folder "MYCIN History, 1972–78," ESP.

109. Clancey, "<CLANCEY>CF.TWOCUTOFF;1."

110. Carli Scott, "6/17/76 meeting summary," email printout, June 18, 1976, box 10, folder "MYCIN–Current, 1975–82," ESP.

111. Shortliffe to Scott, July 8, 1976.

112. Shortliffe to Scott, July 8, 1976.

## *Chapter 6 · "Hidden in the Code"*

1. F. J. Ingelfinger, "Algorithms, Anyone?," *NEJM* 288, no. 16 (1973): 847–848.

2. For examples of secondary works that explore physician and professional identity, see Agnes Arnold-Forster, Jacob D. Moses, and Samuel V. Schotland, "Obstacles to Physicians' Emotional Health—Lessons from History," *NEJM* 386, no. 1 (2022): 4–7; Keith Wailoo, *Drawing Blood: Technology and Disease Identity in Twentieth-Century America* (Baltimore: Johns Hopkins University Press, 1997); John Harley Warner, *The Therapeutic Perspective: Medical Practice, Knowledge, and Identity* (Cambridge, MA: Harvard University Press, 1986).

3. "MYCIN USER'S GUIDE," March 9, 1976, box 10, folder "MYCIN–Current, 1975–82," ESP.

4. Edward H. Shortliffe, "Medical Expert Systems—Knowledge Tools for Physicians," *Western Journal of Medicine* 145, no. 6 (1986): 830–839, p. 833; Edward H. Shortliffe, "Computer Programs to Support Clinical Decision Making," *JAMA* 258, no. 1 (1987): 61–66, p. 64.

5. Gregory Cooper to Edward Shortliffe, Bruce Buchanan, and csd.lenat@SCORE, email printout, March 16, 1982, box 1, folder "Cooper, Gregory, 1979–1996," ESP.

6. Homer Warner to Shortliffe, December 6, 1974, box 12, folder "CMPB (Computer Methods and Programs in Biomed.), 1974–94," ESP.

7. Shortliffe to Warner, December 31, 1974, box 12, folder "CMPB (Computer Methods and Programs in Biomed.), 1974–94," ESP.

8. Shortliffe to Warner, December 31, 1974.

9. William J. Clancey, "Notes on 'Epistemology of a Rule-Based Expert System,'" *Artificial Intelligence* 59, no. 1–2 (1993): 197–204, p. 201.

10. Clancey, "Notes on 'Epistemology of a Rule-Based Expert System,'" 201.

11. Clancey, "Notes on 'Epistemology of a Rule-Based Expert System,'" 201.

12. "The Student Model and the Form of the Knowledge Base," unpublished notes, n.d., box 2, folder "Clancey, William (1), 1978–81," ESP. Michael Polyani, *Personal Knowledge: Towards a Post-Critical Philosophy* (London: Routledge, 1958).

13. Shortliffe to Scott (Yu, Buchanan, David, Van Melle, Clancey, Fagan, Axline, Wraith, and Aikins copied), email printout, July 8, 1976, box 10, folder "MYCIN–Current, 1975–82," ESP.

14. "Critique of the Portal Concept in Mycin," unpublished document, n.d., box 10, folder "MYCIN–Current, 1975–82," ESP.

15. Buchanan, "Summary of 11/17/76 meeting," meeting minutes, printout of email to MYCIN team, November 30, 1976, box 10, folder "MYCIN–Current, 1975–82," ESP.

16. "Critique of the Portal Concept in Mycin."

17. Shortliffe to Scott (Yu et al. copied), July 8, 1976.

18. Shortliffe to Scott (Yu et al. copied), July 8, 1976.

19. Scott H. Podolsky, *The Antibiotic Era: Reform, Resistance, and the Pursuit of a Rational Therapeutics* (Baltimore: Johns Hopkins University Press, 2015), 10–42. This section's discussion of midcentury antibiotic reform is very much beholden to Podolsky's book.

20. Podolsky, *The Antibiotic Era*, 43–72.

21. Podolsky, *The Antibiotic Era*, 73–111. For a brief but rich historical discussion of the Kefauver–Harris amendments, see Jeremy A. Greene and Scott H. Podolsky, "Reform, Regulation, and Pharmaceuticals—The Kefauver–Harris Amendments at 50," *NEJM* 367, no. 16 (2012): 1481–1483. See also Daniel P. Carpenter, *Reputation and Power: Organizational Image and Pharmaceutical Regulation at the FDA* (Princeton, NJ: Princeton University Press, 2010), 228–297.

22. Beginning in 1967, Wisconsin Senator Gaylord Nelson initiated widely publicized hearings on the pharmaceutical industry, which, by 1972, would come to focus on the misuse and overuse of antibiotics. Additional high-profile Congressional hearings into antibiotic overuse, led by Massachusetts Senator Edward Kennedy, continued over the following two years. On the Nelson hearings, see Dominique Tobbell, *Pills, Power, and Policy: The Struggle for Drug Reform in Cold War American and Its Consequences* (Berkeley: University of California Press, 2011), 129–130, 163–192; Jeremy Greene, *Generic: The Unbranding of Modern Medicine* (Baltimore: Johns Hopkins University Press, 2014), 53–55; Carpenter, *Reputation and Power*, 342–345.

23. Podolsky, *The Antibiotic Era*, 2–4, 38.

24. See, e.g., W. E. Scheckler and J. V. Bennett, "Antibiotic Usage in Seven Community Hospitals," *JAMA* 213 (1970): 264–267; K. E. Reztak and R. B. Williams, "A Review of Antibiotic Therapy in Patients with Systematic Infections," *American Journal of Hospital Pharmacy* 29 (1972): 935–941; C. M. Kunin, T. Tupasi, and W. A. Craig, "Use of Antibiotics: A Brief Exposition of the Problem and Some Tentative Solutions," *Annals of Internal Medicine* 79 (1973): 555–560; A. W. Roberts and J. A. Visconti, "The Rational and Irrational Use of Systematic Antimicrobial Drugs," *American Journal of Hospital Pharmacy* 29 (1972): 828–834.

25. Henry H. Simmons and Paul D. Stolley, "This Is Medical Progress? Trends and Consequences of Antibiotic Use in the United States," *JAMA* 227 (1974): 1023–1028, p. 1027. Increasing recognition of unwarranted and widespread variation in medical practices and outcomes during the 1970s and 1980s extended beyond the realm of antibiotics. See David S. Jones, *Broken Hearts: The Tangled History of Cardiac Care* (Baltimore: Johns Hopkins University Press, 2013), 215–218.

26. Edward H. Shortliffe, *Computer-Based Medical Consultations: MYCIN* (New York: Elsevier, 1976), 43

27. Podolsky, *The Antibiotic Era*, 112.

28. Richard DuBois to Stanley N. Cohen, March 30, 1977, box 10, folder "MYCIN History, 1972–78," ESP.

29. Cohen to Geral Rosenthal, May 8, 1977, box 10, folder "MYCIN History, 1972–78," ESP. Emphasis added.

30. Cohen to Rosenthal, May 8, 1977. Emphasis added.

31. Quoted in Podolsky, *The Antibiotic Era*, 123.

32. Quoted in Podolsky, *The Antibiotic Era*, 124.

33. Sharon Wraith, "Meeting of March 9, 1977," meeting minutes, printout of email to MYCIN team, March 15, 1977, box 10, folder "MYCIN–Current, 1975–82," ESP.

34. Encounters like this one prompted Yu to recommend giving all site visitors a bibliography that the MYCIN team had prepared with forty references on the subject of antibiotic misuse.

35. William Clancey to Harold Goldberger (Edward Shortliffe and Victor Yu copied), email printout, July 12, 1978, box 11, folder "MYCIN–General, 1973–82," ESP.

36. Goldberger to Clancey (Shortliffe and Yu copied), email printout, July 17, 1978, box 11, folder "MYCIN–General, 1973–82," ESP.

37. Goldberger to Clancey (Shortliffe and Yu copied), July 17, 1978. Emphasis added.

38. Podolsky, *The Antibiotic Era*, 127, 133–136.

39. Janice Aikins to "MYCIN gang," "On Wednesday's meeting," email printout, February 28, 1976, box 10, folder "MYCIN History, 1972–78," ESP.

40. Jan H. van Bemmel to Shortliffe, email printout, May 23, 1989, box 3, folder "Columbia Presbyterian Med Ctr Retreat, (Arden Homestead, 6/89), 1989," ESP. See also "Comments on the 'Medical Knowledge Base Standard,'" box 3, folder "Columbia Presbyterian Med Ctr Retreat, (Arden Homestead, 6/89), 1989," ESP.

41. Sam Ervin to Aikins and Carli Scott ("MYCIN gang" listserv copied), February 29, 1976, box 10, folder "MYCIN History, 1972–78," ESP.

42. Cohen to John R. Hall, March 14, 1974, box 10, folder "MYCIN History, 1972–78," ESP.

43. "Tentative Evaluation Protocol," March 1974, box 10, folder "MYCIN Evaluation, 1974–79," ESP.

44. Shortliffe, manuscript review for *Annals of Internal* Medicine, May 9, 1984, box 2, folder "Pittsburgh, Univ. of, 1980–95," ESP.

45. Gregory Freiherr, "MYCIN: A Medical and Educational Aid," *Research Resources Reporter* 3, no. 12 (Bethesda, MD: National Institutes of Health, 1979): 1–6, p. 2.

46. Cohen to Thomas Merigan and Stanton Axline, "Proposed Computer Project Involving Antibiotics Therapy," memo, February 25, 1972, box 10, folder "MYCIN History, 1972–78," ESP.

47. Yu and Cohen to Morton N. Swartz, August 9, 1977, box 4, folder "Victor's Letters, 1977–78," ESP.

48. Shortliffe to William Mark, email printout, July 21, 1975, box 10, folder "MYCIN, 1973–77," ESP.

49. Victor L. Yu, Bruce G. Buchanan, Edward H. Shortliffe, Sharon M. Wraith, Randall Davis, A. Carlisle Scott, and Stanley N. Cohen, "Evaluating the Performance of a Computer-Based Consultant," *Computer Programs in Biomedicine* 9, no. 1 (1979): 95–102.

50. Yu et al., "Evaluating the Performance of a Computer-Based Consultant," 98–100.

51. Yu and Cohen to Swartz, August 9, 1977, box 4, folder "Victor's Letters, 1977–78," ESP. The experts the MYCIN team considered reaching out to included: Morton Swartz (Harvard), George McCracken (Parkland), Jay Sanford (United Health Services), Philip Lerner (Case Western), Stuart Levin (Chicago), Ralph Feigin (St. Louis), Robert Petersdorf (University of Washington), John E. Bennett (NIH), Philip Dodge (Harvard), Donald Armstrong (Cornell), James Rahal (NYU).

52. Yu to Axline, Shortliffe, Cohen, Wraith (Scott, Fagan, Van Melle, and Clancey copied), email printout, January 29, 1976, box 5, folder "Bacteremia MYCIN–Patient Runs, 1975," ESP.

53. "<LETSINGER>EVAL.DRAFT;2," unpublished printout, November 28, 1979, box 10, folder "MYCIN Evaluation, 1974–79," ESP.

54. For a more detailed draft protocol for the evaluation study, see "The Meningitis Evaluation," unpublished printout, April 4, 1977, box 5, folder "Bacteremia MYCIN–Patient Runs, 1975," ESP.

55. This physician was Robert Blum. On some early discussions of possible selection criteria, as well as a more thorough discussion of the goals of the study, see "Goals for the Meningitis Evaluation," unpublished printout, April 12, 1977, box 5, folder "Bacteremia MYCIN–Patient Runs, 1975," ESP.

56. Victor L. Yu, L. M. Fagan, Sharon M. Wraith, William J. Clancey, A. Carlisle Scott, J. Hannigan, Robert L. Blum, Bruce G. Buchanan, and Stanley N. Cohen, "Antimicrobial Selection by a Computer: A Blinded Evaluation by Infectious Disease Experts," *JAMA* 242, no. 12 (1979): 1279–1282.

57. Richard S. Jones, "Letters: Use of Computers in Medical Practice," *Canadian Medical Association Journal* 122, no. 4 (1980): 400.

58. Shortliffe to HPP Faculty and Staff, "ONCOCIN: An Oncology Protocol Management Consultation System," memo, February 16, 1982, box 2, folder "ONCOCIN 1977–89 (Fl 1 of 2)," ESP.

59. Peter Keating and Alberto Cambrosio, *Cancer on Trial: Oncology as a New Style of Practice* (Chicago: University of Chicago Press, 2011).

60. "<CLANTON>ONCOCIN.INTERFACE;1," unpublished report (computer printout), February 6, 1980, box 2, folder "ONCOCIN–Logistics, 1978–83," ESP.

61. Edward H. Shortliffe, A. Carlisle Scott, Miriam B. Bischoff, A. Bruce Campbell, William van Melle, and Charlotte D. Jacobs, "An Expert System for Oncology Protocol Management," in *Rule Based Expert Systems*, edited by Bruce G. Buchanan and Edward H. Shortliffe (Reading, CA: Addison-Wesley, 1984), 653–668, pp. 654–655.

62. Shortliffe to HPP Faculty and Staff, "ONCOCIN: An Oncology Protocol Management Consultation System."

63. George Weisz, Alberto Cambrosio, Peter Keating, Loes Knaapen, Thomas Schlich, and Virginie J. Tournay, "The Emergence of Clinical Practice Guidelines," *Milbank Quarterly* 85, no. 4 (2007): 691–727, pp. 695–697; Peter Keating and Alberto Cambrosio, "Cancer Clinical Trials: The Emergence and Development of a New Style of Practice," *Bulletin of the History of Medicine* 81 (2007):197–223, p. 208–213.

64. National Institutes of Health, Office of Budget, "Appropriations History of Institute/Center (1938 to Present)," accessed September 25, 2022, https://officeofbudget.od.nih.gov/approp_hist.html. On the history of the clinical trial, see Harry M. Marks, *The Progress of Experiment: Science and Therapeutic Reform in the United States, 1900–1990* (Cambridge: Cambridge University Press, 2000). On the increase of research spending in medical schools, see Daniel M. Fox, "From Piety to Platitudes to Pork: The Changing Politics of Health Workforce Policy," *Journal of Health Politics, Policy and Law* 21 (1996): 825–44.

65. Marc Berg, Klasien Horstman, Saskia Plass, and Michelle van Heusden, "Guidelines, Professionals and the Production of Objectivity: Standardization and the Professionalism of Insurance Medicine," *Sociology of Health and Illness* 22, no. 6 (2000): 765–791.

66. Ingelfinger, "Algorithms, Anyone?," 847–848.

67. Lewis B. Sheiner, George Brecher, and Lawrence A. Wheeler, "Clinical Laboratory Use in the Evaluation of Anemia," *JAMA* 238, no. 25 (1977): 2709–2714.

68. William H. Crosby, "Chess and Combat: The Algorithm in Medicine," *JAMA* 238, no. 25 (1977): 2721.

69. Crosby, "Chess and Combat," 2721.

70. The UCSF team responded forcefully to Crosby, arguing that he had drawn an unwarranted conclusion (all guidelines are useless if not dangerous) from a reasonable observation (medicine cannot be reduced to guidelines). Lewis B. Sheiner, George Brecher, and Lawrence A. Wheeler, "Letters: The Algorithm in Medicine," *JAMA* 239, no. 19 (1978): 1957.

71. On the Reasoner/Interview model used by ONCOCIN, see Phillip E. Gerring, Edward H. Shortliffe, and William van Melle, "Interviewer/Reasoner Model: An Approach to Improving System Responsiveness in Interactive AI Systems," *AI Magazine* 3, no. 4 (1982): 24–27.

72. Shortliffe et al., "An Expert System for Oncology Protocol Management," 653.

73. "Longer Progress Report, Project 1 (1979–1980)," unpublished report, n.d. (circa 1980), box 2, folder "ONCOCIN 1977–89 (Fl 1 of 2)," ESP.

74. "<CLANTON>ONCOCIN.INTERFACE;1," unpublished report (computer printout), February 6, 1980.

75. Cliff Wulfman, "The Interviewer as Input Device and Archivist's Tool," n.d. (circa 1985), box 7, folder "ONCOCIN, 1979–88," ESP.

76. Daniel K. Harris, "Computer-Assisted Decision Support: A New Available Reality," *JAMA* 258, no. 1 (1987): 86.

77. James E. Levin, "Computer Programs to Support Clinical Decision Making," *JAMA* 258, no. 17 (1987): 2375. For other articles in conversation with these articles, see Shortliffe, "Computer Programs to Support Clinical Decision Making," 61–66; Edward H. Shortliffe, "Computer Programs to Support Clinical Decision Making—Reply," *JAMA* 258, no. 17 (1987): 2375–2376; G. Octo Barnett, James J. Cimino, Jon A. Hupp, and Edward P. Hoffer, "Computer Programs to Support Clinical Decision Making—Reply," *JAMA* 258, no. 17 (1987): 2376; Daniel K. Harris, "Computer Programs to Support Clinical Decision Making—Reply," *JAMA* 258, no. 17 (1987): 2376.

78. Harris, "Computer-Assisted Decision Support," 86.

79. Harris, "Computer-Assisted Decision Support," 86.

80. Paul Chang, "Pertinent Findings from Physician Test Interviews," unpublished report, n.d., box 2, folder "[ONCOCIN], 1979–83," ESP.

81. Chang, "Pertinent Findings from Physician Test Interviews."

82. Chang, "Pertinent Findings from Physician Test Interviews."

83. Chang, "Pertinent Findings from Physician Test Interviews."

84. Chang, "Pertinent Findings from Physician Test Interviews."

85. Chang, "Pertinent Findings from Physician Test Interviews."

86. Chang, "Pertinent Findings from Physician Test Interviews."

87. ONCOCIN Annual Report, unpublished report, n.d. (circa late 1982), p. 4, box 2, folder "ONCOCIN 1977–89 (Fl 1 of 2)," ESP; Shortliffe to Derek Sleeman, email printout, January 25, 1988, box 7, folder "ONCOCIN, 1979–88," ESP.

88. ONCOCIN Annual Report, n.d. (circa late 1982), 5.

89. ONCOCIN Annual Report, n.d. (circa late 1982), 5.

90. "<CLANTON>ONCOCIN.INTERFACE;1," unpublished report (computer printout), February 6, 1980.

91. ONCOCIN Annual Report, n.d. (circa late 1982), 6.

92. ONCOCIN Annual Report, n.d. (circa late 1982), 6.

93. Shortliffe, "Computer Programs to Support Clinical Decision Making," 66.

94. Shortliffe, "Computer Programs to Support Clinical Decision Making," 66.

95. Joan Differding, "A Log of Times in the Oncology Day Care Clinic," unpublished report, March 3, 1982, p. 25, box 2, folder "ONCOCIN–Logistics, 1978–83," ESP; "<SHORTLIFFE>FELLOW.COMMENTS;1," unpublished computer printout, June 8, 1981, box 2, folder "[ONCOCIN], 1979–83," ESP.

96. "<SHORTLIFFE>FELLOW.COMMENTS;1," unpublished computer printout, June 8, 1981.

97. "Feature Interview: Edward Shortliffe on the MYCIN Expert System, *Computer Compacts* 1, no. 6 (December 1983–January 1984): 283–289, p. 286.

98. Judy Foreman, "MGH Unveils Diagnostic Computer," *Boston Globe*, June 23, 1987, p. 1.

99. Foreman, "MGH Unveils Diagnostic Computer," 1.

100. Daniel L. Kent, Edward H. Shortliffe, R. W. Carlson, Miriam B. Bischoff, and Charlotte D. Jacobs, "Improvements in Data Collection through Physician Use of a Computer-Based Chemotherapy Treatment Consultant," *Journal of Clinical Oncology* 3 (1985): 1409–1417.

101. David H. Hickam, Edward H. Shortliffe, Miriam B. Bischoff, A. Carlisle Scott, and Charlotte D. Jacobs, "The Treatment Advice of a Computer-Based Cancer Chemotherapy Protocol Advisor," *Annals of Internal Medicine* 103, no. 6 (1985): 928–936.

102. Len Shustek, "An Interview with Ed Feigenbaum," *Communications of the ACM* 53, no. 6 (2010): 41–45, p. 44. "EMYCIN," short for "empty" MYCIN, referred to the original system shorn of all its domain-specific knowledge. Expert system "shells" like EMYCIN allowed for application of the system's inference methods and representation schemes to other domains.

103. Allen Newell, "Forward" in *Rule-Based Expert Systems: The MYCIN Experiments of the Stanford Heuristic Programming Project*, edited by Bruce G. Buchanan and Edward H. Shortliffe (Reading, CA: Addison-Wesley, 1984), xi–xvi, p. xi

104. Clancey, "Notes on 'Epistemology of a Rule-Based Expert System,'" 197.

105. Charles E. Rosenberg, "The Tyranny of Diagnosis: Specific Entities and Individual Experience," *Milbank Quarterly* 80, no. 2 (2002): 237–260, p. 240.

106. As one anonymous referee would put it to Shortliffe in 1988, "The *major* stumbling blocks (apart from money) have been and will continue to be linguistic, organizational, sociological, ethico-legal, and systematic." Helen Goldstein to Shortliffe, June 20, 1988, box 9, folder "Critique/Reviews, 1984–88," ESP.

## *Conclusion*

1. "FDA Permits Marketing of Artificial Intelligence-Based Device to Detect Certain Diabetes-Related Eye Problems," US Food and Drug Administration News Release, April 11, 2018, https://www.fda.gov/news-events/press-announcements/fda-permits-marketing-artificial-intelligence-based-device-detect-certain-diabetes-related-eye.

2. For the purposes of calibration against human performance, studies have shown that board-certified ophthalmologists using indirect ophthalmoscopy only reach a sensitivity of between 33 percent and 73 percent when compared against the same standard.

3. Michael D. Abràmoff, Philip T. Lavin, Michele Birch, Nilay Shah, and James C. Folk, "Pivotal Trial of an Autonomous AI-Based Diagnostic System for Detection of Diabetic Retinopathy in Primary Care Offices," *NPJ Digital Medicine* 1, 39 (2018).

4. Cade Metz, "AI Helps Indian Doctors Save Eyesight," *New York Times*, March 11, 2019, B1.

5. Dr. R. Kim, quoted in Chris Mills Rodrigo, "Google Launches Effort in India to Screen for Leading Causes of Blindness," *The Hill*, February 26, 2019, https://thehill.com/policy/technology/431591-google-launches-effort-to-screen-for-leading-causes-of-blindness.

6. For helpful reviews of recent developments in medical AI, see Alvin Rajkomar, Jeffrey Dean, and Isaac Kohane, "Machine Learning in Medicine," *NEJM* 380, no. 14 (2019): 1347–1358; Kun-Hsing Yu, Andrew L. Beam, and Isaac S. Kohane, "Artificial Intelligence in Healthcare," *Nature Biomedical Engineering* 2 (2018): 719–731.

7. Andre Esteva, Brett Kuprel, Roberto A. Novoa, Justin Ko, Susan M. Swetter, Helen M. Blau, and Sebastian Thrun, "Dermatologist-Level Classification of Skin Cancer with Deep Neural Networks," *Nature* 542 (2017): 115–118; P. Lakhani and B. Sundaram, "Deep Learning at Chest Radiography: Automated Classification of Pulmonary Tuberculosis by Using Convolutional Neural Networks," *Radiology* 284 (2017): 574–582; G. Litjens, Clara I. Sánchez, Nadya Timofeeva, Meyke Hermsen, Iris Nagtegaal, Iringo Kovacs, Christina Hulsbergen-van de Kaa, Peter Bult, Bram van Ginneken, and Jeroen van der Laak, "Deep Learning as a Tool for Increased Accuracy and Efficiency of Histopathological Diagnosis," *Science Reports* 6 (2016): 26286.

8. K. C. Vranas, Jeffrey K. Jopling, Timothy E. Sweeney, Meghan C. Ramsey, Arnold S. Milstein, Christopher G. Slatore, Gabriel J. Escobar, and Vincent X. Liu, "Identifying Distinct Subgroups of ICU Patients: A Machine Learning Approach," *Critical Care Medicine* 45, no. 10 (2017): 1607–1615. Aymen A. Elfiky, Maximilian J. Pany, Ravi B. Parikh, and Ziad Obermeyer, "Development and Application of a Machine Learning Approach to Assess Short-Term Mortality Risk among Patients with Cancer Starting Chemotherapy," *JAMA Network Open* 1, no. 3 (2018): e180926.

9. Ziad Obermeyer and Ezekiel J. Emanuel, "Predicting the Future—Big Data, Machine Learning, and Clinical Medicine," *NEJM* 375 (2016): 1216–1219.

10. Eric Topol, *The Creative Destruction of Medicine: How the Digital Revolution Will Create Better Health Care* (New York: Basic Books, 2012).

11. Ziad Obermeyer and Thomas H. Lee, "Lost in Thought—The Limits of the Human Mind and the Future of Medicine," *NEJM* 377 (2017): 1209–1211, p. 1209.

12. Eric Topol, *Deep Medicine: How Artificial Intelligence Can Make Health Care Human Again* (New York: Basic Books, 2019).

13. Quoted in "Images Aren't Everything," *The Economist* 427, no. 9095 (June 9, 2018): 15–16, p. 15.

14. Bo Gong, James P. Nugent, William Guest, William Parker, Paul J. Chang, Faisal Khosa, and Savvas Nicolaou, "Influence of Artificial Intelligence on Canadian Medical Students' Preference for Radiology Specialty: A National Survey Study," *Academic Radiology* 26, no. 4 (2019): 566–577.

15. Abraham Verghese, "Culture Shock—Patient as Icon, Icon as Patient," *NEJM* 359, no. 26 (2008): 2748–2751, p. 2749.

16. Abraham Verghese, Nigam H. Shah, and Robert A. Harrington, "What This Computer Needs Is a Physician: Humanism and Artificial Intelligence," *JAMA* 319, no. 1 (2018): 19–20.

17. On AI and bias in medicine, see, e.g., S. Scott Graham, *The Doctor and the Algorithm: Promise, Peril, and the Future of Health AI* (Oxford: Oxford University Press, 2022).

18. Samuel G. Finlayson, Adarsh Subbaswamy, Karandeep Singh, John Bowers, Annabel Kupke, Jonathan Zittrain, Isaac S. Kohane, and Suchi Saria, "The Clinician and Dataset Shift in Artificial Intelligence," *NEJM* 385, no. 3 (2021): 283–286.

19. Ruha Benjamin, *Race After Technology: Abolitionist Tools for the New Jim Code* (Cambridge, UK, and Medford, MA: Polity, 2019); Virginia Eubanks, *Automating Inequality: How High-Tech Tools Profile, Police, and Punish the Poor* (New York: St. Martin's Press, 2018); Safiya Umoja Noble, *Algorithms of Oppression: How Search Engines Reinforce Racism* (New York: New York University Press, 2018).

20. Julia Dressel and Hany Farid, "The Accuracy, Fairness, and Limits of Predicting Recidivism," *Science Advances* 4, no. 1 (2018): eaao5580.

21. Joy Buolamwini and Timnit Gebru, "Gender Shades: Intersectional Accuracy Disparities in Commercial Gender Classification," *Proceedings of Machine Learning Research* 81 (2018): 1–15.

22. Jennifer W. Tsai, Jessica P. Cerdeña, William C. Goedel, William S. Asch, Vanessa Grubbs, Mallika L. Mendu, and Jay S. Kaufman, "Evaluating the Impact and Rationale of Race-Specific Estimations of Kidney Function: Estimations from US NHANES, 2015–2018," *EClinicalMedicine* 42 (2021): 101197; Nwamaka D. Eneanya, L. Ebony Boulware, Jennifer Tsai, Marino A. Bruce, Chandra L. Ford, Christina Harris, Leo S. Morales, Michael J. Ryan, Peter P. Reese, Roland J. Thorpe, Jr., Michelle Morse, Valencia Walker, Fatiu A. Arogundade, Antonio A. Lopes, and Keith C. Norris, "Health Inequities and the Inappropriate Use of Race in Nephrology," *Nature Reviews Nephrology* 18, no. 2 (2022): 84–94; Darshali A. Vyas, Leo G. Eisenstein, and David S. Jones, "Hidden in Plain Sight—Reconsidering the Use of Race Correction in Clinical Algorithms," *NEJM* 383, no. 9 (2020): 874–881. On race correction in pulmonology, see Lundy Braun, *Breathing Race into the Machine: The Surprising Career of the Spirometer from Plantation to Genetics* (Minneapolis: University of Minnesota Press, 2014).

23. Ziad Obermeyer, Brian Powers, Christine Vogeli, and Sendhil Mullainathan, "Dissecting Racial Bias in an Algorithm Used to Manage the Health of Populations," *Science* 366, no. 6464 (2019): 447–453. For a rich discussion, analysis, and framing of this study, see Ruha Benjamin, "Assessing Risk, Automating Racism," *Science* 366, no. 6464 (2019): 421–422.

24. Diana Forsythe, *Studying Those Who Study Us: An Anthropologist in the World of Artificial Intelligence* (Stanford, CA: Stanford University Press, 2001), 178.

25. Forsythe, *Studying Those Who Study Us.*

26. Kevin Wiley, Brian E. Dixon, Shaun J. Grannis, and Nir Menachemi, "Underrepresented Racial Minorities in Biomedical Informatics Doctoral Programs: Graduation Trends and Academic Placement (2002–2017)," *Journal of the American Medical Informatics Association* 27, no. 11 (2020): 1647–1641.

27. Sendhil Mullainathan and Ziad Obermeyer, "Does Machine Learning Automate Moral Hazard and Error?," *American Economic Review* 107, no. 5 (2017): 476–480.

28. Xiaoxuan Liu, Samantha Cruz Rivera, David Moher, Melanie J. Calvert, Alastair K. Denniston, and the SPIRIT-AI and CONSORT-AI Working Group, "Reporting Guidelines for Clinical Trial Reports for Interventions Involving Artificial Intelligence: The CONSORT-AI Extension," *Nature Medicine* 26 (2020): 1364–1374.

29. Bryce Goodman and Seth Flaxman, "European Union Regulations on Algorithmic Decision-Making and a 'Right to Explanation,'" *AI Magazine* 38, no. 3 (2017): 50–57.

30. Effy Vayena, Alessandro Blasimme, and I. Glenn Cohen, "Machine Learning in Medicine: Addressing Ethical Challenges," *PLOS Medicine* 15, no. 11 (2018): e1002689. On the legal issues introduced by black box algorithms, see, e.g., W. N. Price, "Regulating Black-Box Medicine," *Michigan Law Review* 116, no. 1 (2017): 421–474.

31. See, e.g., Elizabeth Holm, "In Defense of the Black Box," *Science* 364, no. 6435 (2019): 26–27.

32. See, e.g., Alex John London, "Artificial Intelligence and Black-Box Medical Decisions: Accuracy versus Explainability," *Hastings Center Report* 49, no. 1 (2019): 15–21.

33. The computer is, to borrow a phrase, "an engine, not a camera." Computer algorithms generate new identities and lines inquiry. Donald MacKenzie, *An Engine, Not a Camera: How Financial Models Shape Markets* (Cambridge, MA: MIT Press, 2006).

34. Allison A. Tillack and Richard S. Breiman, "Renegotiating Expertise: An Examination of PACS and the Challenges to Radiology Using a Medical Anthropologic Approach," *Journal of the American College of Radiology* 9, no. 1 (2012): 64–68.

35. Tillack and Breiman, "Renegotiating Expertise," 66.

36. Tillack and Breiman, "Renegotiating Expertise," 67.

37. See, e.g., Jeremy A. Greene, *Prescribing by Numbers: Drugs and the Definition of Disease* (Baltimore: Johns Hopkins University Press, 2007).

38. S. Lochlann Jain, *Malignant: How Cancer Becomes Us* (Berkeley: University of California Press, 2013), 27.

39. Robert Aronowitz, *Risky Medicine: Our Quest to Cure Fear and Uncertainty* (Chicago: University of Chicago Press, 2015); Robert Aronowitz, "The Converged Experience of Disease and Risk," *Milbank Quarterly* 87, no. 2 (2009): 417–442.

40. Carl Berkley to Vladimir Zworykin, 1967, box 81, folder "Correspondence: 1965–71, undated," VZP.

41. Vladimir Zworykin and Carl Berkley, "Applications of Medical Data Processing," Paper No. VMe-3-57, box 77, folder 69, VZP; Robert Haavind, "Needed: A Medical Technology Institute," April 26, 1965, box 82, folder 15, VZP.

42. Zworykin and Berkley, "Applications of Medical Data Processing."

43. Geoffrey C. Bowker and Susan Leigh Star, *Sorting Things Out: Classification and Its Consequences* (Cambridge, MA: MIT Press, 1999); Anne Kveim Lie and Jeremy A. Greene, "From Ariadne's Thread to the Labyrinth Itself—Nosology and the Infrastructure of Modern Medicine," *NEJM* 382, no. 13 (2020): 1273–1277.

44. Topol, *The Creative Destruction of Medicine*; Eric Topol, *The Patient Will See You Now: The Future of Medicine Is In Your Hands* (New York: Basic Books, 2015).

45. R. J. Baron, "Quality Improvement with an Electronic Health Record: Achievable, but Not Automatic," *Annals of Internal Medicine* 147 (2007): 548–552; Katherine Choi, Yevgeniy

Gitelman, and David A. Asch, "Subscribing to Your Patients—Reimagining the Future of Electronic Health Records," *NEJM* 378 (2018): 1960–1962.

46. Keeve Brodman, A. J. van Woerkom, Albert J. Erdmann, Jr., Leo S. Goldstein, "Interpretation of Symptoms with a Data-Processing Machine," *AMA Archives of Internal Medicine* 103 (1959): 776–782.

47. "Diagnosis by Computer Envisaged for Patients," *New York Times*, February 8, 1958, p. 6.

48. See, e.g., "The Future of Medical AI," *The Economist*, February 15, 2022, https://www.economist.com/films/2022/02/15/the-future-of-medical-ai; Jeremy Hsu, "Can a Crowdsourced AI Medical Diagnosis App Outperform Your Doctor?," *Scientific American*, August 11, 2017; Apoorv Mandavilli, "Enlisting Algorithms in the World's Battle against Tuberculosis," *New York Times*, November 24, 2020, p. 5; Megan Molteni, "Want a Diagnosis Tomorrow, Not Next Year? Turn to AI," *Wired*, August 10, 2017; Siddhartha Mukherjee, "The Algorithm Will See You Now," *New Yorker*, April 3, 2017.

# INDEX

Milton Keynes UK
Ingram Content Group UK Ltd.
UKHW011934130923
428621UK00004B/17/J